Review of Pediatric Critical Care

PATRICIA A. MOLONEY-HARMON, RN, MS, CCRN

Clinical Nurse Specialist
Children's Services
Sinai Hospital of Baltimore
Baltimore, Maryland

SANDRA J. CZERWINSKI, RN, MS, CCRN

Administrative Director
Nursing Education, Research, Program Development
All Children's Hospital
St. Petersburg, Florida

W.B. SAUNDERS COMPANY
A Division of Harcourt Brace & Company
Philadelphia London Toronto Montreal Sydney Tokyo

W.B. SAUNDERS COMPANY
A Division of Harcourt Brace & Company

The Curtis Center
Independence Square West
Philadelphia, Pennsylvania 19106

Library of Congress Cataloging-in-Publication Data

Review of pediatric critical care   /   [edited by] Patricia
    Moloney-Harmon, Sandra Czerwinski.

        p.   cm.
    Includes bibliographical references and index.

    ISBN 0–7216–6159–9

    1. Pediatric intensive care.   I. Czerwinski, Sandra.
    [DNLM: 1. Critical Care—in infancy & childhood—nurses'
instruction. 2. Pediatric Nursing.   WS 366 R458 1997]

    RJ370.R48   1997   618.92'0028—dc20

DNLM/DLC   96-15372

REVIEW OF PEDIATRIC CRITICAL CARE   ISBN 0–7216–6159–9

Printed in the United States of America.

Last digit is the print number: 9   8   7   6   5   4   3   2   1

Review of Pediatric Critical Care

CONTRIBUTORS

Joyce Bansbach-Bailey
RN, MSN
Nursing Supervisor
Riverview Hospital
Noblesville, Indiana
Chapter 11. Immunologic Disorders

Patricia A. Berry
RN, CCRN
Staff Nurse II
Children's Hospital
Boston, Massachusetts
Chapter 6. Pulmonary Disorders

Pamela A. Brown
RN, MS, CCRN
Director
Cardiac Intensive Care Unit
Miami Children's Hospital
Miami, Florida
Chapter 8. Fluid and Electrolyte Disorders

Rita Brosnahan
RN, BSN
Staff Nurse II
Children's Hospital
Boston, Massachusetts
Chapter 17. Transplantation

Elaine A. Caron
RN
Staff Nurse III
Children's Hospital
Boston, Massachusetts
Chapter 6. Pulmonary Disorders

Liane S. Conrad
RN, BSN
Staff Nurse II
Children's Hospital
Boston, Massachusetts
Chapter 6. Pulmonary Disorders

Sandra J. Czerwinski
RN, MS, CCRN
Administrative Director
Nursing Education, Research, Program
   Development
All Children's Hospital
St. Petersburg, Florida
Chapter 15. Shock

Beverly J. D'Angio
RN,C, MS
Adjunct Faculty
University of South Florida, Tampa, and
   University of Tampa, Tampa, Florida
Advanced Education Specialist
ICU Staff Nurse
All Children's Hospital
St. Petersburg, Florida
Chapter 9. Renal Disorders

Patricia Dimick
RN, BSN
Nurse Manager
Burn Intensive Care Unit
Harborview Medical Center
Seattle, Washington
Chapter 19. Thermal Injuries

Peggy Dorr
RN, MS, CCRN
Clinical Educator
Pediatric Intensive Care Unit
University of Maryland Medical Center
Baltimore, Maryland
Chapter 5. Cardiovascular Disorders

Janice M. Doyle
RN, CCRN
Staff Nurse II
Children's Hospital
Boston, Massachusetts
Chapter 6. Pulmonary Disorders

Betsy Fisher
RN, BSN, MA, CETN
Enterostomal Therapy Nurse
Sinai Hospital of Baltimore
Baltimore, Maryland
Chapter 24. Skin Integrity

Karen A. Fraser
RN
Staff Nurse II
Children's Hospital
Boston, Massachusetts
Chapter 6. Pulmonary Disorders

Margaret S. Geller
RN, CCRN
Staff Nurse III
Children's Hospital
Boston, Massachusetts
Chapter 6. Pulmonary Disorders

Cathy Haut
RN, MS, CCRN
Clinical Nurse Specialist
Neonatal Intensive Care and Pediatrics
Franklin Square Hospital Center
Baltimore, Maryland
Chapter 23. Thermoregulation

Elizabeth I. Helvig
RN, MS
Adjunct Faculty
University of Washington
School of Physiological Nursing
Seattle, Washington
Burn/Plastics Clinical Nurse Specialist
Harborview Medical Center
Seattle, Washington
Chapter 19. Thermal Injuries

Jody A. Holland
RN, MN
Pediatric Clinical Nurse Specialist
Oregon Health Sciences University
Doernbecher Children's Hospital
Portland, Oregon
Chapter 10. Gastrointestinal Disorders

Mary Howell
RN, MSN
Clinical Nurse Specialist
Emergency Department
St. Louis Children's Hospital
St. Louis, Missouri
*Chapter 1. The Impact of Critical Care on
the Child*

Cindy Hylton Rushton
DNSc, RN, FAAN
Assistant Professor of Nursing
Johns Hopkins University
Clinical Nurse Specialist in Ethics
The Johns Hopkins Children's Center
Baltimore, Maryland
*Chapter 3. Ethical Issues in Pediatric
Critical Care*

Sharon Y. Irving-Daniels
RN, MSN, CRNP, CCRN
Preceptor
Guest Lecturer at University of
Pennsylvania—Nursing of Children
Critical Care Nurse Practitioner Program
University of Pennsylvania
Philadelphia, Pennsylvania
Pediatric Critical Care Nurse Practitioner
Sinai Hospital of Baltimore
Baltimore, Maryland
Chapter 14. Hematologic Disorders

Margaret A. Jones
RN, MA, PhD(c), CCRN
Director of Education and Professional
Development
Miami Children's Hospital
Miami, Florida
*Chapter 2. The Impact of Critical Care on
the Family*

Nancy M. Kraus
RN, MSN, CCRN
Associate Faculty
Saddleback College
Mission Viejo, California

Pediatric Intensive Care Unit Transport
  Coordinator
Children's Hospital Orange County
Orange, California

*Chapter 20. Human Immunodeficiency
  Virus*

Norma L. Liburd
RN,C, MN
Clinical Nurse Specialist
All Children's Hospital
St. Petersburg, Florida

Chapter 22. Nutrition

Susan Linehan
RN, BSN
Staff Nurse II
Children's Hospital
Boston, Massachusetts

Chapter 17. Transplantation

Aimee C. Lyons
RN, BSN, CCRN
Staff Nurse II
Children's Hospital
Boston, Massachusetts

Chapter 17. Transplantation

Bonnie Lysy-Nestler
RN, BSN, CCRN
Nursing Education Specialist
All Children's Hospital
St. Petersburg, Florida

*Chapter 13. Endocrine Disorders; Chapter
  15. Shock*

Natalie Madar
RN, BS, CCRN
Clinical Educator
Emergency Center
All Children's Hospital
St. Petersburg, Florida

Chapter 18. Toxic Ingestions

Karen Maggio
RN
Staff Nurse II
Children's Hospital
Boston, Massachusetts

Chapter 17. Transplantation

Denise Maguire
RN,C, MS
Nursing Department Director
Neonatal Intensive Care Unit
All Children's Hospital
St. Petersburg, Florida

*Chapter 4. Legal Issues in Pediatric
  Critical Care*

Janiece Maloney
RN, CETN
Enterostomal Therapy Nurse
Sinai Hospital of Baltimore
Baltimore, Maryland

Chapter 24. Skin Integrity

Kathleen A. Marine
RN, BSN
Staff Nurse II
Children's Hospital
Boston, Massachusetts

Chapter 17. Transplantation

Clifford B. Miller
RN,C, BSN
Nursing Education Specialist
All Children's Hospital
St. Petersburg, Florida

*Chapter 4. Legal Issues in Pediatric
  Critical Care*

Kathleen Miller
ARNP, MSN, PhD
Clinical Nurse Specialist
All Children's Hospital
St. Petersburg, Florida

Chapter 13. Endocrine Disorders

Patricia A. Moloney-Harmon
RN, MS, CCRN
Clinical Nurse Specialist
Children's Services
Sinai Hospital of Baltimore
Baltimore, Maryland

Chapter 16. Trauma

Linda Oakes
RN, MSN, CCRN
Intensive Care Clinical Nurse Specialist
St. Jude Children's Research Hospital
Memphis, Tennessee

Chapter 12. Oncologic Disorders

Kerri Oates
RN, MSN, CCRN
Clinical Nurse Specialist for Pediatrics and
    Pediatric Intensive Care
DeVos Children's Hospital at Butterworth
Grand Rapids, Michigan

Chapter 21. Resuscitation

Susan J. Senecal
RN, MSN
Clinical Nurse Specialist
Pain Management Team
All Children's Hospital
St. Petersburg, Florida

Chapter 25. Pain Management

Patricia Srnec
RN, MS, CNA
Director of Nursing, Emergency and
    Ambulatory Services
St. Louis Children's Hospital
St. Louis, Missouri

*Chapter 1. The Impact of Critical Care on
    the Child*

Paula Vernon-Levett
RN, MS, CCRN
Family Care Nurse
Pediatric Intensive Care Unit
The Children's Memorial Hospital
2300 Children's Plaza
Chicago, Illinois

Chapter 7. Neurologic Disorders

PREFACE

Review of Pediatric Critical Care is a state-of-the-art reference guide for nurses caring for critically ill children and their families. This study guide serves as a resource for nurses who are interested in developing their advanced decision-making skills or developing their test-taking skills. In addition, this book can be used as a teaching tool in both the classroom and the clinical setting. The case studies will challenge the learner to apply concepts and synthesize information.

The content of the case studies and the questions are based on the text *Critical Care Nursing of Infants and Children,* edited by Martha A.Q. Curley, Janis B. Smith, and Patricia A. Moloney-Harmon, and published by W.B. Saunders. Each case study is followed by multiple-choice questions. Answers are provided to each question, along with rationales and references. Several vignettes are provided for some cases.

We hope that this book will be a useful tool for all nurses who are seeking to advance their knowledge in pediatric critical care.

PATRICIA A. MOLONEY-HARMON
SANDRA J. CZERWINSKI

NOTICE

Pediatric critical care is an ever-changing field. Standard safety precautions must be followed, but as new research and clinical experience broaden our knowledge, changes in treatment and drug therapy become necessary or appropriate. The editors of this work have carefully checked the generic and trade drug names and verified drug dosages to ensure that the dosage information in this work is accurate and in accord with the standards accepted at the time of publication. Readers are advised, however, to check the product information currently provided by the manufacturer of each drug to be administered to be certain that changes have not been made in the recommended dose or in the contraindications for administration. This is of particular importance in regard to new or infrequently used drugs. It is the responsibility of the treating physician, relying on experience and knowledge of the patient, to determine dosages and the best treatment for the patient. The editors cannot be responsible for misuse or misapplication of the material in this work.

THE PUBLISHER

CONTENTS

CHAPTER 1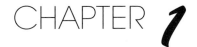

The Impact of Critical Care on the Child

PATRICIA SRNEC, RN, MS, CNA
MARY HOWELL, RN, MSN

CASE 1-1

H., a 4.5-year-old girl, is admitted to the pediatric intensive care unit (PICU) after surgical repair of an atrial septal defect. The atrial septal defect is an ostium secundum, which is an isolated defect in her.

On admission to the PICU, she is intubated, and bilateral chest tubes and arterial and peripheral lines are in place. A Foley catheter and nasogastric tube are also in place. Oxygen saturation levels are 97% to 99% on 40% oxygen, her vital signs and blood pressure are within normal limits, and she is appropriately responsive to painful stimuli.

Within 2 hours of her arrival in the PICU, she is fully alert and stable. She is extubated without difficulty after demonstrating acceptable arterial blood gases. She is placed on oxygen by nasal cannula at 2 L/min. Pain is managed with intravenous morphine sulfate.

1. To assess that H.'s pain is appropriately managed, it is essential that her nurse
   a. Understands that preschool children have a high tolerance for pain.
   b. Realizes that preschoolers are unable to localize pain.
   c. Closely monitors H.'s nonverbal responses and behaviors.
   d. Questions H. frequently about the presence of pain.

The girl's parents are able to stay with her much of the time while she is in the PICU. They ask her primary nurse about ways they can reassure H. and alleviate some of her fears, particularly when they are not able to remain with her during the night.

2. Requesting that parents or family members leave a few familiar items, such as a favorite toy, blanket, or video tape, with their child will help to ease
   a. Fear of painful procedures.
   b. Anxiety related to separation from parents and family.
   c. Mistrust of unfamiliar caregivers.
   d. Discomfort when being restrained.

3. One of the most effective and concrete ways to allow H. to express her fears related to hospitalization is to
   a. Have her tell a story or draw a picture.
   b. Ask her directly if she is afraid of anything.
   c. Wait for her to verbalize any fears.
   d. Safely assume that she is too young to express any fears.

4. During shift change, the day shift nurse reports that H. remained awake all day, without any periods of napping. The night shift nurse assumes that H. will sleep well during the night; however, she notices that H. is still very much awake at 2 A.M. She attributes this to the fact that
   a. H. doesn't realize that her parents have gone home for the night and that she is waiting for them to return.

b. H.'s sleep disturbance is probably related to the high level of sensory input around her (e.g., lights, noises, alarms) and a preschooler's need for bedtime rituals.

c. H. is afraid that she will not wake up or that someone will harm her while she is asleep.

d. The morphine that H. is receiving for pain adversely affects her and causes her to remain awake.

Throughout the night, H. remains stable, her oxygen is weaned to 1 L/min, and chest tube drainage is minimal. After a morning chest x-ray film is obtained, the plan of care (as discussed on rounds) is to discontinue her chest tubes, arterial line, and Foley and nasogastric catheters. H.'s nurse discusses with her parents how H. should be prepared for the planned procedures.

5. Because a preschooler's thinking is concrete,

a. There is no reason to prepare a child of H.'s age for a procedure, because she does not have the ability to understand.

b. A preschooler should be prepared for a planned event several hours before the occurrence.

c. A preschooler must be given the reasons for a planned procedure so the child can better accept it.

d. All procedures must be explained in clear and logical terms.

6. It is essential that preschoolers be protected from disturbing sights, sounds, and conversations that they may not understand. An example may be to avoid describing a "failure to wean" from oxygen in front of the child. The primary reason for such shielding is

a. Developmentally, the preschooler is attempting to overcome a sense of shame and doubt; exposure to such conversations will limit her progress in this regard.

b. The caregiver does not want the preschooler to interpret such conversations to mean that she is going to die.

c. Developmentally, the preschooler understands and interprets things literally and concretely. If she misinterprets a given statement, such as a "failure to wean," she may feel guilty and responsible.

d. Because the preschooler is able to make judgments based on reasoning,

she may interpret "failure to wean" to mean that she is progressing poorly.

During the first postoperative day, H.'s primary nurse notices that H. has wet the bed several times, rather than tell the nurse or her parents that she needs to urinate. Her parents are especially concerned about this behavior, because H. has been toilet trained for the past 2 years.

7. The most probable reason for H.'s bedwetting is that

a. She is exhibiting stress related to her surgery and hospitalization by demonstrating regressive behavior.

b. She has developed a urinary tract infection as a result of an earlier Foley catheter placement.

c. She is experiencing a temporary loss of bladder control postoperatively.

d. She does not want to make her nurse angry by asking for help.

8. A primary reason that a hospitalized preschooler may exhibit regressive behavior is that

a. She is angry and wants to punish her parents.

b. She is attempting to regain mastery of a stressful or anxiety-producing situation.

c. Side effects from pain medication cause her to forget newly learned behaviors or skills.

d. It is her way of attracting sympathy from her parents and caregivers.

During the time that H. is a patient in the PICU, a child across the unit dies as a result of a head injury associated with a motor vehicle accident. H.'s parents are very concerned about her exposure to and understanding of the event.

9. The following best describes a preschooler's concept of death:

a. Death is permanent and irreversible.

b. A preschooler has little awareness of death.

c. Death is temporary and reversible.

d. Death is inevitable.

H. continues to progress throughout the day and experiences a stable postoperative course. She is transferred to the general pediatric unit on the afternoon of her second postoperative day.

CASE 1-2

T., a 12-year-old asthmatic girl, is admitted to the PICU in severe respiratory distress.

On admission, the nurse notices that T. has intravenous lines in both upper extremities, a pulse oximeter probe on one finger, and a cardiac monitor in place and that she is receiving a continuous albuterol aerosol treatment. Continuing with her assessment, the nurse questions T. about her medical history and current medications. T. stares at the nurse and answers in one-syllable words. The nurse continues to press for information.

1. When assessing an adolescent patient, the nurse should
   a. Wait until the parent is at the bedside.
   b. Use very simple language and explanations.
   c. Provide as much privacy as possible.
   d. Allow the patient to start the conversation.

2. The adolescent period that T. is in reflects
   a. A dependence on parents.
   b. Specific goals and plans for life.
   c. Adjustment to pubescent changes.
   d. Individual relationships that are more important than those with peer groups.

T. becomes more withdrawn as the shift progresses. The nurse notices that she makes very little eye contact and no verbal responses. Her vital signs are stable, and her arterial blood gases are within the normal range. A continuous aerosol treatment is in place, although bilateral wheezing is still occurring.

3. Concerned that T. is very anxious, the nurse should
   a. Question T. about why she is upset.
   b. Offer a verbal explanation of her surroundings and treatments.
   c. Ask the doctor for sedation orders.
   d. Have the mother at the bedside.

4. Adolescents tend to solve problems by
   a. Using deductive reasoning from previous experience.
   b. Relying on parental judgment.
   c. Using trial and error.
   d. Denying having any problems.

T.'s mother comes in for a visit and remarks to the nurse that T. looks much better. She explains that although T. has had asthma all of her life, she has never had an attack like this one. The mother then questions T. about her medications, stating that the medications cost a lot of money. T. replies that she does not need the medication. She says, "everyone looks at me strange."

5. The nurse wants to help T. verbalize her feelings to her mother. The best action would be to
   a. Inform the mother that patients who take their medications regularly can still become ill.
   b. Assure T. that she will be fine and that her medications will be reviewed.
   c. Ask the mother for a list of the medications.
   d. Offer to call the physician for the mother.

6. T.'s remarks about the medications indicate that
   a. T. doesn't like to take medicine.
   b. T. may be using the medications in error.
   c. T. feels she is different from her peers when she takes the medications.
   d. T. may be experiencing a reaction to her medications.

7. Peer relationships in the adolescent development stage represent
   a. Added stress to the adolescent's life.
   b. No purpose.
   c. Replacement of the parent's role.
   d. Assistance in avoiding role confusion.

T. starts to complain of a headache and becomes very vocal about getting something for the pain. In a quick assessment of T., the nurse notices a heart rate of 110 beats per minute (bpm) and regular respirations of 24 breaths per minute, with continued mild wheezing and a blood pressure measurement of 100/56 mmHg. T. is alert and responds appropriately to questions. She again verbalizes her need for something for pain. The nurse explains that she must obtain a verbal order from the doctor for pain medication.

8. T.'s demand for pain medication reflects
   a. A worsening respiratory condition.
   b. A low tolerance for pain.
   c. Anger toward the nurse.
   d. Her need to maintain self-control.

9. To assist the adolescent with pain management, the nurse may
   a. Use a patient-controlled analgesia device.
   b. Give only intramuscular injections for pain.
   c. Teach the adolescent relaxation techniques.
   d. Give the adolescent a pain scale to rate her pain.

T. continues to improve and is moved from the intensive care unit the following day.

CASE 1-3

B. is a 1-month-old infant admitted to the PICU with the diagnosis of sepsis. B. has an intravenous line in his right forearm, a pulse oximeter probe, and cardiac monitor, and he is on 1 L/min of oxygen administered by face mask.

B. has a septic workup in the emergency room and receives his first round of intravenous antibiotics. B.'s parents are at his bedside and must wear gloves and mask when they visit. The nurse notices that B.'s parents have not touched him and that they do not approach the crib.

1. Touch is important to the infant because
   a. Touch helps the infant develop physical muscles.
   b. Touch helps the parents relieve stress.
   c. Touch helps comfort and aid the infant in developing trust.
   d. Touch is very negative.

2. The nurse looks for signs that the infant is stressed. These signs include
   a. Crying, agitation, and difficulty in being consoled.
   b. Sleeping more than usual.
   c. Sucking of thumb and fingers.
   d. Turning away from parents.

3. The nurse can reduce stress for the infant by
   a. Reducing noises and lights.
   b. Keeping the infant in a private room.
   c. Turning the infant frequently.
   d. Placing toys and objects in the infant's crib.

The resident approaches and informs the parents that B. needs another lumbar puncture and repeat laboratory work.

4. Because procedures produce stress in the infant, the nurse should
   a. Limit the number of procedures done on the infant.
   b. Have parents present during all procedures.
   c. Plan a rest and recovery time between each procedure.
   d. Plan the procedure during sleep times.

5. The nurse may wish to incorporate other means to reduce stress, such as
   a. Feeding the infant before procedures.
   b. Placing the infant in a large crib.
   c. Giving some sedation before each procedure.
   d. Swaddling the infant, leaving his hands free to reach objects.

B.'s mother expresses concern that she will not be able to continue to breastfeed. She states that she has one other child and that it was beneficial to breastfeed the infant until 6 months of age.

6. B.'s mother's expression of her feelings about breastfeeding reflects
   a. The infant's interaction with the mother.
   b. The mother's need to be a caregiver.
   c. The basis for good physical growth.
   d. An adjustment period for the mother.

B.'s condition deteriorates, and he is placed on a ventilator for support. His parents, although saying they believe everything is going well, become more demanding of the nurse's time.

7. B.'s parents are attempting to cope with his severe illness. To help them through the process, the nurse should
   a. Help the parents identify resources for their use.
   b. Offer to call the physician for the parents.
   c. Provide educational material on sepsis.
   d. Hold all procedures while B.'s parents are at the bedside.

B.'s condition continues to worsen, despite all medical interventions. The physician explains the poor prognosis. B.'s mother continues to state that he will be fine.

8. The mother's statement is an example of
   a. Regression.
   b. Adaptation.
   c. Denial.
   d. Mastery.

B. dies early in the morning; his parents are at his bedside.

9. To help the parents in their bereavement, the nurse should
   a. Instruct the parents that everything will work out for the best.
   b. Offer to find the chaplain for the family.
   c. Take the baby to the morgue.
   d. Support the family by allowing them to express their grief.

10. The nursing staff also needs to cope with the death of an infant. The best way to assist with this is to
    a. Identify the emotions involved and work through them.
    b. Review the medical record with others in the unit.
    c. Ask for light assignments for the rest of the week.
    d. Identify support groups or resources that the nurse could call.

ANSWERS ■ CASE 1-1

1. Answer (c). Recognition and treatment of pain is difficult, because there is no objective measure of pain on which to base clinical decisions. It is therefore essential that the nurse be able to recognize pain behaviors and develop techniques to evaluate the child's nonverbal clues regarding pain.

REFERENCE
Eland, J.M., & Banner, Jr., W. (1992). Assessment and management of pain in children. In M.F. Hazinski (Ed.). *Nursing care of the critically ill child* (pp. 79–100). St. Louis: Mosby–Year Book.

2. Answer (b). Transitional or security objects are valuable to ease distress when the child is separated from parents. Familiar toys, family photos, and video or audio tapes help the preschool child to maintain a sense of contact with parents and siblings.

REFERENCE
Smith, J.B., & Browne, A.M. (1996). The impact of the critical care experience on the child. In M.A.Q. Curley, J.B. Smith, & P.A. Moloney-Harmon (Eds.). *Critical care nursing of infants and children* (pp. 15–46). Philadelphia: W.B. Saunders.

3. Answer (a). Storytelling or puppet play with a child can uncover misconceptions and fantasies about her or his illness and hospitalization. Projective play techniques, such as drawing and storytelling, are useful in eliciting the child's feelings. The feelings of wrongdoing and guilt exhibited can be clarified and dealt with through these techniques.

REFERENCE
Betz, C.L., Hunsberger, M., & Wright, S. (1994). Families with preschoolers. In C.L. Betz, M. Hunsberger, & S. Wright (Eds.). *Family-centered nursing care of children* (pp. 230–273). Philadelphia: W.B. Saunders.

4. Answer (b). The chaotic-appearing environment of the PICU and the lack of H.'s usual bedtime ritual result in her inability to fall asleep. Preschoolers often experience sleep disturbances as a result of sensory input such as lights, sounds, and odors. They are also fairly dependent on bedtime rituals.

REFERENCES
Smith, J.B., & Browne, A.M. (1996). The impact of the critical care experience on the child. In M.A.Q. Curley, J.B. Smith, & P.A. Moloney-Harmon (Eds.). *Critical care nursing of infants and children* (pp. 15–46). Philadelphia: W.B. Saunders.
Stein, M.T. (1992). Children's encounters with illness: Hospitalization and procedures. In S.D. Dixon & M.T. Stein (Eds.). *Encounters with children: Pediatric behavior and development* (2nd ed., pp. 401–409). St. Louis: Mosby–Year Book.

5. Answer (d). Preschool-age children focus on one aspect of a situation rather than on all aspects. The child's reasoning is a reflection of her or his limited viewpoint, and it may seem illogical to others. The preschooler believes that everything has a cause, and the child responds with "why?" to every explanation.

REFERENCE
Ryan-DiSchino, D. (1993). Health assessment, promotion, and maintenance for preschool children. In D.B. Jackson & R. B. Saunders (Eds.). *Child health nursing* (pp. 301–331). Philadelphia: W.B. Saunders.

6. Answer (c). Preschoolers may experience a sense of guilt if they perceive that they have not behaved or acted appropriately. Because preschoolers have a rigid conscience, they frequently have unwarranted guilt feelings about obvious or secret wrongs.

REFERENCES
Betz, C.L., Hunsberger, M., & Wright, S. (1994). Families with preschoolers. In C.L. Betz, M. Hunsberger, & S. Wright (Eds.). *Family-centered nursing care of children* (pp. 230–273). Philadelphia: W.B. Saunders.
Wong, D.L. (1993). Health promotion of the preschooler and family. In D.L. Wong (Ed.). *Whaley and Wong's essentials of pediatric nursing* (pp. 367–381). St. Louis: Mosby–Year Book.

7. Answer (a). Children of all age groups can be expected to demonstrate a loss of some developmental milestones during and after a hospital experience.

REFERENCE
Stein, M.T. (1992). Children's encounters with illness: Hospitalization and procedures. In S.D. Dixon & M.T.

Stein (Eds.). *Encounters with children: pediatric behavior and development* (2nd ed., pp. 401–409). St. Louis: Mosby–Year Book.

8. Answer (**b**). Developmental regression symbolizes a stressor and a protective maneuver to defend against the loss of parents or to allow the preschooler to handle the hospital experience. Parents require reassurance that regressive behavior is the child's temporary way of dealing with a stressful situation and that the child will regain lost skills after recovery. Because the child needs these behaviors, it is important to accept the regressed behaviors and support the child rather than admonish her for bad behavior.

REFERENCE
Lewandowski, L. (1992). Psychological aspects of pediatric critical care. In M.F. Hazinski (Ed.). *Nursing care of the critically ill child* (pp. 19–77). St. Louis: Mosby–Year Book.

9. Answer (**c**). Children between 3 and 5 years of age have usually heard of death, but its meaning is vague. They see death as a departure, possibly as some kind of sleep. They do not understand that death involves the loss of physical abilities, such as eating, breathing, or sleeping. Death is temporary and gradual to them; they believe that life and death can change places with one another.

REFERENCE
Rollins-Holt, J. (1993). Impact of chronic illness, disability, or death on the child and family. In D.L. Wong (Ed.). *Whaley and Wong's essentials of pediatric nursing* (pp. 504–548). St. Louis: Mosby–Year Book.

ANSWERS ■ CASE 1-2

1. Answer (**c**). The adolescent development phase is a time of self-discovery and exploration. The body is developing and changing at a rapid pace. Adolescents become self-conscious about these changes, and they assume everyone around them notices the changes. Privacy becomes a major issue. The clinician should respect this need, whenever possible, by asking questions of the adolescent in private.

REFERENCES
Felice, M.E. (1992). Overview of adolescence. In S.D. Dixon & M.T. Stein (Eds.). *Encounters with children: Pediatric behavior and development* (2nd ed., pp. 341–344). St. Louis: Mosby–Year Book.
Lewandowski, L.A., (1992). Psychosocial aspects of pediatric critical care. In M.F. Hazinski (Ed.). *Nursing*
care of the critically ill child (pp. 19–77). St. Louis: Mosby–Year Book.

2. Answer (**c**). T. is in the early phase of adolescence, one that reflects pubescent changes. These changes include rapid physical, psychosocial, moral, and cognitive growth.

REFERENCE
Felice, M.E. (1992). Overview of adolescence. In S.D. Dixon & M.T. Stein (Eds.). *Encounters with children: Pediatric behavior and development* (2nd ed., pp. 341–344). St. Louis: Mosby–Year Book.

3. Answer (**b**). The nurse may wish to question T., but it is important to remember that T. is only 12 years of age. In the transition period from childhood to adulthood, an adolescent wants to gather the information and then sort through the problem. The nurse can help T. with her anxiety by explaining the surroundings and the procedures to her, allowing T. to become an active member in the health care team.

REFERENCE
Smith, J.B., & Browne, A.M. (1996). The impact of the critical care experience on the child. In M.A.Q. Curley, J.B. Smith, & P.A. Moloney-Harmon (Eds.). *Critical care nursing of infants and children* (pp. 15–46). Philadelphia: W.B. Saunders.

4. Answer (**a**). Adolescents' cognitive development allows them to imagine possibilities and to form and test hypotheses. Testing a hypothesis allows the adolescent to solve problems with deductive reasoning.

REFERENCES
Felice, M.E. (1992). Eleven to thirteen years: Early adolescence—the age of rapid change. In S.D. Dixon & M.T. Stein (Eds.). *Encounters with children: Pediatric behavior and development* (2nd ed., pp. 347–357). St. Louis: Mosby–Year Book.
Smith, J.B., & Browne, A.M. (1996). The impact of the critical care experience on the child. In M.A.Q. Curley, J.B. Smith, & P.A. Moloney-Harmon (Eds.). *Critical care nursing of infants and children* (pp. 15–46). Philadelphia: W.B. Saunders.

5. Answer (**b**). The adolescent wants to be recognized as an adult. By addressing T., the nurse allows her to maintain control. If the adolescent feels in control of the situation, ideas and thoughts can be more freely expressed.

REFERENCE
Felice, M.E. (1993). Eleven to thirteen years: Early adolescence—the age of rapid change. In S.D. Dixon & M.T. Stein (Eds.). *Encounters with children: Pediatric*

behavior and development (2nd ed., pp. 347–357). St. Louis: Mosby–Year Book.

6. Answer (**c**). Adolescents do not want to feel different from their peers. As they separate from their parents, their peer group becomes the measuring stick for physical and psychological growth.

REFERENCE

Smith, J.B., & Browne, A.M. (1996). The impact of the critical care experience on the child. In M.A.Q. Curley, J.B. Smith, & P.A. Moloney-Harmon (Eds.). *Critical care nursing of infants and children* (pp. 15–46). Philadelphia: W.B. Saunders.

7. Answer (**d**). Peer groups help the adolescent avoid role confusion. They serve as safety nets while teens try out social roles and behaviors.

REFERENCE

Smith, J.B., & Browne, A.M. (1996). The impact of the critical care experience on the child. In M.A.Q. Curley, J.B. Smith, & P.A. Moloney-Harmon (Eds.). *Critical care nursing of infants and children* (pp. 15–46). Philadelphia: W.B. Saunders.

8. Answer (**d**). Adolescents relate to pain with a loss of control. They tend to become demanding and angry, and they may grow hostile if their demand for relief is not met.

REFERENCE

Lewandowski, L.A. (1992). Psychosocial aspects of pediatric critical care. In M.F. Hazinski (Ed.). *Nursing care of the critically ill child* (pp. 19–77). St. Louis: Mosby–Year Book.

9. Answer (**a**). The use of a patient-controlled analgesia device reduces the feeling of powerlessness and enhances control. It enables the adolescent to feel in charge of the situation. To an adolescent, any pain rates high on a pain scale, and relaxation techniques may serve no purpose.

REFERENCE

Smith, J.B., & Browne, A.M. (1996). The impact of the critical care experience on the child. In M.A.Q. Curley, J.B. Smith, & P.A. Moloney-Harmon (Eds.). *Critical care nursing of infants and children* (pp. 15–46). Philadelphia: W.B. Saunders.

ANSWERS ■ CASE 1-3

1. Answer (**c**). Touch is one of the first steps a parent takes to form an emotional bond with the newborn. It comforts the infant and helps the infant develop a sense of trust.

REFERENCE

Wong, D.L. (1993). Health promotion of the newborn and family. In D.L. Wong (Ed.). *Whaley and Wong's essentials of pediatric nursing* (pp. 176–210). St. Louis: Mosby–Year Book.

2. Answer (**a**). Signs of stress vary among infants, and the nurse must observe each infant carefully. Signs may include crying and agitation, and the infant may be inconsolable.

REFERENCE

Smith, J.B., & Browne, A.M. (1996). The impact of the critical care experience on the child. In M.A.Q. Curley, J.B. Smith, & P.A. Moloney-Harmon (Eds.). *Critical care nursing of infants and children* (pp. 15–46). Philadelphia: W.B. Saunders.

3. Answer (**a**). The intensive care environment, with all of its noise and lights, contributes to the stress of the infant. By reducing the noise level and light intensity, stress levels can be reduced.

REFERENCE

Smith, J.B., & Browne, A.M. (1996). The impact of the critical care experience on the child. In M.A.Q. Curley, J.B. Smith, & P.A. Moloney-Harmon (Eds.). *Critical care nursing of infants and children* (pp. 15–46). Philadelphia: W.B. Saunders.

4. Answer (**c**). The ill infant sometimes requires several procedures to assist with diagnosis and treatment. Planning a rest and recovery time between procedures allows the infant to better cope with the stress.

REFERENCES

Lewandowski, L.A. (1992). Psychosocial aspects of pediatric critical care. In M.F. Hazinski (Ed.). *Nursing care of the critically ill child* (pp. 19–77). St. Louis: Mosby–Year Book.
Smith, J.B., & Browne, A.M. (1996). The impact of the critical care experience on the child. In M.A.Q. Curley, J.B. Smith, & P.A. Moloney-Harmon (Eds.). *Critical care nursing of infants and children* (pp. 15–46). Philadelphia: W.B. Saunders.

5. Answer (**d**). Swaddling of the infant offers a sense of security. Leaving the hands free allows the infant to continue to explore the environment and maintain hand-to-mouth maneuvers.

REFERENCE

Smith, J.B., & Browne, A.M. (1996). The impact of the critical care experience on the child. In M.A.Q. Curley, J.B. Smith, & P.A. Moloney-Harmon (Eds.). *Critical care nursing of infants and children* (pp. 15–46). Philadelphia: W.B. Saunders.

6. Answer (**b**). Breastfeeding the infant allows the mother to strengthen the bonding process. Breastfeeding also establishes the mother as the caregiver for the infant. When the infant becomes ill, the mother must relinquish the role of caregiver to the health care professionals, but the mother still has a need to be the principal caregiver and should be encouraged to provide as much of the care as possible.

REFERENCES
Lewandowski, L.A. (1992). Psychosocial aspects of pediatric critical care. In M.F. Hazinski (Ed.). *Nursing care of the critically ill child* (pp. 19–77). St. Louis: Mosby–Year Book.
Smith, J.B., & Browne, A.M. (1996). The impact of the critical care experience on the child. In M.A.Q. Curley, J.B. Smith, & P.A. Moloney-Harmon (Eds.). *Critical care nursing of infants and children* (pp. 15–46). Philadelphia: W.B. Saunders.

7. Answer (**a**). The nurse can assist B.'s parents by helping them to identify resources, such as family members, neighbors, or community groups. A strong support system can help the parents comprehend the infant's condition and deal with the outcome.

REFERENCE
Miles, M., & Warner, J. (1992). The dying child in the intensive care unit. In M.F. Hazinski (Ed.). *Nursing care of the critically ill child* (pp. 101–116). St. Louis: Mosby–Year Book.

8. Answer (**c**). Denial is a step in the grief process that reflects shock and disbelief. The other stages include anger, bargaining, depression, and acceptance.

REFERENCE
Wong, D.L. (1993). Impact of chronic illness, disability or death on the child and family. In D.L. Wong (Ed.). *Whaley and Wong's essentials of pediatric nursing* (pp. 504–548). St. Louis: Mosby–Year Book.

9. Answer (**d**). The nurse can best assist the family by allowing them to express their grief.

REFERENCE
Smith, J.B., & Browne, A.M. (1996). The impact of the critical care experience on the child. In M.A.Q. Curley, J.B. Smith, & P.A. Moloney-Harmon (Eds.). *Critical care nursing of infants and children* (pp. 15–46). Philadelphia: W.B. Saunders.

10. Answer (**d**). When a patient dies, the nurse should be allowed to express his or her feelings. This may be done in a formal group discussion or on a one-on-one basis.

REFERENCE
Smith, J.B., & Browne, A.M. (1996). The impact of the critical care experience on the child. In M.A.Q. Curley, J.B. Smith, & P.A. Moloney-Harmon (Eds.). *Critical care nursing of infants and children* (pp. 15–46). Philadelphia: W.B. Saunders.

CHAPTER 2

The Impact of Critical Care on the Family

MARGARET A. JONES, RN, MA, PhD(c), CCRN

CASE 2-1

M., a 13-year-old girl, was struck by a car and taken to the children's hospital. After her parents received the call telling them that their daughter had been involved in a motor vehicle accident, they went to the hospital. When they arrived at the emergency center, they were told that M. had been transferred to the pediatric intensive care unit (PICU), and they were given directions to the PICU.

The father is bilingual. The mother approaches the nurse's desk and identifies herself to the secretary in Spanish. The secretary states that she does not speak Spanish and does not understand the mother. The father approaches the nurse's desk and states in English that they are M.'s parents and that they would like to see her. The secretary calls the PICU and asks for the nurse caring for M. The nurse comes to the desk and introduces herself to the parents.

1. The most appropriate nursing intervention after introducing herself to the parents is to
   a. Take them in to see their daughter and let them have some time alone at the beside.
   b. Tell them about the visitation policy, emphasizing that information is given only to parents.
   c. Explain M.'s status and what the next few days will probably involve.
   d. Tell the parents what M. looks like and about the equipment that is attached to her.

The mother begins to cry at M.'s bedside, and the father stands behind her but does not respond.

2. What should the nurse's response be?
   a. Put her arm around the mother to comfort her.
   b. Stay at the end of the bed and do nothing.
   c. Tell the father to take M's mother out of the unit because she is upset.
   d. Tell the mother not to cry because she needs to be strong for M.

3. The nurse's next intervention should be to
   a. Ask the family to talk about M. and tell what she is like.
   b. Leave the family at the bedside to give them some privacy.
   c. Review the visitation rules of the unit with the family.
   d. Start explaining M.'s condition to the family and ask if they have any questions.

The physician approaches the parents and explains M.'s status. He tells them that she is in critical condition and the next 12 to 24 hours will be very important. He explains that M. has severe head trauma and that her intracranial pressure is being monitored. He states that if M. does survive, "she will have some brain damage, and she will not be the same girl that she was before the accident."

He cannot say, however, how severe the brain damage will be. The physician asks if the parents have any questions. They say that they do not.

4. What will be the most important nursing concern after this discussion with the physician?
   a. Would the parents like to have a priest come in to speak with them?
   b. Because the parents' primary language is Spanish, do they understand what the physician has explained to them?
   c. Will the parents ask the nurse her opinion about M.'s prognosis?
   d. Will the parents want to stay at the bedside for the next 12 to 24 hours?

Two days later, M.'s electroencephalogram is flat. The physician requests that the nurse locate the family so he can explain brain death and potential organ donation.

5. What is the nurse's first priority in this situation?
   a. Arrange for a translator for the parents.
   b. Arrange for a private room for the parents.
   c. Obtain bereavement information for the family.
   d. Request to be with the physician when he explains brain death.

6. What is the nurse's role in a family meeting where brain death and organ donation are discussed?
   a. Bring the appropriate paperwork to the meeting.
   b. Provide support to the family and be their advocate.
   c. Be the witness for the physician.
   d. Give an opinion on whether the family should participate in organ donation.

After the meeting, the family returns to the bedside. The nurse accompanies them. They talk to the nurse about M. and how she was always a giving person. They state that she would probably want them to give her organs to help someone else. However, many of their family members will be upset if they agree to give away parts of M.

7. In this situation, what is the nurse's best response?
   a. Organ donation is a private decision of the family, and it is confidential. No one else in the family will know about

the donation unless M.'s parents decide to tell them.
   b. It is none of the other family members' business, and the parents should just ignore them and do what they want.
   c. It will be a shame if they decide not to donate M.'s organs, because there are so many children who need transplants.
   d. The nurse is willing to meet with the rest of the family and explain all aspects of organ donation and address any concerns.

The family agrees to donate M.'s organs, but they have a special request. They would like M.'s entire junior high school class to be able to visit her in the hospital.

8. What is the nurse's best response to this request?
   a. Explain that it is impossible to have 20 to 30 junior high students come into the PICU.
   b. Tell the parents that it will be necessary to obtain permission from infection control to allow the class into the unit.
   c. Explain that there is not enough time to arrange this type of request.
   d. Clarify for the parents that special arrangements can be made to have the students come in two or three at one time with appropriate support.

One month after M.'s death, the nurse calls the parents to see how they are doing. The family says that they are struggling and that they are having a hard time talking with each other. The husband says that his wife cannot stop crying and that he does not know what to do. He states that he is doing fine and is back at work. He also says that he wants to clean out M.'s room but that his wife has made it like a shrine and spends hours in the room praying. The husband says he would rather just stay at work than come home.

9. A critical intervention at this time would be to
   a. Suggest that the couple attend a support group meeting with other parents whose children have died.
   b. Tell them not to worry about not talking with each other, because that is a common response to grief.
   c. Explain that time heals everything

and that they just need to give it more time.

d. Suggest that they go to a marriage counselor to help with their communication.

CASE 2-2

J., a 5-year-old girl, has had multiple operations for a single-ventricle heart defect. After her sixth operation 1 week ago, she could not be extubated, was extremely weak, and required caloric support with hyperalimentation. The surgeons spoke with the mother and explained that J. needed one more operation because she had too much pulmonary blood flow into her lungs, causing a constant pneumonia. The mother, who is a single parent, felt that J. had been through enough, and she just wanted to take her daughter home. The surgeons told her that J. would not be able to be discharged because of her current status. J.'s mother agreed, with the understanding that this would be the final surgical procedure.

J. survived surgery without complications, but after 1 month, she remains intubated. Her kidneys have failed, and she is on dialysis. J.'s blood pressure is labile, and she is on a dopamine drip. J.'s mother is at her bedside 16 hours each day. J.'s mother asks the surgeon what his plan is for J. The surgeon's response is that everything is being done to try to get J. well.

1. The mother approaches J.'s primary nurse and asks her opinion about whether J. will get better. What is the nurse's best response?
   a. I am not comfortable giving my opinion. The doctor knows what he's talking about, and I trust his opinion.
   b. My opinion is that J. is very sick, but because she came through tough times before, we should maintain hope.
   c. It is very hard for me to answer your question. J. is very sick, and I am not sure if she will be able to survive, but we are trying to do everything to help her.
   d. We work with critically ill children all the time, and I have seen many miracles. Maybe J. will be one, too.

J.'s mother says that she made a mistake in agreeing to this last operation. She hates seeing J. suffer like this.

2. After the mother's statement, what would be the most therapeutic intervention?
   a. Approach the mother and hug her instead of saying anything.
   b. Reinforce the mother by telling her that she had a difficult decision to make and that she did what she thought was best.
   c. Explain to the mother that she should not feel that way and that she is a good mother.
   d. Tell the mother that J. is not suffering, because she is on a continuous fentanyl drip.

After another week, J.'s status deteriorates even more. She is now on several inotropic drips, continuous dialysis, and extremely high ventilator settings. The mother sits at the bedside and asks the nurses to let J. go. She cannot stand to see her like this anymore.

3. When J.'s mother requests to "let J. go," what options does the nurse have?
   a. Call the physician about the mother's statement, and discuss an Ethics Committee referral.
   b. Tell the mother that J. cannot be let go, because she has a functioning brain.
   c. Tell the mother that she should talk to J.'s physician about these feelings.
   d. Tell the mother about the Ethics Committee, and explain that she should discuss her request with her physician.

The physician speaks to the mother and explains that J. has a functioning brain. Because her condition is not considered to be a permanent vegetative state, he is not comfortable with the idea of withdrawing support. The mother continues to cry at the bedside and pray for J. to die.

4. What would be an appropriate nursing intervention at this point?
   a. Contact her immediate supervisor or clinical nurse specialist (CNS), explain the circumstances, and request that the case be reviewed by the Ethics Committee.
   b. Refer the mother to the psychiatry department for help with her grieving.
   c. Tell the mother that it might be better if she did not spend so much time at the bedside.
   d. Tell the physician that it is difficult to work with the mother crying all the time and praying out loud to let the child die.

The nursing staff requests an Ethics Committee meeting to review the case and consider the mother's request to stop everything. The mother states that she does not want to attend the Ethics Committee meeting. She does not want people to think she is a terrible mother who is requesting that her child be allowed to die. She hopes that they allow J. to stop suffering and stop treatments.

5. The nurse should respond to the mother
   a. That it is her option to attend or not to attend the Ethics Committee meeting.
   b. That it is difficult to make a request as she has but that it is important for the Ethics Committee to hear her feelings about the quality of J.'s life now.
   c. That if she is not willing to attend, there is no reason to have the meeting.
   d. That J.'s nurse will be there with her and that it is important for the Ethics Committee to hear her feelings about J.'s quality of life.

The Ethics Committee members meet concerning J.'s status and concur with the mother that the treatment J. is receiving is futile and should be stopped. The physician, however, states that it is against his moral values to stop everything when she still has a functioning brain.

6. What options do the Ethics Committee members have at this point?
   a. Recommend that the physician refer the case to another physician who could follow the mother's request.
   b. Recommend that the case go to court to be resolved, because there is nothing more that the Ethics Committee can do.
   c. Tell the mother that the Ethics Committee is not a decision-making body and that they can only make a recommendation.
   d. Tell the physician that he must follow their recommendations.

While J.'s status is being discussed by the Ethics Committee and the physician, J. dies. The nursing staff turn their attention to supporting the mother.

CASE 2-3

C., a 14-year-old boy, has been admitted to the PICU with septic shock. He is being ventilated at maximum ventilator settings and is on dopamine, epinephrine, dobutamine, and fentanyl drips. Because he is having seizures periodically, his electroencephalographic pattern is monitored continuously. He is not interactive with the environment. His parents are recently divorced, and his father has remarried. C. was living with his mother, but she told one of the nursing staff that he has been rebellious and difficult to manage. The mother and father did not have an amicable divorce.

1. What other history concerning the family dynamics would be important to know?
   a. How the parents have handled decision-making concerning C. since the divorce.
   b. What the custody standing is for the child.
   c. What the culture of the family is.
   d. What disciplinary methods the mother was using with C.

C. has been in the unit 3 days and is progressively deteriorating. The mother comes in and finds the doctor explaining C.'s condition to the father and his new wife. The mother becomes angry and begins to scream at the father and his wife to get out of the unit.

2. What would the nurse's action be at this time?
   a. Approach the family, and request them to step into the conference room to work out the problem.
   b. Ask the father and his wife to leave, because the mother has custody.
   c. Call social services to get clarification on the parental rights.
   d. Call security to the unit to help.

3. What is an important collaborative intervention to prevent this type of problem?
   a. Ensure that everyone on the team is totally aware of the family situation.
   b. Determine who has the right to information about C.'s condition.
   c. Meet with both the parents to set up visitation guidelines and a system for sharing information.
   d. Make sure that the parents are never at the bedside at the same time.

4. After meeting with the family and developing a plan for visitation and information sharing, how does the nurse ensure that the plan is followed?
   a. Make a list of rules and post it at the bedside.
   b. Make a note in the chart.

c. Place the information in the multi-disciplinary plan of care.

d. Tell the next nurse in report about the outcomes from the meeting.

After 6 weeks, C.'s condition slowly improves. He has a tracheostomy and requires support with only 35% oxygen. He no longer requires vasoactive medications. However, he is not really awake and continues to have seizures. The mother sits at his bedside and writes in a journal all day. She records when he has a seizure, what the seizure looks like, and anything else that happens with C.'s care.

5. What could the nurse do to help the mother at this point?
   a. Allow the mother to read the nurses' notes.
   b. Get her involved in caring for C.
   c. Explain to the mother that she needs to have some time for herself.
   d. Take the mother out of the unit, and tell her that her writing makes the nurses uncomfortable.

The ICU staff find the mother difficult to deal with, and they do not want to care for C.

6. How can these feelings be handled?
   a. Design a rotation list so no one has to work with her for more than one shift.
   b. Assign the newer staff so they get experience working with a difficult family.
   c. Assign float staff when possible to give the PICU staff a break.
   d. Have a patient care conference with the PICU staff to discuss the best approach to working with the mother.

The next day, a nurse from another unit comes to the PICU to assist in care, and she is assigned to C.

7. What would be critical to share in a nursing report with the nurse?
   a. Explain about the family dynamics and how information is shared.
   b. Explain that it would be better not to tell the mother anything, because the nurse is here for only one shift.
   c. Explain that a PICU nurse will be at the next bedside if she needs assistance.
   d. Tell her about how difficult the mother is and that she is writing everything in a journal about the care.

The mother approaches the charge nurse and requests that another nurse care for C., because she does not know the nurse who is assigned to him.

8. What is the best way for the charge nurse to handle this situation?
   a. Change the nursing assignments in response to the mother's request.
   b. Explain that the nurse who is assigned to C. is qualified to care for him and that other nurses are available to help if necessary.
   c. Explain that assignments cannot be changed after they are made and that other nurses are available to keep an eye on C.
   d. Tell her that the nursing supervisor will be called and that the supervisor will discuss her request with her.

9. How can a nurse assigned to the PICU from another unit reassure a patient or family that they can provide safe care?
   a. Tell the patient or family about the number of years of pediatric nursing experience he or she has.
   b. Explain that he or she has been cross-trained to this area, even though he or she does not work on the unit regularly.
   c. Review the daily plan of care for C. with the mother.
   d. Explain that there are other nurses on the floor who will assist if help is needed in caring for C.

Several days later, the physician decides that C. can be transferred to the seizure unit.

10. What is important for the nurse to do to coordinate C.'s transfer?
    a. Contact the CNS of the seizure unit and explain C.'s care.
    b. Set up a meeting with the CNS from the seizure unit and the mother to review C.'s care.
    c. Tell the mother that C. is better and will be transferred to the seizure unit tomorrow.
    d. Take the mother to the seizure unit for a tour and to meet some of that unit's nurses.

11. What problems may parents identify when their child is transferred to the floor after a long PICU stay?
    a. An increase in anxiety related to the decrease in monitoring equipment and personnel.
    b. An expectation that they may stay

overnight in the room with their child.

c. An expectation that they may assume more responsibility for care.

d. An expectation that the routines on the unit are similar to the routines in the PICU.

The transfer is completed. After 2 days, the nurses in the PICU notice that the mother has been down in the unit at least twice each shift to complain about the floor nurses.

12. What is the role of the ICU nurse with this mother?

a. Keep talking with the mother to support her so that she has a place to vent her concerns.

b. Take the issue to the nurse manager or CNS of the PICU and let them handle it.

c. Tell the mother that you will talk with the nurse manager or CNS of the seizure unit about her concerns.

d. Tell the mother she should discuss her concerns with the nurse manager or the CNS of that unit.

ANSWERS ■ CASE 2-1

1. Answer (**d**). An orientation should be given to a family whose child has just been admitted to an intensive care unit so they can begin to cope with the crisis. Parents who experience an unexpected admission to a PICU are more stressed than parents who are prepared for their child's admission.

REFERENCES

Curley, M.A.Q. (1988). Effects of the nursing mutual participation model of care on parental stress in the pediatric intensive care unit. *Heart & Lung*, 17 (6), 682–688.

Moloney-Harmon, P.A., Srnec, P., & Muir, R. (1996). Trauma. In M.A.Q. Curley, J. B. Smith, & P.A. Moloney-Harmon (Eds.). *Critical care nursing of infants and children* (pp. 893–923). Philadelphia: W.B. Saunders.

2. Answer (**a**). At this time, the best intervention is to comfort the mother through touch. Touch is an effective intervention for comforting patients and families in times of stress. Some research shows that mothers are frequently more distressed than fathers.

REFERENCES

Hall, T., & Lloyd, C. (1990). Non-verbal communication in a health care setting. *British Journal of Occupational Therapy*, 53 (9), 383–386.

Ingham, A. (1989). A review of the literature relating to touch and its use in intensive care. *Intensive Care Nursing*, 5, 65–75.

Miles, M.S., Carter, M.C., Spicher, C., & Hassanein, R.S. (1984). Maternal and paternal stress reactions when a child is hospitalized in a pediatric intensive care unit. *Issues in comprehensive pediatric nursing*, 7, 333–342.

3. Answer (**d**). One of the most important needs for parents is information. Frequently, information must be repeated because of the stress level of the parents and because the material is often difficult for nonmedical persons to understand.

REFERENCES

Kirschbaum, M.S. (1990). Needs of parents of critically ill children. *Dimensions of Critical Care Nursing*, 9 (6), 344–352.

Moloney-Harmon, P.A., Srnec, P., & Muir, R. (1996). Trauma. In M.A.Q. Curley, J.B. Smith, & P.A. Moloney-Harmon (Eds.). *Critical care nursing of infants and children* (pp. 893–923). Philadelphia: W.B. Saunders.

4. Answer (**b**). When working with families from different cultures, the primary language should be determined to ensure that the information shared is understandable to the family. Even if the family is bilingual, it is better to communicate in a person's primary language in times of stress.

REFERENCES

Garcia Coll, C.T., Meyer, E.C., & Brillon, L. (1995). Ethnic and minority parenting. In M.H. Bornstein (Ed.). *Handbook of parenting* (Vol. II). Hillsdale, NJ: Lawrence Erlbaum Associates.

Hatton, D. (1992). Information transmission in bilingual, bicultural contexts. *Journal of Community Health Nursing*, 9 (1), 53–59.

Meadows, J. (1991). Multicultural communication. *Physical & Occupational Therapy in Pediatrics*, 11 (4), 31–41.

5. Answer (**a**). Speaking the family's primary language is important when giving significant information. Although it is important that the nurse participate in the discussion as much as possible, the first priority is that the parents understand the information presented.

REFERENCES

Rothenburger, R. (1990). Transcultural nursing: Overcoming obstacles to effective communication. *Association of Operating Room Nurses Journal*, 51 (5), 1349–1363.

Turner, M.A., Tomlinson, P.S., & Harbaugh, B.L. (1990). Parental uncertainty in critical care hospitalization of children. *Maternal-Child Nursing Journal*, 19 (1), 45–62.

6. Answer (**b**). A critical nursing responsibility is to provide support to families during their hospital stay. An important component of this responsibility is being the family's advocate, allowing them to ask questions or giving them time to consider the issues they may be facing.

REFERENCES

Fry, S.T. (1987) Autonomy, advocacy and accountability: Ethics at the bedside. In M.D.M. Fowler & J. Levine-Ariff (Eds.). *Ethics at the bedside*. Philadelphia: J.B. Lippincott.

Moloney-Harmon, P.A., Srnec, P., & Muir, R. (1996). Trauma. In M.A.Q. Curley, J.B. Smith, & P.A. Moloney-Harmon (Eds.). *Critical care nursing of infants and children* (pp. 893–923). Philadelphia: W.B. Saunders.

7. Answer (**a**). Organ donation is a private matter for a family. According to the Organ Donation Foundation, organ donation is confidential.

REFERENCES

University of Miami Transplant Consent Form. (1994). *University of Miami transplant team protocols and guidelines*.

Willis, R., & Skelley, L. (1992) Serving the needs of donor families: The role of the critical care nurse. *Critical Care Nursing Clinics of North America*, 4 (1), 63–77.

8. Answer (**d**). Fulfilling a family's special request may help them in their grieving process. It may be necessary to consult with other departments, such as infection control, about this type of request, but meeting the family's needs is the priority. Ancillary services such as child life and social services are able to assist the nurse. They are able to help in providing support for the large number of students, and they can assist with crisis intervention.

REFERENCES

Moloney-Harmon, P.A., Srnec, P., & Muir, R. (1996). Trauma. In M.A.Q Curley, J.B. Smith, & P.A. Moloney-Harmon (Eds.). *Critical care nursing of infants and children* (pp. 893–923). Philadelphia: W.B. Saunders.

Wortman, C.B, & Silver, R.C. (1989). The myths of coping with loss. *Journal of Consulting and Clinical Psychology*, 57 (3), 349–357.

9. Answer (**a**). Support groups are therapeutic for families in grief, because the group shares similar experiences.

REFERENCES

Johnson, P.A., Nelson, G.L., & Brunnquell, D.J. (1988). The development of a comprehensive bereavement program to assist families experiencing pediatric loss. *Journal of Pediatric Nursing*, 8 (3), 142–146.

McClelland, M.L. (1993). Our unit has a bereavement program. *American Journal of Nursing*, 93 (1), 62–68.

ANSWERS ■ CASE 2–2

1. Answer (**c**). It is often difficult to give your opinion, but an honest answer that the child is very sick and may die helps the parent begin to think about the possibility of death. It is also important to explore why the parent is asking the question and to let the parent verbalize his or her fears.

REFERENCES

Barnsteiner, J.H. & Gillis-Donovan, J. (1990). Being related and separate: A standard for therapeutic relationships. *Maternal-Child Nursing Journal*, 15, 223–228.

Ramos, M.C. (1992). The nurse-patient relationship: Theme and variations. *Journal of Advanced Nursing*, 17, 496–506.

2. Answer (**a**). Touch is an effective intervention to provide comfort. In this situation, the mother has a difficult decision to make, and she needs reassurance. Hugging her provides her with comfort and reassurance.

REFERENCES

Estabrooks, C.A., & Morse, J. (1992). Toward a theory of touch: The touching process and acquiring a touching style. *Journal of Advanced Nursing*, 17, 448–456.

Ingham, A. (1989). A review of the literature relating to touch and its use in intensive care. *Intensive Care Nursing*, 5, 65–75.

3. Answer (**a**). The mother needs to be aware of her options. It is also critical that the physician be involved and help the mother with her decisions through the Ethics Committee. According to the Joint Commission on Accreditation of Hospital Organizations (JCAHO) 1995 standards, it is mandatory that families are informed about the process available for resolution of ethical issues. It is also important for nurses at the bedside to be familiar with the process to assist families more readily. The JCAHO standards do not mandate the appropriate person to inform families of their options. This is an important role for nurses as advocates for the children and their families.

REFERENCES

Fry, S.T. (1987) Autonomy, advocacy and accountability: Ethics at the bedside. In M.D.M. Fowler & J. Levine-Ariff (Eds.). *Ethics at the bedside*. Philadelphia: J.B. Lippincott.

Joint Commission for Accreditation of Hospital Organizations (1994). Patient rights and organizational ethics. In *The Joint Commission 1995 accreditation manual for hospitals*. 67 Oakbrook Terrace, IL: JCAHO.

4. Answer (**a**). Anyone can identify a case that may need to go to the Ethics Committee. However, each hospital has a policy about which person takes the case to the Ethics Committee. It is important to inform your supervisor of the issue to ensure support in the handling of the case.

REFERENCES

Doka, K., Rushton, C., & Thorstenson, T. (1994). Caregiver distress: If it is so ethical, why does it feel so bad? *AACN Clinical Issues in Critical Care Nursing,* 5 (3), 346–352.
Joint Commission for the Accreditation of Hospital Organizations. (1994). Patient rights and organizational ethics. In *The Joint Commission 1995 accreditation manual for hospitals.* 67 Oakbrook Terrace, IL: JCAHO.

5. Answer (**d**). Families are often afraid to go before a group of strangers and present their personal feelings. It is helpful for the nurse who has worked with the family to go with them for support. Hearing from the family also allows the Ethics Committee members to make the most informed decision.

REFERENCES

Bartels, D., Youngner, S., & Levine, J. (1994). Ethics committees: Living up to your potential. *AACN Clinical Issues in Critical Care Nursing,* 5 (3), 313–323.
Richmond, T.S., Coolican, M., McKnew, L.B, & Burton, H. (1994) Ethical care from the patient's perspective. *AACN Clinical Issues in Critical Care Nursing,* 5 (3), 308–312.

6. Answer (**a**). The Ethics Committee is not a decision-making body, but the members do make recommendations. The best option would be for the Ethics Committee to recommend that the physician turn the case over to another physician who could fulfill the mother's request. The state laws, which vary from state to state, ultimately govern the decision to withdraw support from a child who is not brain dead.

REFERENCES

Bartels, D., Youngner, S., & Levine, J. (1994). Ethics committees: Living up to your potential. *AACN Clinical Issues in Critical Care Nursing,* 5 (3), 313–323.
Chaney, E.A. (1987) Legal reflections on ethics. In M.D.M. Fowler & J. Levine-Ariff (Eds.). *Ethics at the bedside* (pp. 171–181). Philadelphia: J.B. Lippincott.

ANSWERS ■ CASE 2-3

1. Answer (**b**). It can be very challenging to work with divorced families. It is essential to clarify the custody status as soon as possible. This information confirms who is legally responsible for making decisions regarding the care of the child. Clarification also is provided about who is given information about the status of the child.

REFERENCES

Ahmann, E. (1994). Family-centered care: The time has come. *Pediatric Nursing,* 20 (1), 52–53.
Lewandowski, L.A. (1992) Psychosocial aspects of pediatric critical care. In M.F. Hazinski (Ed.). *Nursing care of the critically ill child* (2nd ed., pp. 19–77). St. Louis: Mosby–Year Book.
Moloney-Harmon, P.A., Srnec, P., & Muir, R. (1996). Trauma. In M.A.Q. Curley, J.B. Smith, & P.A. Moloney-Harmon (Eds.). *Critical care nursing of infants and children* (pp. 893–923). Philadelphia: W.B. Saunders.

2. Answer (**a**). Knowledge of which parent has custody is important, but calming this situation is the priority. A private room for the family can be helpful; there they can be assisted in working through their issues, and guidelines can be established for visitation and the exchange of information.

REFERENCES

Ahmann, E. (1994). Family-centered care: The time has come. *Pediatric Nursing,* 20 (1), 52–53.
Lewandowski, L.A. (1992) Psychosocial aspects of pediatric critical care. In M.F. Hazinski (Ed.). *Nursing care of the critically ill child* (2nd ed., pp. 19–77). St. Louis: Mosby–Year Book.
Moloney-Harmon, P.A., Srnec, P., & Muir, R. (1996). Trauma. In M.A.Q. Curley, P.A. Moloney-Harmon, & J.B. Smith (Eds.). *Critical care nursing of infants and children* (pp. 893–923). Philadelphia: W.B. Saunders.

3. Answer (**c**). Setting guidelines for families who are divorced should be done at the first meeting so that minimal conflict occurs. Developing a plan for visitation and information sharing initially can relieve some of the conflict. This is especially true if the family does not have good coping skills and has a history of problems.

REFERENCES

Broome, M.E. (1985). Working with the family of a critically ill child. *Heart & Lung,* 14 (4), 368–372.
Moloney-Harmon, P.A., Srnec, P., & Muir, R. (1996). Trauma. In M.A.Q. Curley, J.B. Smith, & P.A. Moloney-Harmon (Eds.). *Critical care nursing of infants and children* (pp. 893–923). Philadelphia: W.B. Saunders.
Turner, M. A., Tomlinson, P. S., & Harbaugh, B.L. (1990). Parental uncertainty in critical care hospitalization of children. *Maternal-Child Nursing Journal,* 19 (1), 45–62.

4. Answer (**c**). Sharing information about the family can be challenging, because many disciplines are commonly involved. Having a multidisciplinary plan of care is helpful to everyone involved in the care of the child.

REFERENCES

Kirschbaum, M.S. (1990). Needs of parents of critically ill children. *Dimensions of Critical Care Nursing,* 9 (6), 344–352.
La Montagne, L.L., & Pawlak, R. (1990). Stress and coping of parents of children in a pediatric intensive care unit. *Heart & Lung,* 19 (4), 416–421.

5. Answer (**b**). Families commonly feel they have lost control of their child because they are not the primary caregivers. Encouraging the family members to become involved in the care gives them a sense of control. Involvement reinforces the idea that they are assisting the health care team to get their child well.

REFERENCES

Broome, M.E. (1985). Working with the family of a critically ill child. *Heart & Lung,* 14 (4), 368–372.
Curley, M.A.Q., & Wallace, J. (1992). Effects of the nursing mutual participation model of care on parental stress in the pediatric intensive care unit—A replication. *Journal of Pediatric Nursing,* 7 (6), 377–385.
La Montagne, L.L., Hepworth, J.T., Pawlak, R., & Chiafery, M. (1992). Parental coping and activities during pediatric critical care. *American Journal of Critical Care,* 1 (2), 76–80.

6. Answer (**d**). Continuity of care is important for patients and families. It is beneficial to have a patient care conference with the staff to discuss the issues and have the staff participate in the decision-making. Empowering the staff to develop an action plan helps them participate in the decision and take responsibility for the implementation.

REFERENCES

Leebov, W., & Scott, G. (1990). From directing to empowering your staff. In *Health care managers in transition.* San Francisco: Jossey-Bass Publishers.
Tughan, L. (1992). Visiting in the PICU: A study of the perceptions of patients, parents, and staff members. *Critical Care Nursing Quarterly,* 15 (1), 57–68.
Vachon, M.L.S. (1987). *Occupational stress in the care of the critically ill, the dying, and the bereaved.* New York: Hemisphere Publishing.

7. Answer (**a**). The family dynamics and the system of information sharing must be explained to the nurse assigned from another unit. To effectively communicate with the family, she must also be informed about the child's physiological status.

REFERENCES

Kirschbaum, M.S. (1990). Needs of parents of critically ill children. *Dimensions of Critical Care Nursing,* 9 (6), 344–352.
La Montagne, L.L., & Pawlak, R. (1990). Stress and coping of parents of children in a pediatric intensive care unit. *Heart & Lung,* 19 (4), 416–421.

8. Answer (**b**). At this point, it is important to explain to the mother how qualified the nurse is to manage her child's care. Reassuring the mother that another nurse will be available as a resource also can provide her with some comfort and support.

REFERENCES

Farrel, M. J., & Frost, C. (1993). The most important needs of parents of critically ill children: Parents' perceptions. *Intensive and Critical Care Nursing,* 8, 1–10.
La Montagne, L.L., Hepworth, J.T., Pawlak, R., & Chiafery, M. (1992). Parental coping and activities during pediatric critical care. *American Journal of Critical Care,* 1 (2), 76–80.

9. Answer (**c**). The nurse can demonstrate a knowledge base and confidence to the parents by reviewing the plan of care with them. The family will be assured that there will be continuity in the plan of care.

REFERENCES

Ahmann, E. (1994). Family-centered care: The time has come. *Pediatric Nursing,* 20 (1), 52–53.
Broome, M.E. (1985). Working with the family of a critically ill child. *Heart & Lung,* 14 (4), 368–372.

10. Answer (**b**). Sharing information with the unit that the child is being transferred to is important. Involving the mother helps her in the transition to the new unit and ensures that her concerns are addressed. The mother can be assisted in beginning a relationship with the new group of health care workers.

REFERENCES

Bokinske, J.C. (1993). Family conferences: A method to diminish transfer anxiety. *Journal of Neuroscience Nursing,* 24 (3), 129–133.
Curley, M.A.Q., & Wallace, J. (1992). Effects of the nursing mutual participation model of care and parental stress in the pediatric intensive care unit—A replication. *Journal of Pediatric Nursing,* 7 (6), 377–385.

11. Answer (**a**). When the patient is transferred to the floor, the patient and family can find the lack of equipment and personnel frightening. Preparing the family in advance and pointing out the positive aspects helps the family adjust to these changes.

REFERENCES

Bokinske, J.C. (1993). Family conferences: A method to diminish transfer anxiety. *Journal of Neuroscience Nursing,* 24 (3), 129–133.

12. Answer (**d**). Being honest with the mother is the best way to handle this problem. Directing the mother to the appropriate person who can handle any of her concerns will enable her to begin to work with the new staff.

REFERENCES

Bokinske, J.C. (1993). Family conferences: A method to diminish transfer anxiety. *Journal of Neuroscience Nursing,* 24 (3), 129–133.
Curley, M.A.Q., & Wallace, J. (1992). Effects of the nursing mutual participation model of care and parental stress in the pediatric intensive care unit—A replication. *Journal of Pediatric Nursing,* 7, 377–385.

CHAPTER 3

Ethical Issues in Pediatric Critical Care

CINDY HYLTON RUSHTON, DNSc, RN, FAAN

A CASE STUDY

R. is a 3-week old baby who was diagnosed with complex congenital heart disease (Epstein's anomaly) during the prenatal period. At birth, he was aggressively managed with pharmacologic, ventilatory, and hemodynamic support. A central shunt was performed and postoperatively the baby developed capillary leak syndrome, acute renal failure, and hemodynamic instability. After 2 weeks of intense intervention, the family approached the care team about their concern that their baby was experiencing tremendous suffering and that his condition was not responding to the aggressive interventions. The family requested that no further aggressive treatment be initiated and that he not be resuscitated should he arrest. The cardiology team was hesitant to agree to the parents' request, because they believed that the baby had a reasonable chance for a good outcome and that his condition was reversible. An ethics consultation is requested.

■ Commentary

The central ethical issue in this case involves determining what will promote R.'s well-

being. The primary goal of medical and nursing care is to do good and avoid harm. Choices among alternative treatments should therefore benefit the infant and clearly outweigh the associated burdens and harms. A moral tension exists, however, between benefitting R. by sustaining his life with aggressive interventions and avoiding, or at least minimizing, the burdens that may accompany the treatments necessary to do so. Searching for a clear understanding of what R.'s interests are and how to promote them should be based on the best information that is available at the time. Questions such as the following may be useful in clarifying the range of options and the values that underlie the pursuit of each option.

I. What is known about the treatment and prognosis for R.'s cardiac lesion?

Epstein's anomaly is an uncommon cardiac defect, but R.'s particular cardiac malformation was extremely rare. The outcome of treatment ranges from early death to survival following several surgical reconstructive procedures. None of the survivors reported in the literature with anatomy similar to R.'s have reached adulthood yet, and the degree of morbidity associated with the treatment is described as moderate to severe.

II. What medical and nonmedical goals are possible for R.?

This case study is reprinted (slightly modified) from The Communique, (1994), 3 (3), 6–8, a publication of the Center for Ethics and Human Rights, American Nurses Association, Washington, DC.

The range of medical goals may include the following: 1) aggressive stabilization in preparation for a staged surgical reconstruction of the heart; this would include interventions to reverse the complications that occurred following cardiac surgery (acute renal failure, capillary leak syndrome, hemodynamic instability) in an effort to maximize survival and positive outcome, 2) maintenance of the current level of support and treatment of complications with standard therapies, but no invasive interventions such as dialysis or resuscitation, or 3) allowing R.'s underlying disease process to take its course, and promote a peaceful death. Other relevant goals may include relieving pain and suffering, maximizing opportunities for interaction with family and others, or promoting parent or infant bonding and family integrity.

III. Based on the goals that are possible for R., what is the range of outcomes that could be expected in relation to each goal, and what is the likelihood of each?

Given the medical goals described above, it is important to determine the probable outcomes of pursuing each goal. For example, how likely is it that the proposed treatment will be effective? What degree of risk, intrusiveness, or discomfort is associated with the proposed treatment? Will the proposed treatment alter the natural course of the disease? Is the patient experiencing pain? Is the patient dependent on respirator or other technology or treatment for survival? Does the treatment prolong dying? What is the patient's capacity to experience and enjoy life? If the complications are reversed, what is the likely outcome of each reconstructive surgical procedure? What would happen if treatment was not escalated or withdrawn?

Evaluating the possible goals for R. also involves important values about what makes life meaningful and what sorts of burdens are acceptable to achieve those goals. This case highlights the differences in values between the parents and treatment team about how to promote R.'s interests. The treatment team values the possibility, however small, to promote survival, and therefore it has a high threshold for the burdens it will tolerate to give R. a chance for life. The team believes that the multiple organ system dysfunction is reversible, and because the complications are unusual for this type of surgery, aggressive intervention is warranted.

The parents, in contrast, also value giving R. a chance for life, but their threshold for reasonable burdens to give him a chance for life are somewhat different. They believe that the burdens of his current treatment and the possibility that his life may continue to be significantly burdened even if he does survive are disproportionate in relation to the chance that he may survive now and to adulthood.

A secondary issue concerns whose values are to count in determining what will be done for R. Even though infants are not autonomous or self-determining, an element of respect is still required, because the lives of children also have unique meaning. To treat patients with respect is to acknowledge and value who they are outside of a medical context, rather than to treat them only according to how professional goals and values are advanced. To respect a child is to acknowledge the importance of his or her world and the relationships that are central to it.

Based on the moral framework of shared decision making, it is necessary for someone to represent the interests of the child. There is a strong presumption that parents should make judgments about what is in the best interest of their child. Parents are identified as appropriate surrogates because strong bonds of affection and commitment are likely to yield the greatest concern for the well-being of their children. Parents are obligated to protect their children from harm and to do as much good for them as possible.

Although there are compelling reasons to extend parents' decision-making authority, such authority is not absolute. The interests of the parents and the family must take a high priority but do not override the fundamental respect for the best interest of the infant or child. Parents should be decision makers for their infant unless they are disqualified by decision-making incapacity or unresolvable discontentment between them, or their choice of a course of action that is clearly against the best interest of the infant.

When parental decision making is questioned, it is crucial to assess whether the parents are capable of serving as the child's surrogate and whether their position is morally defensible. The following questions may assist in such an assessment.

- Do the parents meet the standard of reasonable parents? (Do the parents have the capacity to understand the information relevant to the decision? Are the parents capable of making a reasoned decision in accordance with their values and beliefs? Are the parents able to put their child's interests above all others? Are there any serious conflicts of interest that may bias their decision making?)

- Is the parents' request within the range of morally acceptable action?
- What evidence is there that the parents should be disqualified as the decision makers for their child?
- Are there actions that could be taken to enhance the parents' ability to act as the child's surrogate?

In R.'s case, his parents clearly met the criteria of reasonable parents, and it could be argued that, given the uncertainty surrounding his prognosis, their request to forego any further aggressive intervention was a morally acceptable option. Professionals must be cautious, however, not to base their decision to disqualify parents as decision makers merely because the parents disagree with the recommendations of the health care team or because the parents must be protected from future guilt or responsibility.

Nurses involved in the care of infants such as R. may be confronted with conflicting values and obligations. Nurses have a duty to benefit others and prevent and remove harmful conditions. Their duty is to help others to further their important legitimate interests.

In the case of infants, nurses attempt to provide them with the opportunity to become autonomous adults who will realize their own unique life goals. However, the very interventions that sustain life may also cause significant burdens to the patient.

Nurses also have obligations to families. A moral framework for shared decision making requires the balanced involvement of parents and health care professionals. Both are committed to the goal of patient well-being, and both must have enough information from the other to accomplish this goal. As responsible parties in the health care setting, nurses and other professionals are obligated to facilitate and support a collaborative process of caregiving and decision making. Parents are obligated to continue their caregiving role within the critical care setting, and to work with health care professionals to establish the scope of parental caregiving including decision making.

As advocates for patients and families, nurses must have a clear understanding of the facts of the case, the context of the decision, family values and goals, and the family's understanding of their child's condition. Nurses must also clarify their own values and possess an adequate understanding of the ethical dimensions of decisions such as this one. Their advocacy can be enhanced by having mechanisms for resolving disputes, support systems that facilitate advocacy efforts, and direct access to ethics consultants and ethics committee consultation.

CHAPTER 4

Legal Issues in Pediatric Critical Care

DENISE MAGUIRE, RN,C, MS
CLIFFORD B. MILLER, RN,C, BSN

CASE 4-1

A newly licensed registered nurse has completed a 6-month orientation program in the pediatric intensive care unit (PICU). The census and acuity are higher than usual, and the nurse is glad to be finished with orientation so she can help reduce the workload of her peers. On her second night after completion of orientation, she is assigned to care for G., a 12-month-old boy who underwent surgical repair of a cardiac defect earlier that day.

During her orientation period, the nurse cared for intubated patients with vasoactive drips, chest tubes, and ventilators, but she never cared for a child as unstable as this one. At 19:00 hours, she notices that almost 60 mL of blood have drained from the chest tube in the past hour; she continues her hourly assessment of vital signs and makes a mental note to inform the on-call resident about the chest tube drainage. Ten minutes later, the charge nurse checks in to see how she is doing and to deliver the evening laboratory results. All looks well, with the exception of a hematocrit of 32%. The deterioration of a patient in the next room demands the immediate attention of the charge nurse, who assures the new nurse that she will be back to check on her soon.

At 20:10, the resident house officer arrives at the bedside with G.'s chart. He orders one unit of whole blood. The nurse questions the order because it is more blood than she has ever given anyone. The resident says, "The baby's hematocrit is 32, and he needs the whole unit." The nurse checks the blood type, unit number, and patient name with another registered nurse and hangs the blood. She knows that it must infuse over 4 hours. Shortly after 23:00 hours, the patient begins to desaturate, with oxygen saturation levels hovering around 86% to 88%.

As the charge nurse returns to check on the newly assigned nurse and her patient, she apologizes for not being back sooner because the unit became extremely busy. She notices the unit of blood hanging and questions the nurse about the chest tube drainage, the hematocrit, and the transfusion order. The oximeter continues to alarm, and in her brief assessment, the charge nurse finds evidence of volume overload. Later in the shift, despite diuretics and careful titration of the vasopressors, G. sustains a cardiovascular accident; the hematocrit is reported to be 75%.

1. If the family brings a suit against her, G's nurse will
   a. Be protected from litigation because she was following the physician's order.
   b. Be responsible for the consequences of her actions.
   c. Rely on the hospital to protect her.
   d. Need to seek her own legal counsel immediately.

2. Will the charge nurse be implicated in this situation?
   a. Maybe, because she is responsible for ensuring that the assignments are appropriate.
   b. No, because each registered nurse is accountable for her or his own practice.
   c. Maybe, because any number of individuals can be named in a lawsuit.
   d. No, because she wasn't in the room when the incident occurred.

The orientation documentation is reviewed, and it is noted that the competency-based orientation tool does not include the administration of blood products. However, G's nurse has attended classes about blood products and their administration.

3. What responsibility, if any, does the nursing education department have in ensuring the orientation of competent nurses in the nursing service?
   a. All the responsibility, because the hospital assumes accountability for training nurses in specialty areas.
   b. No responsibility, because the nurse is a licensed professional.
   c. The department may be held liable, because any number of individuals may be named in a lawsuit.
   d. The department has no responsibility.

CASE 4-2

J., a 1-year-old girl, has been hospitalized since birth. She was born prematurely with respiratory distress syndrome, and her condition has progressed over the months to severe bronchopulmonary dysplasia. She is currently managed with a tracheostomy, ventilatory support, aerosol treatments, diuretics, and steroids. She continues to have occasional bronchospasms and significant hypoxemia.

Her parents have not visited or made phone contact with the staff or hospital in 2 months. Attempts to reach them have been futile; social work services have contacted the state agency to report an apparent abandonment. J. recently had a prolonged hypoxemic event secondary to bronchospasm that resulted in marked neurologic impairment. Her primary nurses believe their nursing care may be hurting more than helping her and prolonging her inevitable death. They raised their concerns in a multidisciplinary care conference that was convened to discuss the options.

1. Under what circumstances may the health care team remove life support from J.?
   a. Evidence of terminal illness is present.
   b. J.'s parents have signed a consent form.
   c. The hospital Ethics Committee agrees with the decision.
   d. The health care team concludes that J.'s disease is deteriorating and irreversible.

2. If her parents are not available, who advocates J.'s best interest?
   a. A court-appointed advocate.
   b. Her primary nurse.
   c. The hospital social worker.
   d. The family court judge.

J.'s parents appear in the unit unexpectedly. They explain that they had to travel to find work and are back in town "for a little while." During their visit with J., her parents notice that she is not responsive. Her nurse explains what happened and what support J. needs to be kept alive. On their way out the door, the parents mention they "want everything done" for her.

Weeks later, J. remains unresponsive; her body is grossly edematous, and she has right hemiparesis. Her primary nurses find it painful and morally conflicting to care for her, because she seems to be suffering. She has, in their assessment, no reasonable quality of life. Many of the staff refuse to care for her, because they do not agree with the current plan of care.

3. What is a professional nurse's responsibility in accepting or refusing an assignment?
   a. To match her or his moral beliefs for consistency with unique patient care situations before accepting an assignment.
   b. To care for any patient, regardless of personal moral beliefs.
   c. To voice a complaint with a supervisor regarding an assignment.
   d. To assess his or her ability to adequately care for the patient, given the support available.

4. What single issue most often precipitates a lawsuit?
   a. Removal from life support.
   b. Low socioeconomic status.

c. Lack of communication with the health care team.

d. Severe neurologic sequelae.

CASE 4-3

S. was born 5 days ago to a gravida (4) para (0) mother after an uneventful pregnancy. Delivery was complicated by a tight nuchal cord, and Apgar scores were 0, 0, 1, and 7. Resuscitation began within the first minute of life, and the baby boy was rushed to the newborn intensive care unit as soon as possible. Within several hours and after volume expansion, S.'s vital signs stabilize. His eyes are fixed and dilated, and his tone is limp. He does not respond to tactile stimulation and has no spontaneous respirations. Serial neurologic examinations reveal evidence of brainstem function only.

1. For S. to qualify as an organ donor, doctors must be able to demonstrate
    a. An absence of pulse and respiration.
    b. Evidence of brain death.
    c. No spontaneous movement.
    d. The parents' desire to donate organs.

2. What is the legal definition of brain death?
    a. Absence of pulse, respiration, and spontaneous and elicited movements.
    b. No response to deep, painful stimulation.
    c. Irreversible cessation of cardiorespiratory or whole brain function.
    d. Fixed and fully dilated pupils that are unresponsive to light.

CASE 4-4

A nurse had 16 years of pediatric intensive care nursing experience when she returned to graduate school to become a critical care nurse practitioner. After graduation, she was hired by her hospital to develop the first critical care nurse practitioner role in collaboration with the intensivists. The role is new to her nursing and medical colleagues. After 3 months of orientation, she assumes a caseload of patients.

1. What are the licensure requirements for advanced-practice nurses in critical care?
    a. Successful testing on a certification examination.
    b. Application to the state for an advanced practice license.

c. Written formal agreement with a physician or hospital.

d. They differ from state to state.

The nurse admits a 9-year-old boy from the emergency room with seizures. She orders an intravenous line placed and laboratory tests that include complete and differential blood counts, electrolyte levels, and a calcium determination. She prescribes 100 mg of phenobarbital, administered intravenously.

2. Who or what gives the nurse prescriptive authority in this situation?
    a. Her certification as a pediatric nurse practitioner.
    b. The physicians she works for.
    c. The Nurse Practice Act in her state.
    d. The emergent nature of the case.

The seizures do not cease, and the nurse calls the attending physician about the boy. The physician suggests a few more laboratory and diagnostic tests, which the nurse orders. The seizures finally subside after intravenous administration of phenytoin and diazepam. The rest of the hospitalization is uneventful, although no specific cause for the seizures was ever determined. The boy is discharged to his home on phenytoin.

Throughout the hospitalization, the parents never spoke to a physician about their son. They met with his nurse and appreciated her explanations, but whenever they asked to speak to "the doctor," he was busy with another patient. The nurse knew they were frustrated, but she could not convince the attending physician to sit down with them.

One year later, follow-up examination by a pediatric neurologist in the family's new hometown reveals a normal neurologic status, and the phenytoin is discontinued. The neurologist reviews the boy's medical history and raises concerns about his diagnosis and treatment at the time of his "seizure." The parents seek legal advice and decide to file a lawsuit against the hospital for misdiagnosis and inappropriate treatment of their son. They seek damages to cover their son's medical expenses. The nurse and the attending physician are named in the lawsuit.

3. Would it benefit the nurse to carry her own malpractice insurance?
    a. Yes, because she is in practice with a private professional corporation.
    b. Maybe, but she should first investigate insurance issues with her employer

and make the decision that is best for her in this situation.

   c. No, because she is covered by the hospital's malpractice insurance.

   d. No, because she may be sued for a larger monetary award because of her insurance coverage.

The nurse has exchanged Christmas cards with and occasionally receives a phone call from the parents.

4. What action should the nurse take first when she receives notification that the family has named her in a lawsuit?
   a. Call the family to find out more about their concerns.
   b. Review the medical records.
   c. Cut off all communications with the family.
   d. Notify the hospital risk manager.

CASE 4-5

L. is 16-year-old girl admitted to the PICU with a gunshot wound to the abdomen. She is alert, tachycardic, and scared. She responds to questions in single words, never elaborating. Her parents appear at the nurses' station and inform the secretary that L. may not have blood under any circumstances. They are Jehovah's Witnesses. The surgeon is waiting to obtain the informed consent form for the surgery and is introduced to L.'s parents. He explains the critical nature of the wound and that major blood loss has already occurred. The parents give consent to the surgery but not to a transfusion.

1. The appropriate option of the surgeon is to
   a. Gain a court order from a judge to transfuse if medically necessary.
   b. Ask permission from L.
   c. Use fresh-frozen plasma and albumin as volume expanders.
   d. Refer the patient to another surgeon.

Before surgery, L. reveals that she is pregnant. Her parents are shocked, and the surgeon must now consider the consequences to the fetus. At approximately 28 weeks' gestation, the fetus is viable. L. and her parents are devoted to their religious beliefs and still refuse blood products. The surgeon explains that L.'s blood loss may deprive her baby of oxygen and could result in brain damage or death.

The surgery is successful, and the bleeding has stopped. L. is recovering in the PICU. Her nurse is at the bedside taking vital signs when a person introducing himself as an "infectious disease fellow" comes into the room. He explains to the parents that he is conducting a study and would like to include L. The nurse continues her assessment and completes her documentation at the bedside, not paying much attention to what is being said. Because the parents think the study sounds worthwhile and does not put their daughter at any risk, they sign the consent form enrolling L. The physician asks the nurse to witness the consent. She hesitates because she is not sure if the parents fully understand the study.

2. Before the initiation of the proposed study, approval must be obtained from
   a. The medical director of the hospital.
   b. The director of the infectious disease department.
   c. The institutional review board.
   d. Only the patient or parents.

3. The nurse can sign as a witness to the consent because
   a. She was physically present when the study was being explained.
   b. She is not legally responsible for ascertaining whether the parents' consent is truly informed.
   c. She is in a position to initiate recommendations about which studies would benefit L.
   d. She has a legal duty to obtain informed consent.

CASE 4-6

A nurse has been contacted by a defense attorney to be an expert witness in a malpractice trial. She has worked as a staff nurse in pediatric intensive care for 22 years. She is a member of Sigma Theta Tau, has published several articles, and is regarded as an expert by her peers and supervisors. Before her first meeting with the defense attorney, she reviewed the medical records and deposition transcripts. A nurse and a physician were named in a suit because a patient they assessed as normal had a cardiorespiratory arrest about an hour later and suffered severe neurologic sequelae.

1. The purpose of the first meeting with the defense attorney is to

a. Arrive at an unbiased opinion about the cause of the arrest.
b. Review the role of the expert witness.
c. Negotiate professional compensation.
d. Develop a defense strategy.

The nurse has previously testified as an expert witness for the defense, and she feels comfortable supporting her colleagues in this way.

2. The prosecuting attorney can be expected to
   a. Ask the nurse how much money she expects to receive for her services.
   b. Highlight her professional accomplishments for the jury.
   c. Focus on her tendency to support nursing colleagues.
   d. Be gentle when posing questions to her.

3. A deposition is
   a. A process of discovery.
   b. A notice to appear in court.
   c. The plaintiff's written explanation of the events of the case.
   d. "Deposing" testimony to the judge.

The nurse appears to testify at the trial. The prosecuting attorney asks her, under oath, to describe the standard of practice.

4. The nurse's answer should include
   a. The use of medical technical language that is as precise as possible.
   b. The names of source texts used to support her rationale.
   c. Description of how a reasonable nurse caring for the patient carries out his or her duties and responsibilities.
   d. Copies of the current nursing standards from her hospital.

ANSWERS ■ CASE 4-1

1. Answer (**b**). Nurses are always responsible for the legal consequences of their acts, whether or not performed at the direction of a physician. A nurse is obligated to use scientific rationale for the orders that she or he carries out. If a nurse believes an order is wrong or dangerous, she or he must refuse to carry it out and voice concerns to the physician who ordered it. If the concerns continue, she or he must use the appropriate chain of command.

REFERENCES

Legal Questions Editor. (1989). *Nursing 89, 19* (5), 29.

Legal Questions Editor. (1989). *Nursing 89,* 19 (8), 30.
Tammelleo, A.D. (1993). Implementing doctor's orders is no defense. *Regan Report on Nursing Law* 34 (7), 4.

2. Answer (**c**). Any number of individuals may be named in a lawsuit. A charge nurse is not responsible for another nurse's practice, but she does have the responsibility of ensuring that the assignment is appropriate for a particular nurse's skill level. This emphasizes the importance of documentation of competency. The hospital may also be held responsible for a nurse's negligence, especially if competency of that practice cannot be established with complete documentation.

REFERENCES

Creighton, H. (1986). *Law every nurse should know* (5th ed.). Philadelphia: W.B. Saunders.
Legal Questions Editor. (1989). *Nursing 89,* 19 (4), 26.
May, K.A., & Mahlmeister, L.R. (1994). *Maternal and neonatal nursing family centered care* (pp. 43–44). Philadelphia: J.B. Lippincott.

3. Answer (**c**). If the nursing education department has assumed responsibility for establishing and maintaining competency for the nursing service, they may also be found negligent in this case. However, if this role is decentralized to the individual units, the education department may have no responsibility.

REFERENCES

Creighton, H. (1986). *Law every nurse should know* (5th ed.). Philadelphia: W.B. Saunders.
Legal Questions Editor. (1989). *Nursing 89.* 19 (4), 26.

ANSWERS ■ CASE 4-2

1. Answer (**a**). It is not required that brain death be established to remove life support. The Baby Doe Guidelines uphold the rights of parents of terminally ill infants to remove extraordinary life support in the circumstance of irreversible and virtual terminal illness. The health care team must demonstrate that J.'s disease meets this criterion by whatever means necessary.

REFERENCES

Creighton, H. (1989). *Law every nurse should know* (5th ed.). Philadelphia: W.B. Saunders.
Driscoll, K. M. (1993). Legal aspects of perinatal care. In C. Kenner, A. Brueggemeyer, & L. Gunderson (Eds.). *Comprehensive neonatal nursing: A physiologic perspective* (pp. 36–51). Philadelphia: W.B. Saunders.

2. Answer (**a**). The court appoints an advocate for any patient who does not have a family. Such appointees often have no medical background, which may assist them in advocating what is best for the child.

REFERENCES
Feutz-Harter, S. (1989). *Nursing and the law* (3rd ed., pp. 64–65). Eau Claire, WI: M.G. Publishing.

3. Answer (**d**). Professional nurses have the responsibility to recognize patient situations that they are unable to adequately handle and to negotiate the appropriate support or another patient assignment with their supervisor. With one exception, it is not appropriate to refuse assignments based on the nurse's personal values. The one exception that has been upheld in state court is the right of an individual not to assist in an abortion in keeping with his or her moral, ethical, or religious beliefs. When nurses do not believe the course of treatment is appropriate, they are obligated to seek alternatives through an appropriate course of action.

REFERENCES
Creighton, H. (1986). *Law every nurse should know* (5th ed.). Philadelphia: W.B. Saunders.

4. Answer (**c**). Lack of communication with the patient or family is the most common cause of litigation. When family members believe the health care team is not being truthful or not telling them everything, they become suspicious that an error has been made.

REFERENCES
Brent, N.J. (1990). Avoiding professional negligence: A review. *Home Health Nurse,* 8, 45–47.
Creighton, H. (1986). *Law every nurse should know* (5th ed.). Philadelphia: W.B. Saunders.

ANSWERS ■ CASE 4-3

1. Answer (**b**). Before approaching a family to consider organ donation, doctors must be able to demonstrate evidence of brain death. Research indicates that the physiologic symptoms of brain death include absence of spontaneous respirations and absence of response to stimuli such as pain, touch, sound, or light. The lack of reflexes, lack of movement, flat electroencephalogram, and lack of blood flow to the brain also are required, and all must occur without evidence of hypothermia or central nervous system depressants. All tests must be repeated in 24 hours and show no change. The American Academy of Pediatrics reports the unique and difficult issues in confirming brain death in children. They recommend two examinations with electroencephalograms obtained at least 48 hours apart for patients 7 days to 2 months of age. The American Academy of Pediatrics Task Force concluded that clinical criteria were not useful in newborns younger than 7 days of age.

REFERENCES
Annas, G.J., Bray, P.F., Bennett, D.R., et al. (1987). Guidelines for the determination of brain death in children. *Pediatrics,* 80 (2), 298–300.
Ashwal, S. (1989). Brain death in the newborn. *Clinics in Perinatology,* 16 (2), 501–518.
Ashwal, S., & Schneider, S. (1989). Brain death in the newborn. *Pediatrics,* 84 (3), 429–437.
Creighton, H. (1986). *Law every nurse should know* (5th ed.). Philadelphia: W.B. Saunders.

2. Answer (**c**). The legal definition of brain death is the irreversible cessation of cardiorespiratory or whole brain function.

REFERENCES
Creighton, H. (1986). *Law every nurse should know* (5th Ed.) Philadelphia: W.B. Saunders.

ANSWERS ■ CASE 4-4

1. Answer (**d**). Each state regulates the licensure of its health care personnel. Most state Nurse Practice Acts have minimum requirements for entry, define the scope of the practice, and regulate the conduct of clinicians with their requirements for licensure and relicensure.

REFERENCES
Creighton, H. (1986). *Law every nurse should know* (5th ed). Philadelphia: W.B. Saunders.

2. Answer (**c**). Each state defines professional practice in the Nurse Practice Act. Many states require certification as an advanced practice nurse, but some do not. Some states require specific course material on pharmacology. Most states require an agreement with a supervising physician, although they define those agreements differently.

REFERENCES
Betz, C.L. Hunsberger, M., & Wright, S. (1994). Child health issues, ethics, and nursing process. In C.L.

Betz, M. Hunsberger, & S. Wright (Eds.). *Family centered nursing care of children* (2nd ed., pp. 3–34). Philadelphia: W.B. Saunders.

Cohn, S.D. (1984). Prescriptive authority for nurses. *Law, Medicine and Health Care,* 12, 72–75.

Curtain, L. (1992). Advanced licensure: personal plum or public shield? *Nursing Management,* 23 (8), 7–8.

3. Answer (**b**). A definitive answer does not exist for all situations. Employers approach liability issues differently and individually. An employer may deny coverage if it believes that the nursing action was outside the scope of the job description.

REFERENCES

Colburn, V. (1991). The nurse as an expert witness: A new expanded role. *Journal of Perinatal and Neonatal Nursing,* 5 (3), 16–24.

Driscoll, K. M. (1993). Legal aspects of perinatal care. In C. Kenner, A. Brueggemeyer, & L. Gunderson (Eds.). *Comprehensive neonatal nursing: A physiologic perspective* (pp. 36–51). Philadelphia: W.B. Saunders.

Feutz-Harter, S.A. (1991). *Nursing and the law.* Eau Claire, WI: M.G. Publishing.

4. Answer (**d**). The first thing any nurse should do if she is named in a lawsuit is to notify the hospital risk manager of the legal action. The risk manager begins an investigation and notifies the hospital attorney. The nurse should terminate all communications with the persons who have filed the lawsuit. Because anything said or written could potentially be used as evidence to support the litigation, all opportunities for communication should be avoided. Later, it would help to review the medical records and develop a list of nursing experts for the defense, but these are not usually the first thing a nurse would do.

REFERENCES

Quinley, K.M. (1990). Legal side: Twelve tips for defending yourself in a malpractice suit. *American Journal of Nursing,* 90 (1), 37–38.

ANSWERS ■ CASE 4-5

1. Answer (**a**). Although adult Jehovah's Witnesses may legally refuse treatment with blood, the court has held that temporarily depriving the parents of a minor child of consent for the purpose of giving a blood transfusion is not depriving them of religious freedom or parental rights. The court will seek to protect the child and not permit him or her to be deprived of the right to life because the parents hold specific religious beliefs.

REFERENCES

Creighton, H. (1986). *Law every nurse should know* (5th ed.). Philadelphia: W.B. Saunders.

2. Answer (**c**). The institutional review board is a committee consisting of physicians, nurses, and lay representatives who review all research proposals for the protection of human subjects. They ensure that the risks are reasonable, the benefits are worthwhile, and the explanation is simple enough for a patient to understand. Institutional review boards must follow federal guidelines that set a national standard for medical research.

REFERENCES

Callaway, S.D. (1986). *Nursing ethics & the law.* Eau Claire, WI: Professional Education Systems.

National Commission for the Protection of Human Subjects of Biomedical and Behavioral Research (1978). *The Belmont Report: Ethical principles and guidelines for the protection of human subjects of research.* Department of Education and Welfare, Pub. No. 105, pp. 78–0012.

3. Answer (**b**). The nurse is not legally responsible for ascertaining whether the parent's consent is truly informed. By law, the responsibility for obtaining the informed consents for treatments or research protocols belongs to the physician or the principal investigator. However, the nurse can work with the physician and the patient or family to ensure that the patient and family understand the information presented.

REFERENCE

Driscoll, K. M. (1993). Legal aspects of perinatal care. In C. Kenner, A. Brueggemeyer, & L. Gunderson (Eds.). *Comprehensive neonatal nursing: A physiologic perspective* (pp. 36–51). Philadelphia: W.B. Saunders.

Wong, D. (1993). *Essentials of pediatric nursing* (4th ed). St. Louis: Mosby–Year Book.

ANSWERS ■ CASE 4-6

1. Answer (**a**). The purpose of the first meeting with the defense attorney is to arrive at an unbiased opinion about the cause of the arrest after careful review of the records. The attorney will want to know if the nurse followed or deviated from the standard of care. The nurse who serves as an expert witness should know what the role entails before accepting any materials from the attorneys. Negotiating professional compensation can occur at any time during the process. It is the role of the attorney to develop a defense strategy.

REFERENCES

Colburn, V. (1991). The nurse as an expert witness: A new expanded role. *Journal of Perinatal and Neonatal Nursing,* 5 (3), 16–24.

2. Answer (**a**). When the nurse works for the defense, she can expect the prosecution to highlight for the jury how much money she is receiving to testify. Although accepting compensation is ethical and acceptable, the expert witness should not demand an exorbitant amount of money, because it would only serve to illustrate the point the prosecution is sure to make. The prosecution will not highlight the nurse's professional accomplishments for the jury; rather, they may ask if she has testified on behalf of the defense numerous times, building a case of witness bias. The prosecuting attorney may try to confuse the expert witness by applying her "general" responses to specific situations.

REFERENCES

Colburn, V. (1991). The nurse as an expert witness: A new expanded role. *Journal of Perinatal and Neonatal Nursing,* 5 (3), 16–24.
Driscoll, K. M. (1993). Legal aspects of perinatal care. In C. Kenner, A. Brueggemeyer, & L. Gunderson (Eds.). *Comprehensive neonatal nursing: A physiologic perspective* (pp. 36–51). Philadelphia: W.B. Saunders.

3. Answer (**a**). A deposition is a process of discovery that usually occurs before the trial begins. It gives both sides an opportunity to know what the witnesses will say during their testimony. Witnesses are sworn before the deposition begins, as in court. Both sides may ask the witness questions, and transcripts are made available to both sides.

REFERENCES

Colburn, V. (1991). The nurse as an expert witness: A new expanded role. *Journal of Perinatal and Neonatal Nursing,* 5 (3), 16–24.
Feutz-Harter, S. (1989). *Nursing and the law* (3rd ed.). Eau Claire, WI: M.G. Publishing.

4. Answer (**c**). When the nurse testifies at the trial, she should describe how a reasonable nurse caring for the patient carries out her duties and responsibilities. The questions are asked so the jury will gain an understanding of the standard in question and eventually come to a decision. The nurse should direct her responses to the jury in language they can understand. Citing or bringing current nursing standards is probably not applicable, because cases often come to court years after the incident.

REFERENCES

Colburn, V. (1991). The nurse as an expert witness: A new expanded role. *Journal of Perinatal and Neonatal Nursing,* 5 (3), 16–24.
Driscoll, K. M. (1993). Legal aspects of perinatal care. In C. Kenner, A. Brueggemeyer, & L. Gunderson (Eds.). *Comprehensive neonatal nursing: A physiologic perspective* (pp. 36–51). Philadelphia: W.B. Saunders.

ACKNOWLEDGMENTS

The authors and editors thank Marty Clayton, RN, Administrative Director, Quality Management Services, at All Children's Hospital for her careful review of this chapter.

CHAPTER 5

Cardiovascular Disorders

PEGGY DORR, RN, MS, CCRN

CASE 5–1

S. is a 10-month-old, term infant with Down's syndrome and a complete atrioventricular septal defect (AVSD). He was diagnosed at 1 month of age as a result of his tachypnea and consistent tiring with feedings. His most recent visit to the cardiology clinic revealed increases in the heart and respiratory rates, failure to thrive, and a history of four upper respiratory infections during the past 3 months. His chest x-ray film showed gross cardiomegaly and increased pulmonary vascular markings. Based on these data, cardiac catheterization was performed. Relevant data obtained from the catheterization included a pulmonary vascular resistance (PVR) of 4.6 Wood's units, with a pulmonary: systemic blood flow ratio (Q_p/Q_s) of 1.9. A complete repair of his defect is scheduled for next week.

1. Which of the following best describes the physiology of blood flow in an AVSD?
   a. There is increased blood flow only to the right atrium and right ventricle because of the atrial septal defect (ASD) and ventricular septal defect (VSD).
   b. There is increased systemic blood flow, because the common atrioventricular (AV) valve allows flow to all chambers, with a preferential right-to-left shunt.
   c. There is no alteration in blood flow, because the common AV valve allows flow to all chambers.
   d. There is increased pulmonary blood flow, because the common AV valve

allows flow to all chambers, with a preferential left-to-right shunt.

2. Which of the following nursing diagnoses is most appropriate for S. as his primary diagnosis?
   a. Potential for injury related to hypertension caused by increased systemic flow.
   b. Potential for decreased cardiac output related to diminished flow to the left side of the heart.
   c. Potential for injury related to pulmonary vascular disease caused by increased pulmonary blood flow.
   d. Potential for injury related to congestive heart failure caused by poor contractility of the myocardium.

3. S. goes to surgery for repair of his AV canal. After the operation, the anesthesiologist reports that the cardiopulmonary bypass (CPB) time was 115 minutes, with a circulatory arrest time of 55 minutes. How does this affect postoperative nursing care?
   a. There is no need for a deviation in care. The pump times are well within normal limits, and no changes are expected from a standard postoperative course.
   b. The pump times are not important to the bedside nurse. They have some influence on the intraoperative care but do not affect the child's postoperative status in any way.
   c. The reported times are prolonged, and as a result, the nurse expects to see significant fluid shifts and hema-

30

tologic abnormalities. She must monitor for altered end-organ function.

d. The reported times are dangerously prolonged. The nurse expects this child to experience severe neurologic deficits and warns parents of this potential.

Postoperatively, S.'s pulmonary artery catheter shows pressures of 55/35 mmHg, and his radial arterial line shows pressures of 98/55 mmHg. He is receiving dopamine (3 μg/kg/min), dobutamine (5 μg/kg/min), and prostaglandin E_1 (0.02 μg/kg/min).

4. Prostaglandin E_1 is indicated for S. because prostaglandin
   a. Helps to maintain ductal patency, which can prevent cardiac overload in the initial postoperative period.
   b. Primarily produces afterload reduction, allowing the heart to pump against less systemic vascular resistance.
   c. Enhances cardiac contractility through its positive inotropic action.
   d. Produces pulmonary vasodilation, decreasing PVR and the potential for pulmonary hypertension.

5. What other interventions aid in decreasing S.'s high pulmonary pressures?
   a. Active cooling to 35°C, initiation of a nitroprusside (Nipride) drip, and administration of muscle relaxants and sedatives.
   b. Administration of muscle relaxants and sedatives and production of an alkalotic environment through manipulation of the ventilator settings.
   c. Vigorous diuresis with mannitol to produce a hematocrit of 50%.
   d. Hyperventilation on the ventilator, a positive end-expiratory pressure (PEEP) of 10 cmH$_2$O, and a normothermic environment.

6. The nurse explains to S.'s parents that it is critical to prevent pulmonary pressures from increasing in the postoperative period because
   a. An increase in pulmonary pressures can lead to a pulmonary hypertensive crisis if circulating blood flow decreases dramatically. This impedes oxygenation.
   b. An increase in pulmonary pressures causes increased pulmonary blood flow, initiating events that lead to more pulmonary tissue damage.
   c. As pulmonary pressures rise, so do systemic pressures, which places the patient at risk for a stroke or intracranial bleeding.
   d. Any increase in pulmonary pressures increases oxygen consumption and metabolic demands.

7. Twelve hours after surgery, S.'s blood pressure begins to decrease and his electrocardiographic rhythm indicates a complete heart block. Is this an expected response after his surgery?
   a. Yes, but it is usually seen much later in the postoperative course as the myocardial tissues begin to heal.
   b. Yes, this is the expected time frame to see this dysrhythmia, because the repair was close to or through the conduction system.
   c. No, one would expect to see an atrial dysrhythmia such as paroxysmal atrial tachycardia or atrial flutter.
   d. No, the repair was not performed near the conduction system.

S.'s transthoracic pacing wires are attached to the bedside pacemaker. The settings are appropriate for his age and condition and have been checked against the postoperative orders. The cardiovascular surgeon requests that the pacemaker be on to enhance S.'s cardiac output. Figure 5–1 indicates the rhythm that appears on the cardiac monitor.

8. What type of pacemaker activity is occurring?
   a. Failure to capture.
   b. Failure to sense.
   c. Atrial and ventricular pacing with good capture.
   d. Atrial sensing and ventricular pacing with good capture.

S.'s parents go home to sleep for the night. When they return, they are shocked at S.'s

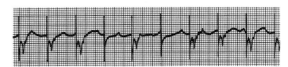

Figure 5-1 Electrocardiogram strip depicting failure to capture. (From Park, M.K., & Guntheroth, W.G. (1992). Analysis of arrhythmias and atrioventricular conduction disturbances. In M.K. Park & W.G. Guntheroth (Eds.). *How to read pediatric ECGs* (3rd ed., p. 218). St. Louis: Mosby–Year Book.)

appearance. His eyes, face, hands, and feet are very swollen. They also notice he is getting a platelet transfusion and want to know why.

9. How does the nurse explain these changes and therapies to them?
   a. S.'s heart is very "sick," and these symptoms are a result of poor myocardial function in the immediate postoperative period.
   b. The edema may be related to the fluids he received in surgery. The platelet transfusion is necessary because his platelets are being destroyed by the VSD patch.
   c. These are common occurrences after such extensive surgery. The capillaries of the vessels weaken and leak fluids into the tissues. Because many blood cells are injured during the CPB operation, transfusions are necessary.
   d. S. lost a lot of blood in surgery that needs to be replaced. The extremities are swollen because his urine output has dropped and he is experiencing acute renal failure.

Twenty-four hours after surgery, S.'s breath sounds are coarse and his Pao_2 is 85 mmHg, with an oxygen saturation of 92%. His pulmonary artery pressures are 50/30 mmHg, and the systemic arterial pressures are 75/40 mmHg. His heart rate is 180 beats per minute (bpm), the right atrial pressure is 8 mmHg, and the left atrial pressure is 15 mmHg. His urine output has decreased to 0.5 mL/kg per hour. His extremities are cool, with a 4- to 5-second capillary refill time.

10. The nurse suspects
    a. Decreased cardiac output secondary to increased systemic vascular resistance.
    b. Decreased left heart function secondary to complete heart block.
    c. Right-sided overload secondary to tricuspid valve dysfunction.
    d. Left-sided failure secondary to mitral valve dysfunction.

CASE 5-2

An 18-month-old boy presents in the pediatric unit with an 8-day history of fever and irritability. Vital signs include a heart rate

of 135 bpm, blood pressure of 95/50 mmHg, and a respiratory rate of 40 breaths per minute. Other relevant physical features include erythema of the lips, a strawberry tongue, and generalized peripheral edema. Significant laboratory data include a platelet count of 850,000/mm³, a hemoglobin concentration of 10 g/dL, a hematocrit of 35%, and an increased sedimentation rate. All serum chemistry determinations are within normal limits, except the elevated liver function test results. The physicians' discussion leads them to a primary diagnosis of Kawasaki disease.

1. Based on the diagnosis of Kawasaki disease, which physiologic changes are of primary concern when developing the nursing plan of care?
   a. Altered cardiac function, altered hematologic status, and altered comfort.
   b. Altered neurologic status, altered cardiac function, and altered renal function.
   c. Altered immunologic processes, altered fluid and electrolyte balance, and altered comfort.
   d. Altered renal function and altered acid-base balance.

2. On initial assessment, the nurse notices an increased heart rate, shortness of breath, rales on auscultation, and a capillary refill time of 4 seconds, with weak but palpable pulses. In view of the potential diagnosis, these findings are interpreted as
   a. Fluid overload secondary to mild acute renal failure.
   b. Congestive heart failure secondary to myocardial inflammation.
   c. Left ventricular dysfunction secondary to mitral valve incompetence.
   d. Pulmonary embolism secondary to thrombocytopenia.

3. The child's primary nurse is with the family as the physician discusses this disease process and the typical course of treatment. He mentions the need to obtain an echocardiogram approximately 10 to 14 days after the initial onset of the fever. At that time, they will be looking for
   a. Pericardial tamponade.
   b. Coronary artery aneurysms.
   c. Persistent right and left ventricular dysfunction.
   d. Aortic stenosis.

The echocardiogram confirms the cardiac catheterization finding, and the child is admitted to the pediatric intensive care unit for continuous cardiorespiratory monitoring.

4. The echocardiogram results, combined with the laboratory data, are of special concern because
   a. The thrombocytopenia places the child with aortic stenosis at risk for thrombus formation around the valve.
   b. The decreased cardiac output is enhanced by the low hemoglobin and hematocrit levels.
   c. The tamponade only contributes to the decreased circulating amount of red blood cells.
   d. Thrombocytopenia, along with a coronary artery aneurysm, places children at risk for myocardial ischemia or infarction.

5. Initial medical therapy for patients with Kawasaki disease is aimed at
   a. Enhancing cardiac output and increasing the hemoglobin and hematocrit.
   b. Decreasing the fever and identifying the causative organism for appropriate antibacterial treatment.
   c. Reducing inflammation and preventing coronary thrombosis.
   d. Enhancing cardiac output and decreasing the fever.

6. The child has an order for intravenous immunoglobulin (IVIG) and a high dose of aspirin. What is the purpose of this drug regimen in the initial stages of Kawasaki disease?
   a. IVIG in combination with aspirin has been shown to resolve inflammation significantly and decrease the likelihood of coronary artery abnormalities.
   b. IVIG is purely an experimental therapy aimed at decreasing systemic mediator actions. The aspirin is given for its antithrombotic properties.
   c. These two drugs are not to be given together. The research has shown that they are more effective when given independently of one another, 1 week apart.
   d. IVIG with aspirin has been shown to resolve the fever and irritability rapidly, although it has no effect on the inflammatory responses.

Two days later, the child's condition appears to be worsening. His heart rate is 185 bpm, his blood pressure is 70/35 mmHg, the respiratory rate is 65 breaths per minute, and the Pa_{O_2} is 93%. Arterial blood gas results indicate respiratory and metabolic acidosis. He remains irritable, his extremities are cool, and pulses are demonstrated by Doppler only. His capillary refill time is 5 to 6 seconds. He is intubated, and a right internal jugular double-lumen catheter is placed. The central venous pressure from the internal jugular is 15 mmHg. These clinical findings support a diagnosis of worsening congestive heart failure (CHF) secondary to the myocardial inflammation.

7. Therapy at this stage is aimed at
   a. Increasing contractility and decreasing preload.
   b. Decreasing preload and increasing afterload.
   c. Increasing afterload and increasing contractility.
   d. Increasing preload and decreasing afterload.

8. Based on the patient's clinical presentation, which of the following interventions is anticipated?
   a. Epinephrine infusion administered at 0.2 μg/kg per minute.
   b. A bolus of 25% albumin administered at 4 mL/kg and an epinephrine infusion administered at 0.2 μg/kg per minute.
   c. Dopamine infusion administered at 3 μg/kg per minute.
   d. Furosemide (Lasix) administered at a dose of 1.0 mg/kg as an intravenous push and dobutamine infusion administered at 6 μg/kg per minute.

ANSWERS ■ CASE 5–1

1. Answer (**d**). An AVSD results from incomplete fusion of the endocardial tissues. A complete defect results in an ostium primum ASD, a VSD located in the upper ventricular septum, and one common AV valve, with no delineation between the tricuspid and mitral valves. Left-to-right shunting occurs because systemic pressures (left sided) are greater than pulmonary pressures (right sided). The free communication among all four chambers results in increased blood flow to the right side of the heart,

which produces an increase in pulmonary blood flow.

REFERENCES

Moynihan, P.J., & King, R. (1989). Caring for patients with lesions increasing pulmonary blood flow. *Critical Care Nursing Clinics of North America,* 1(2), 195–213.

Smith, J.B., Baker, A.L., Moynihan, P.J., et al. (1996). Cardiovascular critical care problems. In M.A.Q. Curley, J.B. Smith & P.A. Moloney-Harmon (Eds.). *Critical care nursing of infants and children* (pp. 557–618). Philadelphia: W.B. Saunders.

2. Answer (**c**). Cardiac lesions such as an AVSD that permit blood to flow from the high-pressure left-sided to the lower-pressure right-sided chambers increase the flow of blood to the lungs. Because of the increased flow, pressure is increased in the pulmonary vessels and tissues. Muscularization of the small pulmonary arteries contributes to sustained elevation of PVR, and pulmonary vascular disease eventually develops in the pulmonary bed. Pulmonary vascular disease results in pathologic changes in the pulmonary vessels and a subsequent constant elevation of PVR.

REFERENCES

Medicus, L., & Thompson, L. (1995). Preventing pulmonary hypertensive crisis in the pediatric patient after cardiac surgery. *American Journal of Critical Care,* 4(1), 49–53.

Moynihan, P.J., & King, R. (1989). Caring for patients with lesions increasing pulmonary blood flow. *Critical Care Nursing Clinics of North America,* 1(2), 195–213.

3. Answer (**c**). CPB provides perfusion and oxygenation to the body's tissues during cardiac surgery. Three methods of CPB are used in pediatrics: moderate hypothermia (25°C–32°C), deep hypothermia (15°C–20°C), and deep hypothermic circulatory arrest (DHCA). Moderate hypothermia maintains a high flow rate to meet the metabolic demands of the patient. This method of CPB is used for older children and adolescents and can also be used for infants with uncomplicated ASD or simple VSD repairs. Deep hypothermic CPB is reserved for neonates and infants requiring complex cardiac repairs. Because of the use of nonpulsatile flow and the need for reduced perfusion flow rates to minimize blood return to the heart, hypothermia is required to prevent end-organ ischemia. This method of CPB allows a low-flow state, which provides an almost bloodless field for the surgeon. With DHCA, the surgeon can remove the atrial and aortic cannulas, thus allowing better visualization of the cardiac anatomy. Although CPB has proven instrumental in advancing our ability to repair complex congenital cardiac defects, it remains an unphysiologic state and has a number of deleterious effects.

Many organ-specific and global pathophysiologic changes occur during and after CPB. One such response is the release of mediators that initiate systemic inflammation. The main target of many of these mediators is vascular endothelium. Results of these mediator actions include altered microcirculation, impaired release of vasodilators, and alterations in the regulation of water and solute transport. Dysfunction of the endothelial lining also occurs. This promotes increased capillary permeability and interstitial edema.

Clinical experience with DHCA has shown that periods of 30 to 45 minutes of circulatory arrest are safe and appear to be well tolerated by patients. Beyond this time, the incidence of permanent and transient neurologic sequelae may be increased. Hypothermia seems to protect the brain from ischemic injury, but the duration of the arrest period and the quality of perfusion techniques influence the subsequent development of problems.

REFERENCES

Kern, F.H., Greely, W.J., & Ungerleider, R.M. (1995). Cardiopulmonary bypass. In D.G. Nichols et al. (Eds.). *Critical heart disease in infants and children* (pp. 499–507). St. Louis: Mosby–Year Book.

Mayer, J.E. (1992). Cardiopulmonary bypass for repair of congenital heart disease in infants and children. In B.P. Fuhrman & J.J. Zimmerman (Eds.). *Pediatric critical care* (pp. 339–344). St. Louis: Mosby–Year Book.

4. Answer (**d**). Alprostadil (prostaglandin E_1) has a direct relaxant effect on the smooth muscles throughout the body. Although it is frequently and effectively used to maintain patency of the ductus arteriosus in neonates with cyanotic, ductal-dependent lesions, this patient had no patent ductus before surgery. Patients with AVSDs are not necessarily ductal dependent, even at birth, because they have no obstruction to pulmonary blood flow. In this case, prostaglandin E_1 is used to decrease PVR by dilating

arterioles in the bronchioles and in the trachea, causing a direct relaxant effect on the pulmonary bed. Prostaglandin E_1 is considered most effective when infused directly through a pulmonary artery catheter.

REFERENCES

Hultgren, M.S. (1991). Pulmonary management of children after cardiac surgery. *Critical Care Nurse,* 11 (8), 55–69.

Taketomo, C.K., Hodding, J.H., & Kraus, D.M. (1992). *Pediatric dosage handbook.* Hudson, OH: Lexi-Comp.

5. Answer (**b**). There are several interventions that directly affect pulmonary physiology and circulation, and they are implemented to reduce the risk of increasing PVR. Acidosis, which causes vessel constriction and an increase in PVR, is prevented by hyperventilation to a Pco_2 of 25 to 35 mmHg. By maintaining an alkalotic environment, as seen with a Pco_2 of 25 to 35 mmHg and a pH of 7.45 to 7.55, lower pulmonary artery pressures and PVR result. The use of sedatives and muscle relaxants aids in controlling respirations mechanically and in decreasing the episodic PVR elevations associated with agitation or fear.

Oxygen itself is a potent vasodilator. Maintaining the partial pressure of oxygen at greater than 100 mmHg is essential to ensure vasodilation and to reduce the risk of hypoxia, in which smooth muscles of the arterioles contract and increase the PVR. Hypoxia alone can initiate the cascade of a hypertensive crisis.

Although PEEP can enhance oxygenation and ventilation in mechanically ventilated patients, it also has negative effects. PEEP has been shown to increase intrathoracic pressures and decrease cardiac output at any level. A high PEEP (>8 cmH_2O) has distended the lungs and caused an increase in PVR. The risk-benefit ratio must be addressed when setting PEEP values. The ideal PEEP setting for children at risk for pulmonary hypertension is less than 6 cmH_2O.

If the hematocrit rises too high ($>40\%$), blood viscosity may increase, with an equal increase in resistance to blood flow (i.e., increased PVR). If the hematocrit drops too low, the oxygen carrying capacity is diminished. Oxygen availability can also be affected by body temperature. As temperature decreases, the solubility of oxygen and carbon dioxide increase, and they become inaccessible for the body's use. Cooler body temperatures also lead to vasoconstriction, which can progress to acidosis and potentiate pulmonary vasoconstriction. The optimal temperature postoperatively is normothermic to warm.

REFERENCES

Hultgren, M.S. (1991). Pulmonary management of children after cardiac surgery. *Critical Care Nurse,* 11 (8), 55–69.

Medicus, L., & Thompson, L. (1995). Preventing pulmonary hypertensive crisis in the pediatric patient after cardiac surgery. *American Journal of Critical Care,* 4 (1), 49–53.

6. Answer (**a**). Postoperatively, children with defects that caused significant left-to-right shunting of blood flow before correction are at potential risk for pulmonary hypertensive crisis. During a pulmonary hypertensive crisis, the pulmonary artery pressures rise and become equal to or greater than systemic pressures. Right atrial and ventricular pressures rise, and as they do, left atrial and ventricular output decreases. The result is a decrease in systemic pressure, Pao_2, and oxygen saturation, with an increase in the $Paco_2$ and peak airway pressures. A pulmonary hypertensive crisis that is not controlled or halted can be lethal.

REFERENCE

Medicus, L., & Thompson, L. (1995). Preventing pulmonary hypertensive crisis in the pediatric patient after cardiac surgery. *American Journal of Critical Care,* 4 (1), 49–53.

7. Answer (**b**). Surgical repair for an AVSD includes patching the ASD and VSD, as well as repairing the mitral and tricuspid valves. The AV valves are reconstructed with available tissue from the common AV valve leaflets. Anatomically, the AV node divides the atria from the ventricles and lies just above the tricuspid valve. The bundle of His is a further extension of the AV node; it passes between the tricuspid and mitral valves and traverses parallel to the interventricular septum. All of the work done for an AVSD repair involves areas that are close to the conduction system. It is easy for direct injury to occur to the conduc-

tion system or for damage related to edema and inflammation to occur.

REFERENCES

Duszynski, S. (1992). *Pediatric ECG interpretation: A self-study text* (pp. 32–33). Milwaukee: Maxishare Corporation.

Smith, J.B., Baker, A.L., Moynihan, P.J., et al. (1996). Cardiovascular critical care problems. In M.A.Q. Curley, J.B. Smith & P.A. Moloney-Harmon (Eds.). *Critical care nursing of infants and children*. Philadelphia: W.B. Saunders.

8. Answer (**a**). Capture refers to the ability of the electrical discharge of the pacemaker to stimulate the myocardium. This stimulus causes contraction, and the wave is depicted on the electrocardiographic complex. The strip shows tall, very narrow pacer spikes followed by smaller, wide complex ventricular depolarization waves for the first three beats. The QRS complex is expected to be wide, because the electrical stimulus is originating from a site other than the AV node, and the stimulus takes longer to spread across the ventricles. The fourth and sixth beats are pacer spikes, but they are not followed by any ventricular response. The electrical charge is emitted from the pacemaker but fails to cause a stimulus within the heart itself, explaining the occasional failure to capture. Troubleshooting for this situation may include evaluating the threshold set on the pacemaker. The threshold is the minimum stimulus required to excite the myocardium. With myocardial inflammation or edema, the myocardial threshold may increase, and a greater electrical charge is necessary to cause the same response.

REFERENCES

Moses, H.W., Schneider, J.A., Miller, B.D., & Taylor, G.J. (1991). *A practical guide to cardiac pacing* (3rd ed.). Boston: Little, Brown.

Park, M.K., & Guntheroth, W.G. (1992). Analysis of arrhythmias and atrioventricular conduction disturbances. In M.K. Park & W.G. Guntheroth (Eds.). *How to read pediatric ECGs* (3rd ed., p. 218). St. Louis: Mosby–Year Book.

9. Answer (**c**). The dependent edema observed in S. results from the third spacing of intravascular fluids through permeable or "leaky" capillaries. Because the blood is hemodiluted during bypass to decrease the viscosity and to augment capillary perfusion at low flow rates, there is a fall in the protein concentration of the blood. This produces a fall in the oncotic pressures, which leads to tissue edema. The impact of surgery, the stress and length of time of the operation, and the use of CPB with hypothermic circulatory arrest contribute to the occurrence of leaky capillaries.

Contact of the circulating red blood cells and platelets with the inner surfaces of the bypass tubing and oxygenator results in thrombus formation unless the coagulation system is inhibited with heparin. All patients are anticoagulated during CPB and reversed at the end of the procedure with protamine sulfate. The numbers of platelets and their function are also impaired by CPB. The integrity of the platelets is disrupted by the cardiotomy suction and adhesion to the pump surfaces, and platelets are destroyed by the trauma of CPB. Concerns have been raised that platelets are activated in the bypass circuit. They may aggregate and lodge in the microcirculation, leading to further organ dysfunction. Despite some experimental use of platelet-inhibiting agents to reduce the effects of the bypass pump on platelets, the accepted course of treatment for destroyed platelets is to replace them as necessary.

REFERENCES

Craig, J. (1991). The postoperative cardiac infant: Physiologic basis for neonatal nursing interventions. *Journal of Perinatal and Neonatal Nursing, 5* (2), 60–70.

Mayer, J.E. (1992). Cardiopulmonary bypass for repair of congenital heart disease in infants and children. In B.P. Fuhrman & J.J. Zimmerman (Eds.). *Pediatric critical care* (pp. 339–344). St. Louis: Mosby–Year Book.

10. Answer (**d**). The clinical presentation and hemodynamic data indicate a decrease in left-sided heart function, probably due to mitral valve problems. Right atrial pressures are appropriate for the postoperative condition and do not indicate right-sided heart failure. Although the urine output and systemic perfusion indicate decreased cardiac output, it is not secondary to increased systemic vascular resistance because the arterial pressures are low. The left atrial catheter provides a measurement of pulmonary venous pressure, indicating systemic volume, left ventricular preload, and left ventricular function. An increase in left atrial pressure indicates hypervolemia, mitral valve insuffi-

ciency, loss of AV conduction, or global ventricular dysfunction.

The pulmonary congestion and the increased left atrial pressures indicate that some left-sided failure is occurring, probably caused by mitral valve damage. Mitral valve dysfunction is thought to be a major cause of morbidity and mortality for AVSD patients, and these patients occasionally need to return to surgery for mitral valve replacement.

REFERENCES

Elixson, E.M. (1989). Hemodynamic monitoring modalities in pediatric cardiac surgical patients. *Critical Care Nursing Clinics of North America, 1* (2), 263–273.

Smith, J.B., Baker, A.L., Moynihan, P.J., et al. (1996). Cardiovascular critical care problems. In M.A.Q. Curley, J.B. Smith & P.A. Moloney-Harmon (Eds.). *Critical care nursing of infants and children* (pp. 557–618). Philadelphia: W.B. Saunders.

ANSWERS ■ CASE 5-2

1. Answer (**a**). The primary nursing diagnosis addresses the patient's altered cardiac function, altered hematologic status, and altered comfort. Kawasaki disease is an acute vascular inflammatory process. There is widespread release of inflammatory mediators, including acute-phase reactants and leukocytes. During the initial acute phase of illness, some degree of myocarditis is present in all children. The myocardium is directly affected by the inflammatory process. The resulting myocellular hypertrophy, degeneration of myocytes, and endocardial changes lead to myocarditis and decreased ventricular function. Inflammation of the myocardium commonly manifests as CHF.

Altered cardiac function occurs as the result of myocarditis but can also be related to dysrhythmias or coronary artery aneurysms. Electrocardiographic changes may include a prolonged PR interval because of myocardial inflammation, which results in slowed conduction. Nonspecific ST and T wave changes may also be observed. Local areas of ischemia may occur and predispose the child to atrial or, more commonly, ventricular dysrhythmias.

Normochromic, normocytic anemia and thrombocytosis cause alterations in the patient's hematologic status. Patients with Kawasaki disease typically present with decreased hemoglobin and hemato-

crit concentrations, although the exact cause is unknown. Hemoglobin concentrations of more than two standard deviations below the mean for age are found for about one half of patients. Thrombocytosis typically occurs in the subacute phase of the illness, during which platelet counts can reach almost 1 million/mm^3. Elevated platelet counts cause sluggish, swirling blood flow and increase the risk of thrombosis in patients with aneurysms. This elevation places all children at risk for myocardial ischemia or infarction.

The diagnosis of altered comfort reflects a persistent fever, irritability, and the potential for arthritis. Fever is a hallmark of Kawasaki disease and is frequently the reason for seeking further treatment when the fever does not resolve after a standard antibiotic regimen. The fever may continue and be high despite antipyretic interventions throughout the acute phase (i.e., first 14 days). Irritability is another hallmark symptom of children with Kawasaki disease and can continue throughout the entire course of the disease. Arthritis or arthralgia can occur during the first week of the illness and is usually polyarticular, involving the knees, ankles, and hands. This pattern may continue into the second or third week of the illness and then become isolated to one joint.

REFERENCES

Dajani, A.S., Taubert, K.A., Gerber, M.A., et al. (1993). Diagnosis and therapy of Kawasaki disease in children. *Circulation, 87* (5), 1776–1780.

Smith, J.B., Baker, A.L., Moynihan, P.J., et al. (1996). Cardiovascular critical care problems. In M.A.Q. Curley, J.B. Smith & P.A. Moloney-Harmon (Eds.). *Critical care nursing of infants and children* (pp. 557–618). Philadelphia: W.B. Saunders.

2. Answer (**b**). The inflammation of the myocardium frequently manifests as CHF, which is defined as the inability of the heart to pump blood to meet the body's metabolic demands. Kawasaki disease is documented as one of the causes of acquired CHF in older infants and children. In the presence of inadequate cardiac output, several compensatory mechanisms are initiated to maintain adequate blood flow. These mechanisms include stimulation of baroreceptors, stretch receptors, and the sympathetic nervous system in an effort to increase the heart rate and force of myocardial contraction. Sympa-

thetic stimulation also decreases blood flow to the skin and splanchnic areas in an effort to optimize blood flow to the myocardium and brain. Venous smooth muscle tone increases in an attempt to enhance blood return to the heart. These compensatory mechanisms adequately sustain perfusion for a short time but eventually cause failure of the heart. Hypertrophy and excess stretch due to the fluid overload exhaust the myocardium. CHF in infants and children is manifested as tachycardia, even at rest. Blood flow to all peripheral organs, including the skin, diminishes and causes peripheral hypotension and cool extremities. The failing heart eventually experiences venous congestion, which can manifest as hepatomegaly, edema, or dyspnea. Changes in pressures cause fluid to leak from the pulmonary veins into the surrounding tissue, leading to dyspnea.

REFERENCES

Sims, S.L. (1990). Alterations of cardiovascular function in children. In K.L. McCance & S.E. Huether (Eds.). *Pathophysiology—The biologic basis for disease in adults and children* (pp. 1015–1016). St. Louis: C.V. Mosby.

Smith, J.B., Baker, A.L., Moynihan, P.J., et al. (1996). Cardiovascular critical care problems. In M.A.Q. Curley, J.B. Smith & P.A. Moloney-Harmon (Eds.). *Critical care nursing of infants and children* (pp. 557–618). Philadelphia: W.B. Saunders.

Sundel, R.P., & Newburger, J.W. (1993). Kawasaki disease and its cardiac sequelae. *Hospital Practice, 28* (11), 51–66.

3. Answer (**b**). The most important sequela of Kawasaki disease is coronary artery aneurysm. Coronary artery abnormalities typically do not develop until the second week after the onset of fever. One of five children develops damage to the coronary arteries in the form of aneurysms or dilatation. In the acute phase, damage to the coronary arteries causes weakness in the vessel wall. In the following weeks, the damaged vessel increases in diameter, resulting in dilatation or aneurysm formation. The affected vessels can continue to enlarge through the fourth week of the illness, at which time the maximum dimension usually is reached. Over time, the aneurysms usually regress.

REFERENCE

Smith, J.B., Baker, A.L., Moynihan, P.J., et al. (1996). Cardiovascular critical care problems. In M.A.Q. Curley, J.B. Smith & P.A. Moloney-Harmon (Eds.). *Criti-*
cal care nursing of infants and children (pp. 557–618). Philadelphia: W.B. Saunders.

4. Answer (**d**). Thrombocytosis causes sluggish blood flow throughout the body. When this type of flow encounters enlarged coronary vessels, there is an increased risk of thrombosis. Clot formation is more likely to occur because blood can pool in enlarged spaces, and it can readily clump because of the high platelet count. Any thrombosis places these children at significant risk for myocardial ischemia or infarction. Patients with giant aneurysms (≥8 mm in diameter) are at greatest risk for clot development.

REFERENCE

Smith, J.B., Baker, A.L., Moynihan, P.J., et al. (1996). Cardiovascular critical care problems. In M.A.Q. Curley, J.B. Smith & P.A. Moloney-Harmon (Eds.). *Critical care nursing of infants and children* (pp. 557–618). Philadelphia: W.B. Saunders.

5. Answer (**c**). Initial therapy for Kawasaki disease is directed at reducing inflammation, particularly in the coronary arterial wall and myocardium. Later, therapy is directed toward preventing coronary thrombosis by inhibiting platelet aggregation. To prevent long-term morbidity or mortality, it is imperative that treatment be initiated early in the illness, mandating a prompt and accurate diagnosis.

Specific pharmacologic therapy depends on identifying the etiology, but there is no known etiologic agent or organism for Kawasaki disease. Enhancing cardiac output or correcting an anemic state is beneficial to the patient, but to avert long-term cardiac sequelae, initial medical therapy must be directed at prevention of coronary artery aneurysms and possible development of thromboses.

REFERENCES

Dajani, A.S., Taubert, K.A., Gerber, M.A., et al. (1993). Diagnosis and therapy of Kawasaki disease in children. *Circulation, 87* (5), 1776–1780.

Sundel, R.P., & Newburger, J.W. (1993). Kawasaki disease and its cardiac sequelae. *Hospital Practice, 28* (11), 51–66.

6. Answer (**a**). High-dose aspirin alone hastens the resolution of acute manifestations of Kawasaki disease, particularly fever. However, the combination of aspirin and IVIG has a more rapid anti-inflammatory effect than aspirin alone and appears to decrease the rate of devel-

opment of coronary abnormalities. Studies show that dosing with a single dose of 2 g/kg of IVIG has better results than the previously prescribed 400 mg/kg per day for 4 days. After the fever subsides, the dose is reduced for 2 weeks to 30 mg/kg per day and then to 10 mg/kg per day. Low-dose aspirin therapy is continued for 3 months. Aspirin can be stopped if no aneurysm is identified, but if an aneurysm is present, aspirin should be continued until the coronary artery appears normal by echocardiogram.

REFERENCES

Dajani, A.S., Taubert, K.A., Gerber, M.A., et al. (1993). Diagnosis and therapy of Kawasaki disease in children. *Circulation*, 87 (5), 1776–1780.

Park, M.K. (1991). *The pediatric cardiology handbook* (pp. 129–131). St. Louis: Mosby–Year Book.

7. Answer (**a**). This patient's clinical presentation demonstrates a state of low-output heart failure. Systemic perfusion is markedly decreased, ventricular filling pressures are elevated, and pulmonary congestion has developed. Heart failure is regulated by several adaptive mechanisms that attempt to maintain vital organ tissue perfusion. Initially, the mechanisms are beneficial, but with sustained heart failure, the effects can be detrimental. The factors that control cardiac output are preload, afterload, contractility, and heart rate. The associations among these determinants of stroke volume provide the physiologic basis for therapeutic interventions directed toward improving the cardiac function in the failing heart.

Pharmacologic interventions in this phase of CHF are aimed at improving the inotropic state of the heart, decreasing preload, and decreasing afterload. Efforts to increase inotropic action of the heart are aimed at augmenting the contractility of the heart and enhancing cardiac output to the systemic tissues.

Preload is defined as the degree of stretch on the myocardial muscle fibers just before systole and is most accurately estimated by left ventricular end-diastolic pressures. In this case, the central venous pressure gives an approximation of the preload or filling pressures. Preload needs to be decreased, because excess circulating blood volume strains the heart. Preload can be decreased with diuretics or vasodilators. Diuresis decreases preload and moves cardiac function into a more favorable position on the Starling curve. The Frank-Starling law describes contractility as a function of preload.

Afterload is the resistance to blood flow out of the left ventricle into the systemic circulation. This is measured as systemic vascular resistance but can be subjectively assessed by a patient's clinical features, such as pulse strength, capillary refill time, extremity temperature, and urine output. All of these are indicators of tissue and end-organ perfusion adequacy. Afterload can be reduced to enhance tissue perfusion with vasodilators. Phosphodiesterase inhibitors such as amrinone (Inocor) are useful in CHF because they increase contractility and decrease afterload.

REFERENCES

Ruggerie, D.P. (1990). Congestive heart failure. In J.L. Blumer (Ed.). *A practical guide to pediatric intensive care* (3rd ed., pp. 114–118). St. Louis: Mosby–Year Book.

Smith, J.B., Baker, A.L., Moynihan, P.J., et al. (1996). Cardiovascular critical care problems. In M.A.Q. Curley, J.B. Smith & P.A. Moloney-Harmon (Eds.). *Critical care nursing of infants and children* (pp. 557–618). Philadelphia: W.B. Saunders.

8. Answer (**d**). Diminished blood flow to the kidney causes the kidneys to conserve sodium and fluid. Diuretics play a fundamental role in the treatment of the congestive elements of cardiac failure in all pediatric patients. Furosemide is frequently the first diuretic chosen, because it inhibits the active reabsorption of chloride anions and thus the passive reabsorption of sodium and water. The initial dose is usually 1.0 mg/kg, which is given intravenously or intramuscularly.

Dobutamine is a synthetic sympathomimetic that is capable of β_1- and β_2-adrenergic receptor stimulation. It primarily has an inotropic effect on the heart, increasing cardiac output, but it also causes some systemic vasodilation, which decreases afterload. Because of myocardial inflammation and CHF symptoms, the heart requires pharmacologic support to maintain adequate cardiac output to meet the body's metabolic demands. Dobutamine is a proven agent.

Dopamine administered at 3 μg/kg per minute is primarily a renal vasodilator. Although the added effect of renal vasodilation is advantageous, it does not address the underlying problem of myocardial inflammation and decreased contractility. A bolus of 25% albumin is unnecessary at this point, because there are no signs of third space fluid. With a central venous pressure of 15 mmHg, most of the excess fluid is still within the circulating vascular spaces, and a diuretic can appropriately manage this.

An infusion of epinephrine increases the systemic vascular resistance and afterload, making adequate cardiac output even more difficult.

REFERENCE

Ruggerie, D.P. (1990). Congestive heart failure. In J.L. Blumer (Ed.). *A practical guide to pediatric intensive care* (3rd ed., pp. 114–118). St. Louis: Mosby–Year Book.

CHAPTER 6

Pulmonary Disorders

LIANE S. CONRAD, RN, BSN
MARGARET S. GELLER, RN, CCRN
KAREN A. FRASER, RN
PATRICIA A. BERRY, RN, CCRN
ELAINE A. CARON, RN
JANICE M. DOYLE, RN, CCRN

CASE 6-1

J. was born prematurely at 32 weeks' gestation and was diagnosed with hyaline membrane disease at birth. He was intubated and ventilated for 4 weeks, requiring supplemental oxygen and intermittent use of bronchodilators after extubation. J. was discharged home at 7 weeks of age with oxygen delivered through a nasal cannula at 0.5 L/min and nebulized albuterol given as needed. He was admitted to the pediatric intensive care unit (PICU) at 5 months of age with an increased oxygen requirement, increased work of breathing, and copious nasal discharge.

1. An obstructive, restrictive pulmonary disease resulting in oxygen dependency beyond 1 month of age can be defined as
   a. Adult respiratory distress syndrome (ARDS).
   b. Asthma.
   c. Bronchopulmonary dysplasia (BPD).
   d. Emphysema.

2. Which factors in J.'s history contribute to the development of BPD?
   a. An anatomic defect and the use of bronchodilators after extubation.
   b. Age of 5 months and nebulized albuterol administered at home.

   c. Prematurity, oxygen therapy, and ventilation.
   d. Increased oxygen requirements at 5 months of age and nasal discharge.

3. Because J. has BPD, the nurse caring for him is likely to see which of the following signs and symptoms?
   a. Failure to thrive and dehydration.
   b. Hyperinflation and prolonged inspiratory phase.
   c. Hypoxemia and hypocarbia.
   d. Rapid, shallow respirations with crackles and bronchial sounds.

J. is started on oxygen at 2 L/min supplied by nasal cannula and on aerosolized albuterol. Although perfusion is adequate, his extremities are slightly cool and mottled. His oxygen saturation is 90%.

4. Which factor compromises J.'s oxygen tissue delivery?
   a. Aerosolized bronchodilators.
   b. An HCO_3 level between 22 and 26 mEq/L.
   c. A serum pH greater than 7.50.
   d. Supplemental oxygen therapy.

In addition to oxygen and bronchodilators, J.'s treatment includes placement of an intravenous line and intravenous delivery of methylprednisolone. His vital signs include a rectal temperature of 37.5°C., heart rate of

170 beats per minute (bpm), respiratory rate of 68 breaths per minute, and blood pressure of 110/60 mmHg. His physical examination reveals increased work of breathing, with rales and inspiratory and expiratory wheezing. His chest x-ray film shows increased pulmonary markings and an enlarged heart. His weight is increased 0.5 kg above baseline, and his liver is palpated at 4 cm below the right costal margin.

5. Based on these findings, the nurse suspects that J. has developed
   a. Left-sided heart failure.
   b. Hepatic failure.
   c. Right-sided heart failure.
   d. Renal failure.

6. The most appropriate treatment for J. at this point is
   a. Antihypertensives.
   b. Bronchodilators.
   c. Diuretics.
   d. Volume expanders.

J. is intubated and placed on a positive-pressure ventilator with settings of peak inspiratory pressure of 32 cmH_2O, peak end-expiratory pressure (PEEP) of 3 cmH_2O, intermittent mandatory ventilation (IMV) rate of 12 breaths per minute, and fraction of inspired oxygen (FIO_2) of 0.50.

7. An inappropriate outcome in J.'s care plan for ventilator management is
   a. Achievement of adequate gas exchange.
   b. Prevention of barotrauma.
   c. Normalization of arterial blood gases.
   d. Prevention of hyperinflation.

8. Nursing interventions to avoid hypoxemia and bronchospasm in J. include
   a. Adequate nutrition through continuous feedings.
   b. Developmental stimulation and play therapy.
   c. Stress reduction and structured care.
   d. Supplemental oxygen therapy and scheduled pulmonary toilet.

J. remains intubated for 5 days. On day 2, gastrostomy feedings are initiated.

9. Nutritional needs can be difficult to meet in J. because of
   a. Fluid restriction, increased caloric demands, and poor feeding tolerance.
   b. Increased gastric motility, fluid overload, and a dislike of certain foods.

   c. Small gastric residuals, gastric distention, and aggressive sucking.
   d. Use of nasogastric feedings, decreased caloric demands, and the parents' presence.

J.'s condition gradually improves, and he is slowly weaned from the ventilator.

10. J.'s readiness for weaning from mechanical ventilation is demonstrated by
   a. A reduction in the baseline spontaneous respiratory rate and the baseline $Paco_2$ value.
   b. An increase in the infant's tendency to become agitated when cares are done.
   c. A reduction in tracheal secretions and the frequency of suctioning.
   d. Sustained weight loss over a period of several weeks.

J. is successfully extubated. He is transferred to the pediatric medical unit on supplemental O_2 and scheduled aerosolized bronchodilators.

CASE 6-2

B. is a 20-month-old boy with a history of possible aspiration of gastric contents. When he presents in the emergency department, he is lethargic, pale, and tachypneic, with circumoral cyanosis. An arterial blood gas analysis on room air reveals the following results: pH of 7.48, $Paco_2$ of 30 mmHg, Pao_2 of 64 mmHg, HCO_3 level of 20 mEq/L. His O_2 saturation is 91%. Oxygen therapy is started with a face mask at an FIO_2 of 0.50. He is admitted to the PICU with a diagnosis of respiratory failure.

1. These arterial blood gas values are indicative of
   a. Metabolic acidosis.
   b. Metabolic alkalosis.
   c. Respiratory acidosis.
   d. Respiratory alkalosis.

B's chest x-ray film reveals bilateral diffuse pulmonary infiltrates. Coarse rales are heard on auscultation. B. experiences increased respiratory distress, including intercostal retractions, fatigue, and worsening hypoxemia that is unresponsive to an increased FIO_2.

ARDS is suspected. B. is intubated and placed on a conventional ventilator.

2. ARDS is best described as
  a. Hypoxemia, congestive heart failure, and bilateral diffuse infiltrates.
  b. Hypoxemia, elevated pulmonary wedge pressure, and bilateral diffuse infiltrates.
  c. Hypoxemia, hyperinflation, and bilateral diffuse infiltrates.
  d. Hypoxemia, normal pulmonary wedge pressure, and bilateral diffuse infiltrates.

3. Which of the following are considered risk factors for ARDS?
  a. Aspiration of gastric contents, sepsis, and trauma.
  b. BPD and diaphragmatic hernia.
  c. Congestive heart failure and pulmonary hypertension.
  d. Asthma, Guillain-Barré syndrome, and seizures.

B. is placed on a volume ventilator with a tidal volume of 180 cc, PEEP of 8 cmH$_2$O, IMV of 12 breaths per minute, and F$_{IO_2}$ 0.70. After 24 hours, his arterial blood gas values deteriorate to a pH of 7.29, Pa$_{CO_2}$ of 54 mmHg, Pa$_{O_2}$ of 56 mmHg, HCO$_3$ level of 22 mEq/L, and O$_2$ saturation of 86%, with peak inspiratory pressures elevated to the mid-40s (cmH$_2$0).

4. Based on this information, the nurse would expect further treatment to include
  a. Paralysis and decreased PEEP.
  b. Paralysis and pressure-control ventilation.
  c. Sedation and decreased rate.
  d. Sedation and increased tidal volume.

5. An important nursing intervention for B. after neuromuscular blocking agents and sedatives or anxiolytics have been administered is to
  a. Closely monitor for pain and agitation by observing the physiologic parameters.
  b. Avoid the use of sedatives and anxiolytics to prevent hemodynamic instability.
  c. Keep visitors away from the bedside, because having someone talk to the child may cause anxiety.
  d. Ensure that the neuromuscular blockade does not wear off until the child is ready for extubation.

Parenteral nutrition is started to meet the appropriate caloric requirements for B.

6. Appropriate nutritional support is of vital importance to B.'s recovery because
  a. Nutritional adequacy is necessary for the development of new type II alveolar cells.
  b. Nutritional support can reverse any infections that develop.
  c. Nutritional support is mandatory for appropriate oxygenation.
  d. Poor nutritional status negatively affects diaphragmatic mass and strength.

Nursing assessment reveals an acute change in the physical examination findings, including tachycardia, decreased breath sounds on the left side, elevated blood pressure, and a decrease in oxygen saturation.

7. The nurse caring for B. suspects
  a. Inadvertent extubation.
  b. Pneumonia.
  c. Pneumothorax.
  d. Pulmonary edema.

Despite appropriate treatment for this complication, B. continues to deteriorate, with continued hypoxemia. His chest x-ray film shows significant bilateral infiltrates. His PEEP is increased to 15 cmH$_2$O.

8. The nurse should be aware that the potential complications associated with the use of increased PEEP include
  a. Barotrauma and decreased cardiac output.
  b. Increased cardiac output and hypertension.
  c. Increased oxygen delivery and oxygen toxicity.
  d. Pulmonary edema and decreased oxygen delivery.

9. Which of the following measures may be instituted to minimize tissue oxygen demand in B.?
  a. Administration of neuromuscular blocking agents, sedatives, and anxiolytics.
  b. Allowance of hyperthermia to treat any pulmonary infections.
  c. Provision of frequent chest physiotherapy and suctioning.
  d. Prevention of parents or other visitors at B.'s bedside.

A pulmonary artery catheter is placed to measure pulmonary wedge pressures and to determine oxygen delivery. The cardiac index is measured as 2.85 L/minute/m^2, and B.

is started on vasopressors to increase contractility and systemic perfusion.

10. The nurse should observe for which signs of decreased systemic perfusion in B.?
    a. Capillary refill of less than 2 seconds, central cyanosis, and bradycardia.
    b. Capillary refill of more than 2 seconds, cool and mottled extremities, and decreased urine output.
    c. Fever, tachycardia, and decreased systolic blood pressure.
    d. Tachycardia, warm extremities, and decreased urine output.

11. The approach to fluid therapy in B. will include
    a. Administration of vasopressin and fluids at maintenance plus one-half level.
    b. Restriction of fluids and diuretic therapy.
    c. Ionotropic agents and vasopressin.
    d. Fluids at maintenance plus one-half level and vasodilators.

B. continues to deteriorate, and his PaO_2 is 50 mmHg on an FIO_2 of 1.0. He develops a persistent air leak and requires placement of additional chest tubes. As hypoxia progresses, B. develops multiorgan failure, including renal failure, hepatic failure, and disseminated intravascular coagulation. Despite maximal medical intervention, B. dies.

CASE 6-3

G. is a 20-kg, 5-year-old boy with known reactive airway disease that is treated with albuterol by inhalation as needed at home. He presents to the emergency department with a 3-day history of rhinorrhea, low-grade fever, decreased oral intake, and an increased respiratory rate with cough and wheezing that is unresponsive to home albuterol treatments.

His physical examination reveals that he is pale, restless, and fatigued, with grunting, nasal flaring, and retractions. On auscultation, he has scattered inspiratory and expiratory wheezes, with a marked decrease in aeration bilaterally. Vital signs include an axillary temperature of 38°C, heart rate of 155 bpm, respiratory rate of 44 breaths per minute, and blood pressure of 94/58 mmHg. His oxygen saturation is 88% on room air.

1. Based on G.'s history and presenting symptoms, the initial intervention is to
    a. Administer an inhalation bronchodilator.
    b. Begin O_2 therapy.
    c. Administer aminophylline.
    d. Intubate immediately.

In response to therapy, G. has an oxygen saturation of 92%. His chest x-ray film reveals bilateral hyperinflation but no focal findings. The percutaneous arterial blood gas analysis shows a pH of 7.48, $PaCO_2$ of 29 mmHg, PaO_2 of 62 mmHg, O_2 saturation of 93%, and HCO_3 level of 25 mEq/L.

2. These arterial blood gas values are indicative of
    a. Metabolic alkalosis.
    b. Normal blood gas.
    c. Respiratory acidosis.
    d. Respiratory alkalosis.

G. receives a bolus of aminophylline, followed by an aminophylline infusion. He receives parenteral corticosteroids, continuous albuterol nebulizers are begun, and a normal saline bolus of 10 mL/kg is given twice to correct dehydration.

3. The appropriate dose for G.'s aminophylline bolus is
    a. 40 mg administered over 5 minutes.
    b. 100 mg administered over 20 minutes.
    c. 200 mg administered over 30 minutes
    d. 300 mg administered over 60 minutes.

4. The nurse observes for which of the following side effects when administering the aminophylline bolus to G.?
    a. Bradycardia, hypotension, and vomiting.
    b. Bradycardia, seizures, and ventricular arrhythmias.
    c. Tachycardia, hypotension, and vomiting.
    d. Tachycardia, seizures, and constipation.

5. Corticosteroids are indicated for G. because they
    a. Liquefy his thick, tenacious sputum and allow him to cough more effectively.
    b. Increase the number of β-adrenergic receptors and reduce mucosal inflammation.

c. Facilitate alveolar emptying and promote alveolar reinflation.

d. Reduce lung water and prevent the development of pulmonary edema.

With limited response to the therapy received in the emergency department, G. is transferred to the PICU. After admission, he is observed to have decreased aeration, increased work of breathing, and an oxygen saturation of 90% on an FIO_2 of 1.0 through a non-rebreathing mask. An arterial line is placed; arterial blood gases, a complete blood count, electrolyte concentrations, and theophylline and creatine phosphokinase levels are determined. His theophylline level is therapeutic. The results of a 12-lead electrocardiogram are normal.

6. Knowing that G. is receiving sympathomimetics, the nurse should monitor for which of the following significant adverse effects?
a. Bronchospasm.
b. Myocardial ischemia.
c. Nausea and vomiting.
d. Tachycardia.

7. The nurse anticipates which therapy for G. at this point?
a. Chest physical therapy.
b. Facial CPAP (continuous positive airway pressure).
c. Intubation.
d. Terbutaline infusion.

8. The anticipated approach to intravenous therapy in this child is
a. Maintenance fluids.
b. One-half maintenance fluids.
c. Three-fourths maintenance fluids.
d. Twice maintenance fluids.

9. Chest physical therapy is contraindicated in G. because of possible
a. Aggravation of bronchospasm.
b. Increased agitation.
c. Induction of vomiting.
d. Interruption of inhalation therapy.

10. Intubation and positive-pressure ventilation are high-risk therapies for G. because of the risk of
a. Infection.
b. Oxygen toxicity.
c. Pneumothorax.
d. Ventilator dependence.

After 48 hours of therapy, G.'s arterial blood gas values show a pH of 7.40, $PaCO_2$ of 40 mmHg, PaO_2 of 98 mmHg, and HCO_3 level of 27 mEq/L on an FIO_2 of 0.40. His vital signs are an axillary temperature of 36.6°C, heart rate of 94, respiratory rate of 22, and blood pressure of 108/54 mmHg. He continues to have mild, occasional wheezes without retractions. The terbutaline is slowly tapered over 24 hours, and he is then transferred to the general pediatric unit on intermittent inhalation therapy.

ANSWERS ■ CASE 6-1

1. Answer (**c**). BPD is a chronic respiratory disease occurring in premature infants who have been exposed to treatment for respiratory failure. Characteristic abnormalities in BPD include increased airway resistance and decreased compliance. BPD is truly a "mixed" disorder that is obstructive and restrictive in nature. Typically, these children demonstrate physical and radiologic evidence of lung disease at 1 month of age and require continuous oxygen therapy.

REFERENCES
Few, B. (1996). Pulmonary critical care problems. In M.A.Q. Curley, J.B. Smith, & P.A. Moloney-Harmon (Eds.). *Critical care nursing of infants and children* (pp. 619–655). Philadelphia: W.B. Saunders.
Zander, J., & Hazinski, M. (1992). Pulmonary disorders. In M. Hazinski (Ed.). *Nursing care of the critically ill child* (2nd ed., pp. 395–497). St. Louis: Mosby–Year Book.

2. Answer (**c**). Theories regarding BPD have suggested that it is the response of the immature lung to early injury. Positive-pressure ventilation along with high concentrations of inspired oxygen have been implicated as contributing to this insult.

REFERENCE
Zander, J., & Hazinski, M. (1992). Pulmonary disorders. In M. Hazinski (Ed.). *Nursing care of the critically ill child* (2nd ed., pp. 395–497). St. Louis: Mosby–Year Book.

3. Answer (**d**). Infants with BPD typically have tachypnea, mild retractions, rales, and wheezing on examination of the chest.

REFERENCE
Burchfield, D., Neu, J. (1993). Neonatal parenchymal diseases. In P. Koff, D. Eitzman, & J. Neu (Eds.). *Neonatal and pediatric respiratory care* (2nd ed., pp. 75–91). St. Louis: Mosby–Year Book.

4. Answer (**c**). Factors that impair the release of oxygen to the tissues by shifting the oxyhemoglobin dissociation curve to the left include hypothermia and metabolic or respiratory alkalosis.

REFERENCE

Few, B. (1996). Pulmonary critical care problems. In M.A.Q. Curley, J.B. Smith, & P.A. Moloney-Harmon (Eds.). *Critical care nursing of infants and children* (pp. 619–655). Philadelphia: W.B. Saunders.

5. Answer (**c**). With prolonged respiratory failure, some infants develop signs of right-sided heart failure secondary to pulmonary hypertension with cardiomegaly and fluid retention.

REFERENCE

Bancalari, E., & Gerhardt, T. (1986). Bronchopulmonary dysplasia. *Pediatric Clinics of North America, 33* (1), 1–23.

6. Answer (**c**). Diuretics are indicated in infants with BPD to eliminate excess water. In addition, diuretics can improve pulmonary compliance and reduce airway resistance.

REFERENCE

Burchfield, D., & Neu, J. (1993). Neonatal parenchymal diseases. In P. Koff, D. Eitzman, & J. Neu (Eds.). *Neonatal and pediatric respiratory care* (2nd ed., pp. 75–91). St. Louis: Mosby–Year Book.

7. Answer (**c**). During the early stages of acute respiratory failure, the goal of ventilator management is to achieve adequate gas exchange while minimizing barotrauma. This is accomplished by limiting peak inspiratory pressures and hyperinflation. Normalization of arterial blood gas tensions is often attempted, but strategies that allow a lower Pao_2 and higher $Paco_2$ may decrease barotrauma and improve outcome by minimizing the toxic effects of ventilation.

REFERENCE

Abman, S., & Groothius, J. (1994). Pathophysiology and treatment of bronchopulmonary dysplasia: Current issues. *Pediatric Clinics of North America, 41* (2), 277–315.

8. Answer (**c**). Minimizing agitation and the hypoxemia and bronchospasm that often accompany it is a primary goal in the care of children with BPD. The infant's individual temperament directs nursing measures to reduce stress. Sedation may sometimes be required. Necessary procedures are spaced throughout the day to permit time for recovery, and unnecessary interventions are avoided. Clinical assessment, not time alone, guides the frequency of chest physical therapy and suctioning.

REFERENCE

Few, B. (1996). Pulmonary critical care problems. In M.A.Q. Curley, J.B. Smith, & P. A. Moloney-Harmon (Eds.). *Critical care nursing of infants and children* (pp. 619–655). Philadelphia: W.B. Saunders.

9. Answer (**a**). Nutritional needs are difficult to meet in patients with BPD because of poor feeding tolerance, the necessity to restrict fluids, and increased caloric demands due to the excessive work of breathing.

REFERENCE

Bancalari, E., & Gerhardt, T. (1986). Bronchopulmonary dysplasia. *Pediatric Clinics of North America, 33* (1), 1–23.

10. Answer (**a**). Attempts to rapidly reduce mechanical ventilation often meet with acute decompensation 24 to 48 hours later, when the infant tires and the $Paco_2$ climbs. It is important to move slowly and allow adequate time for the infant to adjust. Readiness for weaning from mechanical ventilation is demonstrated by a persistent reduction in baseline spontaneous respiratory rate and $Paco_2$, accompanied by a sustained weight gain.

REFERENCE

Few, B. (1996). Pulmonary critical care problems. In M.A.Q. Curley, J.B. Smith, & P.A. Moloney-Harmon (Eds.). *Critical care nursing of infants and children* (pp. 619–655). Philadelphia: W.B. Saunders.

ANSWERS ■ CASE 6-2

1. Answer (**d**). When respiratory alkalosis develops, a primary increase in alveolar ventilation lowers the $Paco_2$ and raises the arterial pH. Acute respiratory alkalosis in children may result from acute hyperventilation caused by severe hypoxemia.

REFERENCE

Zander, J., & Hazinski, M. (1992). Pulmonary disorders. In M. Hazinski (Ed.). *Nursing care of the critically ill child* (2nd ed., pp. 395–497). St. Louis: Mosby–Year Book.

2. Answer (**d**). Early signs of ARDS are

dyspnea and profound hypoxemia that fail to respond to supplemental oxygen. Bilateral diffuse infiltrates seen on the chest x-ray film strongly suggest the diagnosis. The pulmonary capillary wedge pressure is low to normal, suggesting the absence of cardiac dysfunction, contributing to pulmonary disease. A clinical diagnosis of ARDS means that congestive heart failure must be unequivocally ruled out.

REFERENCE

Lillington, G., & Redding, G. (1988). What you need to know about ARDS. *Patient Care, 22* (5), 67–78.

3. Answer (**a**). The medical risk factors for ARDS are sepsis, aspiration of gastric contents, trauma, and near-drowning. Children with asthma, BPD, cystic fibrosis, Kawasaki disease, and Guillain-Barré syndrome do not seem to be at increased risk for ARDS.

REFERENCES

Hudson, L. (1990). The predictors and preventions of ARDS. *Respiratory Care* 35 (2), 161–173.
Lillington, G., & Redding, G. (1988), What you need to know about ARDS. *Patient Care, 22* (5), 67–78.

4. Answer (**b**). Pressure control with inverse-ratio ventilation is a method that reverses the conventional inspiratory-expiratory ratio to greater than 1. This strategy has been reported to improve oxygenation with lower peak pressures. The use of pressure control has reduced the peak inspiratory pressure, PEEP requirements, and minute ventilation. Mean airway pressure is increased, and oxygenation is improved. Pharmacologic paralysis eliminates the work of breathing and increases chest wall compliance, This may result in a fall in the peak inspiratory pressure.

REFERENCES

Vidal, R., Kissoon, N., & Denicola, L. (1993). Adult respiratory distress syndrome in children. In P. Koff, D. Eitzman, & J. Neu (Eds.). *Neonatal and pediatric respiratory care* (2nd ed., pp. 212–223). St. Louis: Mosby–Year Book.
Zander, J., & Hazinski, M. (1992). Pulmonary disorders. In M. Hazinski (Ed.). *Nursing care of the critically ill child* (2nd ed., pp. 395–497). St. Louis: Mosby–Year Book.

5. Answer (**a**). Sedatives or analgesic drugs are used in conjunction with muscle relaxants to ensure that the child is free of pain and comfortable during treatment. Because the child can still hear, fre-

quent, comforting words, explanations, and reassurances must be provided.

REFERENCE

Zander, J., & Hazinski, M. (1992). Pulmonary disorders. In M. Hazinski (Ed.). *Nursing care of the critically ill child* (2nd ed., pp. 395–497). St. Louis: Mosby–Year Book.

6. Answer (**d**). Adequate nutritional status is of vital importance in treating ARDS. Poor nutritional status can adversely affect respiratory system function by impairing diaphragmatic mass and strength, ventilatory drive, and immune mechanisms, resulting in a failure to wean from mechanical ventilation. Although nutritional support is necessary to sustain immune mechanisms, it cannot reverse an infection.

REFERENCE

Vidal, R., Kissoon, N., & Denicola, L. et al. (1993). Adult respiratory distress syndrome in children. In P. Koff, D. Eitzman, & J. Neu (Eds.). *Neonatal and pediatric respiratory care* (2nd ed., pp. 212–225). St. Louis: Mosby–Year Book.

7. Answer (**c**). Patients receiving supportive care for ARDS must be carefully monitored for development of complications. If the patient suddenly deteriorates, asymmetry of the chest may indicate pneumothorax. A chest x-ray film, if time permits, can confirm a pneumothorax. However, obtaining a chest radiograph should not delay treatment.

REFERENCE

Idell, S. (1989). The deadly danger of ARDS. *Emergency Medicine, 21* (7), 67–72.

8. Answer (**a**). Patients have an increased risk of barotrauma and pneumothorax with high levels of PEEP. High levels of PEEP also can reduce cardiac output, resulting in a paradoxical decrease in oxygen delivery.

REFERENCE

Raffin, T.A. (1987). ARDS: Mechanisms and management. *Hospital Practice, 22* (11), 65–80.

9. Answer (**a**). Fever and pain are treated in the child with ARDS, because both conditions increase oxygen requirements. Pharmacologic paralysis may reduce oxygen consumption by the respiratory muscles. The hypoxemic child is likely to be irritable and frightened, and any child should be sedated when paral-

ysis is necessary. Because hypoxemia is a primary feature of ARDS, measures to reduce oxygen consumption are critical. In patients with very large intrapulmonary shunts, fever, anxiety, and physical activity can increase oxygen demand.

REFERENCES

Few, B. (1996). Pulmonary critical care problems. In M.A.Q. Curley, J.B. Smith, & P.A. Moloney-Harmon (Eds.). *Critical care nursing of infants and children* (pp. 619–655). Philadelphia: W.B. Saunders.

Zander, J., & Hazinski, M. (1992). Pulmonary disorders. In M. Hazinski (Ed.). *Nursing care of the critically ill child* (2nd ed., pp. 395–497). St. Louis: Mosby–Year Book.

10. Answer (**b**). If the child has pale mucous membranes, cool mottled extremities, and sluggish capillary refill, cardiac output may be inadequate, compromising systemic and renal perfusion.

REFERENCE

Kennedy, J. (1992). In M. Hazinski (Ed.). *Nursing care of the critically ill child* (2nd ed., pp. 629–713). St. Louis: Mosby–Year Book.

11. Answer (**b**). Although there are many controversies regarding fluid requirement and restriction, it is generally advisable to restrict fluids. The ultimate goal of fluid therapy is to maintain an adequate cardiac output, but fluid therapy in the child with ARDS is aimed at reducing intravascular volume. If the pulmonary capillary wedge pressure (PCWP) increases in the acute stage of ARDS, diuretics may be indicated. Diuretics may be helpful in shifting extravascular water into the intravascular space if volume overload has occurred, as indicated by an increased PCWP. Inotropic agents may be indicated to treat systemic hypotension and to increase cardiac output, but fluid administration must still occur judiciously.

REFERENCES

Bradley, R. (1987). Adult respiratory distress syndrome. *Focus on Critical Care,* 14 (5), 48–57.

Few, B. (1996). Pulmonary critical care problems. In M.A.Q. Curley, J.B. Smith, & P.A. Moloney-Harmon (Eds.). *Critical care nursing of infants and children* (pp. 619–655). Philadelphia: W.B. Saunders.

ANSWERS ■ CASE 6-3

1. Answer (**b**). Oxygen is administered immediately to all seriously ill or injured patients with respiratory insufficiency, shock, or trauma. Oxygen delivery may be limited in these patients by inadequate pulmonary gas exchange or by inadequate circulatory volume or function.

REFERENCE

Lundberg, G. (1992). Pediatric advanced life support, Guidelines for cardiopulmonary resuscitation and emergency cardiac care. *The Journal of the American Medical Association,* 2199, 2262.

2. Answer (**d**). When respiratory alkalosis develops, a primary increase in alveolar ventilation lowers the $Paco_2$ and raises the arterial pH. Acute respiratory alkalosis in children may result from acute hyperventilation caused by severe hypoxemia.

REFERENCE

Zander, J., & Hazinski, M. (1992). Pulmonary disorders. In M. Hazinski (Ed.). *Nursing care of the critically ill child* (2nd ed., pp. 395–497). St. Louis: Mosby–Year Book.

3. Answer (**b**). The appropriate dose for an aminophylline bolus is 5 mg/kg.

REFERENCE

Taketomo, C., Hodding. J., & Kraus, D. (1993). *Pediatric dosage handbook* (2nd ed., pp. 38–39). Hudson, OH: Lexi-Comp.

4. Answer (**c**). Rapid administration of aminophylline can cause severe hypotension, premature ventricular contractions, and cardiac arrest. Toxicity can cause nausea, vomiting, cardiac arrhythmias, and seizures.

REFERENCES

Orsi, A. (1991). Asthma—The danger is real. *RN,* 4, 58–63.

Taketomo, C., Hodding. J., & Kraus, D. (1993). *Pediatric dosage handbook* (2nd ed., pp. 38–39). Hudson, OH: Lexi-Comp.

5. Answer (**b**). Corticosteroids shorten the duration and severity of severe asthma attacks. Although the exact mechanism of action remains unknown, they restore β-adrenergic responsiveness, decrease mucus secretion, and suppress the inflammatory response.

REFERENCE

Kurth, C., & Goodwin, S. (1992). Obstructive airway diseases in infants and children. In P. Koff, D. Eitzman, & J. Neu (Eds.). *Neonatal and pediatric respiratory care* (2nd ed., pp. 102–127). St. Louis: Mosby–Year Book.

6. Answer (**b**). Myocardial ischemia is a known adverse effect of sympathomimetics.

REFERENCE

Kurth, C., & Goodwin, S. (1992). Obstructive airway diseases in infants and children. In P. Koff, D. Eitzman, & J. Neu (Eds.). *Neonatal and pediatric respiratory care* (2nd ed., pp. 102–127). St. Louis: Mosby–Year Book.

7. Answer (**d**). It has been the practice in most children's centers to use intravenous isoproterenol in patients with impending respiratory failure to avoid the need for mechanical ventilation. Although this has been considered a safe practice in the pediatric population, several reports of myocardial ischemia in this population have prompted trials of intravenous selective β_2-adrenergic agents, such as terbutaline, which have fewer cardiovascular side effects. If the child still fails to improve after the β_2-adrenergic agents, a continuous intravenous infusion of terbutaline can be administered. Before this therapy is used, theophylline is discontinued to prevent dysrhythmias.

REFERENCE

Kurth, C., & Goodwin, S. (1992). Obstructive airway diseases in infants and children. In P. Koff, D. Eitzman, & J. Neu (Eds.). *Neonatal and pediatric respiratory care* (2nd ed., pp. 102–127). St. Louis: Mosby–Year Book.

8. Answer (**a**). Fluid replacement and maintenance of a euvolemic state in the child with status asthmaticus are important to minimize the tenacity of secretions. Increased hydration in acute asthma may be detrimental, because it may increase intrathoracic hydrostatic pressure, leading to pulmonary edema.

REFERENCES

Orsi, A. (1991). Asthma—The danger is real. *RN, 4,* 58–63.
Stempel, D., & Redding, G. (1992). Management of acute asthma in children. *Pediatric Clinics of North America,* 39 (6), 1320.

9. Answer (**a**). Routine maneuvers to maintain airway patency may irritate airway receptors and trigger bronchospasm and hypoxia. Chest physiotherapy may aggravate bronchospasm during status asthmaticus and is avoided until clinical improvement occurs.

REFERENCES

Bechler-Karsch, A. (1994). Assessment and management of status asthmaticus. *Pediatric Nursing,* 20 (3), 217–223.
Few, B. (1996). Pulmonary critical care problems. In M.A.Q. Curley, J.B. Smith, & P. Moloney-Harmon (Eds.). *Critical care nursing of infants and children* (pp. 619–655). Philadelphia: W.B. Saunders.

10. Answer (**c**). High airway pressures are usually required to move gas through severely narrowed lower airways. These high pressures can cause pneumothorax, pneumomediastinum, and subcutaneous emphysema, complications that occur in 10% to 15% of mechanically ventilated asthmatic children.

REFERENCE

Kurth, C., & Goodwin, S. (1992). Obstructive airway diseases in infants and children. In P. Koff, D. Eitzman, & J. Neu (Eds.). *Neonatal and pediatric respiratory care* (2nd ed., pp. 102–127). St. Louis: Mosby–Year Book.

CHAPTER 7

Neurologic Disorders

PAULA VERNON-LEVETT, RN, MS, CCRN

CASE 7-1

T., a 5-year-old boy, fell from an apartment fourth floor window. When the paramedics arrived, he was unconscious but responded to pain. He was breathing spontaneously (respiratory rate of 22 breaths per minute), his heart rate was 125 beats per minute (bpm), and his blood pressure was normal. The cervical spine was immobilized, an intravenous line started, and oxygen administered.

In the emergency department, he has periods of irritability alternating with unresponsiveness and apnea. The initial Glasgow Coma Scale (GCS) score is 6. He is orally intubated, stabilized, and sent to the radiology department for a computed tomography (CT) scan. The CT scan reveals an anterior basilar fracture, bilateral diffuse swelling, and a large left temporal epidural hematoma.

1. What is the treatment of choice at this time?
   a. Keep the patient in the emergency department for immediate insertion of an intracranial pressure (ICP) catheter.
   b. Transfer the patient to the operating room for evacuation of the hematoma.
   c. Transfer the patient to the pediatric intensive care unit (PICU) for observation.
   d. Transfer the patient to the radiology department for chest and abdominal x-ray films.

After surgical evacuation of the hematoma and placement of an intraventricular fiberoptic ICP catheter, arterial line, and central venous pressure line in the superior vena cava, the patient is sent to the PICU. The baseline ICP is 12 mmHg, heart rate is 100 bpm, blood pressure is 100/55 mmHg (mean arterial pressure of 85 mmHg), central venous pressure is 18 mmHg, and hemoglobin is 8.0 g/dL.

2. Which of the following signs are commonly seen with basilar skull fractures?
   a. Battle's sign.
   b. Dependent edema.
   c. Retinal hemorrhage.
   d. Scleral hemorrhage.

3. What initial independent nursing intervention should be used to maintain cerebral perfusion?
   a. Administer mannitol and furosemide.
   b. Maintain the head in the midline.
   c. Transfuse with packed red blood cells.
   d. Sedate with morphine and valium.

4. The calculated cerebral perfusion pressure (CPP) in this patient is
   a. 60 mmHg.
   b. 67 mmHg.
   c. 73 mmHg.
   d. 88 mmHg.

The patient remains stable for 12 hours, but on day 2, the ICP increases to between

50 and 100 mmHg and remains there for 10 minutes, followed by a rapid decrease in the ICP to baseline.

5. The previous description of the ICP represents
   a. *A* waves.
   b. *B* waves.
   c. *C* waves.
   d. *P* waves.

6. The best place to level this ICP transducer is at
   a. A reference point that approximates the lateral ventricles.
   b. A reference point that approximates the left atrium.
   c. A reference point located at the angle of Louis.
   d. A reference point located at the lower mandible.

7. Which of the following ICP monitoring systems has the greatest potential for infection?
   a. A fiberoptic intraventricular catheter.
   b. A fluid-coupled epidural catheter.
   c. A fluid-coupled intraventricular catheter.
   d. A fluid-coupled subarachnoid bolt.

Several hours later, T. is more agitated and is given continuous infusions of morphine and vecuronium.

8. The nurse assesses the neurologic status of T. by
   a. Assessing the oculovestibular response.
   b. Checking the pupils for a direct light response.
   c. Monitoring for abnormal respiratory patterns.
   d. Using the modified GCS.

Despite sedation, paralysis, hyperventilation, and diuretics, T.'s ICP remains above 25 mmHg. A decision is made to begin pentobarbital as a continuous infusion to induce a clinical coma.

9. To recognize burst suppression in T., the nurse knows which of the following neurodiagnostic tools will be used?
   a. Brain scan.
   b. Cerebral blood flow study.
   c. CT scan.
   d. Electroencephalogram.

10. A common side effect of pentobarbital that may be seen in T. is
    a. Hypertension.
    b. Hypotension.
    c. Seizures.
    d. Tremors.

On day 3, T.'s baseline ICP remains below 10 mmHg, and his vital signs normalize. However, his urine output decreases dramatically, serum Na^+ is 128 mEq/L, urine Na^+ is 30 mEq/L, and serum osmolality is 265 mOsm.

11. Based on the laboratory data, what does the nurse suspect is occurring at this time?
    a. Adrenal insufficiency.
    b. Central diabetes insipidus.
    c. Effects of mannitol therapy.
    d. Syndrome of inappropriate antidiuretic hormone secretion (SIADH).

12. What is the treatment of choice for T.?
    a. Administer aqueous vasopressin.
    b. Administer furosemide of 1 mg/kg.
    c. Increase maintenance fluids.
    d. Restrict fluids.

After day 7, T. is hemodynamically stable, fluid and electrolytes are normal, and the ICP baseline is less than 10 mmHg.

13. After T.'s ICP is stable, which of the following interventions to control his elevated ICP will be discontinued first?
    a. Elevation of the head of the bed.
    b. Intubation.
    c. Maintaining the Pa_{CO_2} between 30 and 35 mmHg.
    d. Continuous pentobarbital infusion.

The pentobarbital coma is discontinued, followed 2 days later by extubation. T. is sent to the ward the following day.

CASE 7–2

M., a 2.5-year-old girl, presents to the emergency room after a 1- to 2-minute episode at home, described as body stiffening, eyes rolling back, and unresponsiveness. She has a 2-day history of fever (maximum temperature 40°C), runny nose, and cough. On admission, she is febrile (39.5°C) and has mild respiratory distress, a heart rate of 120 bpm, and a blood pressure of 96/54 mmHg. She appears lethargic and irritable and has a positive Brudzinski sign. Routine chemistries, blood counts, serum and urine cultures, and a lumbar tap are obtained. An intravenous line is placed, and maintenance fluids are started.

1. Which of the following cerebrospinal fluid (CSF) values represent untreated bacterial meningitis?
   a. Decreased leukocyte count, elevated protein, and decreased glucose.
   b. Decreased leukocyte count, decreased protein, and decreased glucose.
   c. Increased leukocyte count, decreased protein, and increased glucose.
   d. Increased leukocyte count, elevated protein, and decreased glucose.

2. Which of the following pathogens causes meningitis most frequently in M.'s age group?
   a. Group b streptococci.
   b. *Haemophilus influenzae.*
   c. *Listeria monocytogenes.*
   d. Respiratory syncytial virus.

3. Bacterial meningitis most often results from
   a. Bacteremia from a distant site of infection.
   b. Basilar skull fractures.
   c. Direct penetrating trauma to the central nervous system.
   d. Spina bifida.

4. The best description of a positive Brudzinski sign is
   a. Increased irritability during feeding with the head lowered.
   b. Involuntary flexion of the knees and hips with passive flexion of the child's neck while the patient is supine.
   c. Resistance or complaints of neck pain with passive flexion of the lower leg while the patient is supine with hips flexed.
   d. Resistance or complaints of back pain with passive extension of the leg at the knee while the patient is supine with hips flexed.

5. Which of the following nursing interventions has the highest priority at this time?
   a. Administer broad-spectrum antibiotics.
   b. Administer corticosteroids.
   c. Begin 24-hour urine collection for chemistries.
   d. Start a second intravenous line.

M. is admitted to the PICU, and on arrival, she has a grand mal seizure. Her pulse oximeter shows an oxygen saturation of 85%.

6. The nurse should immediately
   a. Administer oxygen.
   b. Administer Valium.
   c. Intubate.
   d. Insert a bite block.

7. Which of the following anticonvulsants is rapidly acting and is recommended as initial therapy to stop a seizure?
   a. Carbamazepine.
   b. Lorazepam.
   c. Paraldehyde.
   d. Valproic acid.

M. continues to have seizure activity for 10 minutes and is given several doses of anticonvulsants.

8. The nurse anticipates that she will be assisting with
   a. Arterial catheter placement.
   b. ICP catheter placement.
   c. Bag-valve-mask ventilation.
   d. Repeat lumbar puncture.

M. is manually ventilated with a resuscitation bag for 5 minutes, after which spontaneous respirations resume. The seizure activity ceases, and she is stabilized.

CASE 7-3

J., a 6-year-old boy, is admitted to the PICU after a craniotomy and gross resection of a medulloblastoma. The patient is hemodynamically stable, intubated, and breathing through a volume ventilator at a rate of 25 breaths per minute. His dressing is dry and intact, and his neurologic examination is within normal limits.

1. Medulloblastomas are most frequently located in the
   a. Cerebral hemispheres.
   b. Chiasmal region.
   c. Fourth ventricle.
   d. Posterior fossa.

2. The most common complication seen in a child with a medulloblastoma is
   a. Cerebral aneurysm.
   b. Cerebral edema.
   c. Obstructive hydrocephalus.
   d. Quadriplegia.

J. has an uneventful postoperative course. Follow-up plans include chemotherapy and irradiation.

3. In general, chemotherapy has been less effective in treating central nervous sys-

tem tumors than neoplasia in other parts of the body because
a. Children are usually not diagnosed until the tumor is in an advanced stage.
b. Intrathecal catheters are not available for children.
c. The blood-brain barrier provides a physiologic barrier for many chemotherapeutic agents.
d. There are not enough trained pediatric neurologists who specialize in oncology.

CASE 7-4

F., a 3-year-old girl, was found floating face down in her backyard pool. The estimated length of time of submersion was 15 minutes. The paramedics arrived 5 minutes later and found the patient pulseless and apneic. She was immediately intubated and hyperventilated. An intraosseous line was placed, and chest compressions begun. The paramedics then transported her to the emergency department.

After 15 minutes in the emergency department, the patient has a sinus rhythm. She is unresponsive (GCS 3), her core temperature is 32°C, and her pupils are fixed and dilated.

1. The nurse should use which of the following techniques for external rewarming?
a. Administration of warm intravenous fluids.
b. Administration of warm, humidified oxygen.
c. Application of warm blankets.
d. Cardiopulmonary bypass.

After rewarming to 36°C, F. remains unresponsive, with fixed and dilated pupils. The family is approached with a potential diagnosis of brain death.

2. A diagnosis of brain death is confirmed by
a. Apnea testing.
b. Cold calorics.
c. Electroencephalogram.
d. Pupillary light response.

After 24 hours, F. remains in a coma and is unresponsive to painful stimuli. A pediatric neurologist is called to confirm a clinical diagnosis of brain death.

3. If F. is brain dead, which of the following ocular responses would be seen after in-stillation of cold water into her right ear canal?
a. Eyes remain midposition and fixed.
b. The left eye remains fixed, and the right eye moves slowly toward the right.
c. Slow conjugate movement of the eyes toward the left ear canal.
d. Slow conjugate movement of the eyes toward the right ear canal.

ANSWERS ■ CASE 7-1

1. Answer (**b**). Epidural hematomas are relatively uncommon in young children, but when they do occur, they are a true neurosurgical emergency. Epidural hematomas occur between the dura and the inner table of the skull, usually from a linear fracture of the temporal bone and laceration of the middle meningeal artery. Because the bleeding is arterial in origin and under significant pressure, dissection of the dura from the bone can occur rapidly, producing a mass effect and herniation.

REFERENCES
Dhellemmes, P., Lejeune, J., Christiaens, J., & Combelles, G. (1985). Traumatic extradural hematomas in infancy and childhood. *Journal of Neurosurgery, 62,* 861–864.
White, R.J., & Likavec, M.J. (1992). The diagnosis and initial management of head injury. *New England Journal of Medicine, 327,* 1507–1511.

2. Answer (**a**). Basilar fractures are less common in children than in adults. However, when they do occur, common signs include otorrhea or rhinorrhea, Battle's sign (i.e., subcutaneous hematoma surrounding the mastoid process), the Raccoon or Panda sign (i.e., extensive hemorrhage around the orbits in the absence of direct orbital trauma), and cranial nerve palsies.

REFERENCES
Kitchens, J.L., Groff, D.B., Nagaraj, H.S., & Fallat, M.E. (1991). Basilar skull fractures in childhood with cranial nerve involvement. *Journal of Pediatric Surgery, 26,* 992–994.
Zimmerman, R.A., & Bilaniuk, L.T. (1983). Radiology of pediatric craniocerebral trauma. In K. Shapiro (Ed.). *Pediatric head trauma* (pp. 69–142). Mount Kisco, NY: Futura Publishing.

3. Answer (**b**). Beyond resuscitation, controlling cerebral hypertension is critical. Keeping the head in a neutral plane pro-

motes venous drainage and prevents an increase in intracerebral blood volume. It is a simple maneuver that should be instituted immediately. A nurse may initiate it without a physician's order. Although all of the listed interventions may be used to control cerebral hypertension, keeping the head in a neutral plane is the only intervention that would be used for all patients regardless of the type of intracranial injury.

REFERENCE
Chudley, S. (1994). The effect of nursing activities on intracranial pressure. *British Journal of Nursing,* 3, 454–459.

4. Answer (**b**). CPP is related to the inflow pressure (i.e., carotid arterial pressure) and the outflow pressure (i.e., jugular pressure or intracranial pressure). In most situations when the ICP exceeds the jugular pressure, CPP is calculated by subtracting ICP from carotid arterial pressure. However, in this situation, when the jugular pressure exceeds the ICP, CPP is calculated by subtracting jugular pressure from carotid arterial pressure. Clinically, we use mean arterial pressure to represent carotid arterial pressure and central venous pressure to represent jugular venous pressure.

REFERENCE
Dean, J.M., Rogers, M.C., & Traystman, R.J. (1992). Pathophysiology and clinical management of the intracranial vault. In M.C. Rogers (Ed.). *Textbook of pediatric intensive care* (2nd ed., Vol. 1, pp. 639–666). Baltimore: Williams & Wilkins.

5. Answer (**a**). *A* waves are spontaneous, rapid, irregular increases in ICP ranging between 50 and 100 mmHg over the baseline and that last approximately 5 to 20 minutes, followed by a rapid decrease in ICP.

REFERENCES
Curley, M.A.Q., & Vernon-Levett, P. (1996). Intracranial dynamics. In M.A.Q. Curley, J.B. Smith & P.A. Moloney-Harmon (Eds.). *Critical care nursing of infants and children* (pp. 336–384). Philadelphia: W.B. Saunders.
McQuillan, K.A. (1991). Intracranial pressure monitoring: Technical implications. *AACN Clinical Issues in Critical Care Nursing,* 2, 623–638.

6. Answer (**a**). In the clinical setting, most practitioners believe the ICP and mean arterial pressure transducers should be placed at a location that approximates

the lateral ventricles. This position is usually approximated by placing the ICP transducer at the external auditory meatus or at the top of a triangle formed by the external auditory meatus, the outer canthus of the eye, and the area behind the hairline. Although consistency of a reference point is the most important factor when trending ICP, the other three options given for this question are not clinically recognized reference points.

REFERENCE
Curley, M.A.Q., & Vernon-Levett, P. (1996). Intracranial dynamics. In M.A.Q. Curley, J.B. Smith & P.A. Moloney-Harmon (Eds.). *Critical care nursing of infants and children* (pp. 336–384). Philadelphia: W.B. Saunders.

7. Answer (**c**). Intraventricular monitoring of ICP is believed to be the most accurate and reliable method. Unfortunately, it is the most invasive and carries the highest infection rates. Meticulous, aseptic technique is used when maintaining this device.

REFERENCES
Lehman, L.B. (1990). Intracranial pressure monitoring and treatment: A contemporary view. *Annals of Emergency Medicine,* 19, 295–303.
McQuillan K.A. (1991). Intracranial pressure monitoring: Technical implications. *AACN Clinical Issues in Critical Care Nursing,* 2, 623–638.

8. Answer (**b**). Vecuronium (Norcuron) is a nondepolarizing paralytic agent that binds to the postsynaptic receptors and prevents binding of acetylcholine at these receptors. The end result is a lack of movement of the skeletal muscles. Because of the peripheral skeletal muscle paralysis, standard neurologic tests of motor function, reflexes, and sensation are not possible. However, the pupillary light reflex can be assessed, and abnormal responses have the same significance as in the nonparalyzed patient.

REFERENCES
Curley, M.A.Q., & Vernon-Levett, P. (1996). Intracranial dynamics. In M.A.Q. Curley, J.B. Smith & Moloney-Harmon (Eds.). *Critical care nursing of infants and children* (pp. 336–384). Philadelphia: W.B. Saunders.
Sickel, A.D., & Spadaccia, K. (1991). Muscle relaxants and reversal agents. *Critical Care Nursing Clinics of North America,* 3 (1), 151–158.

9. Answer (**d**). Theoretically, barbiturates decrease ICP by reducing the cerebral metabolic rate, which results in depression of cerebral electrical activity. Continuous bedside monitoring of the electroencephalogram is used to titrate the effects of barbiturates.

REFERENCE

Hill, J. (1990). Reye's syndrome. In J. Blumer (Ed.). *A practical guide to pediatric intensive care* (pp. 256–270). St. Louis: Mosby–Year Book.

10. Answer (**b**). Pentobarbital has negative inotropic properties, and the major non-respiratory side effect of pentobarbital is acute hypotension. Consequently, barbiturate comas are reserved for patients who are hemodynamically stable, and even in those patients, inotropic infusions may be necessary to support circulation.

REFERENCE

Dean, J.M., Rogers, M.C., & Traystman, R.J. (1992). Pathophysiology and clinical management of the intracranial vault. In M.C. Rogers (Ed.). *Textbook of pediatric intensive care* (2nd ed., Vol. 1, pp. 639–666). Baltimore: Williams & Wilkins.

11. Answer (**d**). Central nervous system disorders have been associated with excessive secretion of antidiuretic hormone. There are no objective data that define SIADH. However, general guidelines include serum hypo-osmolality, hyponatremia, elevated urine osmolality and sodium concentration, and decreased urine output.

REFERENCES

Hill, J.H. (1990). SIADH, cerebral salt wasting, and central diabetes insipidus. In J. Blumer (Ed.). *A practical guide to pediatric intensive care* (pp. 535–545). St. Louis: Mosby–Year Book.
Wood, E.G., & Lynch, R.E. (1992). Fluid and electrolyte balance. In B.P. Fuhrman & J.J. Zimmerman (Eds.). *Pediatric critical care* (pp. 671–687). St. Louis: Mosby–Year Book.

12. Answer (**d**). Management of SIADH involves correcting the underlying neurologic disorder, followed by fluid restriction. Intake and output must be calculated hourly, the patient weighed twice daily, and frequent neurologic assessments performed. Serum sodium levels and osmolality are usually checked several times each day during the acute period.

REFERENCE

Shinimdki-Maher, T. (1991). Diabetes insipidus and syndrome of inappropriate secretion of antidiuretic hormone in children with midline suprasellar brain tumors. *Journal of Pediatric Oncology Nursing, 8,* 106–111.

13. Answer (**d**). After stabilization of ICP with a patient in a barbiturate coma, therapy needs to be withdrawn slowly. In general, the last therapy instituted is withdrawn first, and in this case, it is the barbiturate-induced coma. After the barbiturates are removed and paralyzing agents discontinued, respiratory function and protective reflexes should return, and the patient can be safely extubated.

REFERENCE

Pascucci, R.C. (1988). Head trauma in the child. *Intensive Care Medicine, 14,* 185–195.

ANSWERS ■ CASE 7-2

1. Answer (**d**). Beyond 2 months of age, the normal CSF is free of leukocytes, the protein concentration is less than 40 mg/dL, and the glucose level should be greater than two thirds of the serum glucose. In response to bacterial invasion of the meninges, the immune response is activated, and the leukocyte count increases. The CSF glucose level is depressed, and the CSF protein level is elevated.

REFERENCE

Feigin, R.D., McCracken, G.H., & Klein, J.O. (1992). Diagnosis and management of meningitis. *Pediatric Infectious Disease Journal, 11,* 785–814.

2. Answer (**b**). The highest age-specific attack rates for bacterial meningitis (beyond the newborn period) occur between 3 and 8 months of age. The Centers for Disease Control and Prevention reports *Haemophilus influenzae* type b, *Neisseria meningitidis,* and *Streptococcus pneumoniae* (in decreasing order) as the responsible meningitides for most cases of meningitis in previously well children. Since the approval of a conjugated polysaccharide vaccine in 1990, the number of reported cases of *Haemophilus* disease has decreased. However, the exact decline in incidence remains to be reported.

REFERENCES

Feigin, R.D., McCracken, G.H., & Klein, J.O. (1992). Diagnosis and management of meningitis. *Pediatric Infectious Disease Journal, 11,* 785–814.
Wenger, J.D., Hightower, A.W., Facklam, R.R., et al. (1990). Bacterial meningitis in the United States,

1986: Report of a multistate surveillance study. *Journal of Infectious Disease, 162,* 1316–1323.

3. Answer (**a**). In most cases, bacterial meningitis is a systemic disease, with the meninges' becoming seeded (infected) from the bloodstream. Pathogens gain access to the bloodstream through the nasal mucosa, where they are absorbed through small vessels. The conditions that predispose the mucosa to invasion from colonization are not completely understood.

REFERENCES
Quagliarello, V., & Scheld, W.M. (1992). Bacterial meningitis: Pathogenesis, pathophysiology, and progress. *New England Journal of Medicine, 327,* 864–872.
Rubenstein, J.S. (1992). Acute pediatric CNS infections. In B.P. Fuhrman & J.J. Zimmerman (Eds.). *Pediatric critical care* (pp. 613–620). St. Louis: Mosby–Year Book.

4. Answer (**b**). When meningeal irritation exists, the Brudzinski and Kernig signs may be elicited. Brudzinski's sign represents involuntary bending of the child's knees and hips when the child's neck is passively flexed. Kernig's sign may be demonstrated by placing the child in a supine position with the hips flexed and passively extending the leg at the knee. During this maneuver, the child often resists or complains of back pain. Signs of meningeal irritation are more nonspecific in the infant, and these signs are usually not present.

REFERENCE
Vulcan, B.M. (1987). Acute bacterial meningitis in infancy and childhood. *Critical Care Nurse, 7* (5), 53–65.

5. Answer (**a**). Without question, initial treatment of bacterial meningitis is administration of rapidly acting bactericidal therapy. Even before the specific bacterium is identified, broad-spectrum antibiotics are started. Antibiotic therapy usually includes ampicillin in combination with chloramphenicol or one of the second-generation cephalosporins. Although administration of corticosteroids has been beneficial as adjunctive therapy, antibiotic therapy should not be delayed to administer steroids.

REFERENCES
Klein, J.O., Feigin, R.D., & McCracken, G.H. (1986). Diagnosis and management of meningitis. *Pediatrics, 78* (suppl.), 959–982.
Quagliarello, V., & Scheld, W.M. (1992). Bacterial meningitis: Pathogenesis, pathophysiology, and progress. *New England Journal of Medicine, 327,* 864–872.

6. Answer (**a**). The major complication of a seizure is hypoxia, and the therapeutic priority in management of a seizure is the maintenance of oxygenation and ventilation. The first step in managing a patient with a seizure, even before attempting to stop the seizure, is providing oxygenation. Priority interventions to follow are ensuring adequate ventilation and circulation and protecting the patient from harm. The next management steps are establishing an intravenous line, drawing samples for laboratory studies, and administering anticonvulsants. If intravenous access is delayed, some anticonvulsants may be administered rectally.

REFERENCE
Orlowski, J.P., & Rothner, A.D. (1992). Diagnosis and treatment of status epilepticus. In B.P. Fuhrman & J.J. Zimmerman (Eds.). *Pediatric critical care* (pp. 595–604). St. Louis: Mosby–Year Book.

7. Answer (**b**). The most commonly used anticonvulsants for the treatment of seizures in children are benzodiazepines, phenytoin, and barbiturates. The desired route of administration is intravenous. Of the choices presented, lorazepam acts the fastest, and of the possible answers, it is the only choice that is available for intravenous use. Like diazepam, lorazepam has a rapid onset of action, but it controls seizures for a longer period than diazepam.

REFERENCES
Orlowski, J.P., & Rothner, A.D. (1992). Diagnosis and treatment of status epilepticus. In B.P. Fuhrman & J.J. Zimmerman (Eds.). *Pediatric critical care* (pp. 595–604). St. Louis: Mosby–Year Book.
Rosenberg, D.I. (1990). Status epilepticus. In J.L. Blumer (Ed.). *A practical guide to pediatric intensive care* (pp. 227–234). St. Louis: Mosby–Year Book.

8. Answer (**c**). Most first-line anticonvulsant drugs have respiratory depression as a major side effect. The risk of respiratory depression increases as the duration of the seizure increases and when a combination or multiple doses of anticonvulsants are used. The nurse needs to be continually prepared to intervene with supporting ventilation. Airway equipment should be readily available for "rapid sequence" intubation. The other options listed may be needed, but they do not have priority over the airway.

REFERENCE
Orlowski, J.P., & Rothner, A.D. (1992). Diagnosis and treatment of status epilepticus. In B.P. Fuhrman &

J.J. Zimmerman (Eds.). *Pediatric critical care* (pp. 595–604). St. Louis: Mosby–Year Book.

ANSWERS ■ CASE 7-3

1. Answer (**d**). Medulloblastomas are located in the posterior fossa and represent approximately 15% of all pediatric brain tumors. They enlarge very rapidly, and the tumor is usually detected within 3 months of the onset of the patient's symptoms.

REFERENCE

Albright, A.L. (1993). Pediatric brain tumors. *CA: A Cancer Journal for Clinicians, 43,* 272–288.

2. Answer (**c**). A medulloblastoma is a common tumor type seen in children. It arises from midline cerebellar tissue and frequently causes compression of the fourth ventricle. Consequently, the patient usually develops the symptoms of obstructive hydrocephalus. Typical signs and symptoms include nausea, vomiting, papilledema, headache, and ataxia.

REFERENCE

Smith, R.W. (1988). Tumors. In W.C. Wiederholt (Ed.). *Neurology for non-neurologists* (pp. 320–327). Philadelphia: Grune & Stratton.

3. Answer (**c**). The blood-brain barrier provides a physiologic barrier for many chemotherapeutic agents. It prevents drug penetration in amounts necessary to be effective against the tumor without causing lethal systemic effects. Advances are being made with intrathecal, intraarterial, and intraventricular routes, but these routes are not without complications.

REFERENCE

Mulligan, C.M., & Wittman, B.K. (1990). Nursing care of the child with a brainstem glioma. *Journal of Pediatric Nursing, 5,* 375–386.

ANSWERS ■ CASE 7-4

1. Answer (**c**). Of all the options presented, covering the patient with warm blankets is the only method of external rewarming. The other options are all examples of active internal rewarming. Regardless of the type of rewarming, the nurse needs to observe the patient for hypotension from peripheral vasodilation.

REFERENCES

Beyda, D.H. (1991). Prehospital care of the child with a submersion incident. *Critical Care Nursing Clinics of North America, 3,* 281–285.

Elixson, E.M. (1991). Hypothermia: Cold-water drowning. *Critical Care Nursing Clinics of North America, 3,* 287–292.

2. Answer (**c**). Although many authorities do not believe confirmatory testing is necessary for establishing a diagnosis of brain death in the child, the electroencephalogram is still recognized as a confirmatory test. Others include various types of cerebral blood flow studies. The pupillary light reflex, cold caloric testing, and apnea testing are considered to be part of the clinical examination and are required when determining brain death in a child.

REFERENCE

Vernon-Levett, P. (1996). Neurology. In M.A.Q. Curley, J.B. Smith & P.A. Moloney-Harmon (Eds.). *Critical care nursing of infants and children* (pp. 336–384). Philadelphia: W.B. Saunders.

3. Answer (**a**). The oculovestibular reflex (cold calorics) establishes the integrity of the brainstem ocular pathways. Four cranial nerves (III, IV, VI, and VIII) are involved in this response. If the brainstem is completely dysfunctional, there is no movement of the eyes, and they cannot respond to the pupillary light reflex. The oculocephalic reflex (i.e., doll's eye) may also be used as part of the clinical examination; however, some believe it is extinguished before the oculovestibular reflex and that the cervical spine needs to be free of injury to perform it.

REFERENCE

Zegeer, L.J. (1989). Oculocephalic and vestibulo-ocular responses: Significance for nursing care. *Journal of Neuroscience Nursing, 21*(1), 46–55.

CHAPTER 8

Fluid and Electrolyte Disorders

PAMELA A. BROWN, RN, MS, CCRN

CASE 8-1

A., an 8-month-old infant, is admitted to the pediatric intensive care unit (PICU) with an initial diagnosis of diarrhea and dehydration. Her mother reports that she has been having liquid brown stools for the last several days. On the day of admission, A. has been increasingly irritable and has had only occasional sips of fluid.

1. The initial assessment and treatment of A. should focus on
   a. Determining the degree of dehydration.
   b. Obtaining blood for electrolyte analysis.
   c. Assessing for signs and symptoms of hypovolemic shock.
   d. Determining the type of dehydration.

The initial assessment reveals the following data: heart rate of 185 beats per minute (bpm), respiratory rate of 38 breaths per minute, blood pressure of 92/59 mmHg, and mean arterial pressure of 70 mmHg; the pulses are slightly weak but equal in all four extremities; extremities are cool, with a capillary refill time of less than 3 seconds; and the diaper is dry. Based on this assessment, the nurse determines that A. is exhibiting signs of fluid volume deficit but is not in hypovolemic shock.

2. The degree of dehydration is determined by

a. The calculated fluid requirements minus the calculated fluid losses.
b. Weight loss and the clinical assessment findings.
c. The estimated output minus the estimated fluid intake.
d. Vital signs and the estimated output.

The mother reports that A. weighed 11.8 kg (26 lb) at her last doctor visit. Today, on the scale in the PICU, A. weighs 10.63 kg. The difference calculates to a 10% weight loss.

3. What degree of dehydration does A. have, and what clinical signs and symptoms are consistent with the degree of dehydration?
   a. Moderate dehydration, characterized by a rapid, weak pulse; a sunken fontanelle, normal blood pressure, no tears, and dry mucous membranes; small quantities of dark urine; irritability in response to touch; and drowsiness when left alone.
   b. Mild dehydration, characterized by a rapid pulse; a normal fontanelle, normal blood pressure, no tears but moist mucous membranes; normal-looking urine in reduced quantities; and an alert but restless manner.
   c. Severe dehydration, characterized by rapid, feeble pulses; a very sunken fontanelle, unrecordable blood pressure, no tears, and very dry mucous membranes; no urine output for several hours; and difficult arousal.

d. Moderate dehydration, characterized by a rapid, weak pulse; a sunken fontanelle, normal blood pressure, tears present, and moist mucous membranes; small quantities of dark urine; and an alert but restless manner.

While waiting for the serum analysis to return from the laboratory, the physician asks for a urine specific gravity determination.

4. The nurse would expect the specific gravity to be
   a. 1.035.
   b. An unreliable tool for assessment.
   c. 1.000 to 1.010.
   d. 1.020 to 1.035.

Levels are determined for sodium (Na^+), potassium (K^+), chloride (Cl^-), carbon dioxide (CO_2), glucose (Glu), blood urea nitrogen (BUN), creatine (Cr), hemoglobin (Hgb), and the hematocrit (Hct). The initial laboratory tests reveal the following results:

Na^+: 132 mEq/L	Glu: 115 mg/dL
K^+: 4.5 mEq/L	BUN: 15 mg/dL
Cl^-: 102 mEq/L	Cr: 1 mg/dL
CO_2: 24 mEq/L	Hgb: 13.3 g/dL
	Hct: 39%

5. Combining the history, clinical assessment, and laboratory findings, what type of dehydration does A. have?
   a. Isonatremic.
   b. Hyponatremic.
   c. Hypernatremic.
   d. Hypotonic.

After reviewing the laboratory findings, the nurse prepares to rehydrate A.

6. How is the deficit calculated, and what is the calculated total fluid loss?
   a. Current weight (kg) × % dehydration = kg (1 kg weight = 1000 mL fluid).

   10.63 × 0.1 = 1.063 kg × (1000 mL/ 1 kg) = 1063 mL fluid loss

   b. % dehydration × 100 mL:

   10 × 100 mL = 1000 mL fluid loss

   c. Calculated maintenance fluids for 24 hours = 1090 mL fluid loss.
   d. Actual weight (kg) × % dehydration = kg (1 kg weight = 1000 mL fluid):

11.8 kg × 0.1 = 1.18 kg × (1000 mL/ 1 kg) = 1180 mL fluid loss

7. Excluding the need for resuscitation fluid, how is fluid administered for rehydration over the first 24 hours?
   a. Replace the calculated fluid loss evenly over 24 hours.
   b. Replace the calculated fluid loss evenly over 24 hours in addition to the normal maintenance rate.
   c. Replace one half of the fluid loss plus the maintenance fluid over 8 hours. Over the next 16 hours, replace the second half of the fluid loss plus the maintenance rate.
   d. Replace one half of the fluid loss plus the maintenance fluid over 12 hours. Over the next 16 hours, replace the second half of the fluid loss plus the maintenance rate.

A. arrived from the emergency department with a 22-gauge Angiocath infusing into her right hand at a rate of 45 mL/hour. The intravenous site is flat and soft. The correct intravenous rate is 119 mL/hour.

8. What nursing actions are most appropriate to ensure proper administration of the intravenous fluids?
   a. Start a second intravenous line before beginning the rehydration to ensure intravenous access in case a severe infiltration problem develops.
   b. Begin the rehydration at one half of the calculated rate while a second intravenous line is being started. After the second intravenous line is in, infuse the 119 mL/hour equally between the two intravenous sites.
   c. Begin the rehydration with the current line while a second intravenous line is being started. After the second intravenous line is in, infuse the 119 mL/hour equally between the two lines.
   d. Begin the rehydration with the current line, and frequently assess the intravenous site to ensure it is not becoming infiltrated. When the child's hydration status improves, start a second intravenous line.

9. Which clinical assessment parameters are most important to evaluate to determine if the rehydration therapy is successful?

a. Level of consciousness, heart rate, and urine output.
b. Heart rate, blood pressure, and skin turgor.
c. Peripheral perfusion, urine output, and level of consciousness.
d. Peripheral perfusion, heart rate, and blood pressure.

Nine hours after admission to the unit, A.'s vital signs and assessment are as follows: heart rate of 134 bpm, respiratory rate of 32 breaths per minute, blood pressure of 96/58 mmHg, and mean arterial pressure of 83 mmHg; pulses are strong and equal in all four extremities; extremities are warm, with a capillary refill time of less than 3 seconds; the fontanelle is slightly sunken and soft; mucous membranes are moist; skin turgor is fair; she is alert when awake; and her urine output is 0.5 mL/kg per hour.

10. In order of priority, what are the nursing care needs now?
a. Continue fluid replacement therapy; monitor vital signs; monitor intake and output, including insensible water loss; assess the clinical status for fluid volume deficit or overload; and evaluate electrolyte status.
b. Continue fluid replacement therapy; evaluate electrolyte status; monitor vital signs; assess the clinical status for fluid volume deficit or overload; monitor intake and output, including insensible water loss.
c. Monitor intake and output, including insensible water loss; continue replacement therapy; monitor vital signs; assess the clinical status for fluid volume deficit or excess; and evaluate electrolytes.
d. Continue fluid replacement therapy; monitor intake and output, including insensible water loss; evaluate electrolytes; monitor vital signs; and assess the clinical status for fluid volume deficit or excess.

CASE 8-2

J. is a 2-year-old, 15-kg boy who was admitted yesterday to the PICU with respiratory failure due to pneumonia. He was intubated and ventilated with settings of F_{IO_2} of 0.5; tidal volume of 200 mL; respiratory rate of 30 breaths per minute; peak inspiratory pressure of 30 cmH$_2$O; and positive end-expiratory pressure (PEEP) of 5 cmH$_2$O. Today, because of a deterioration in oxygenation status, the PEEP has been increased to 8 cmH$_2$O. J. is receiving an intravenous administration of 10% dextrose in 0.2 NS with 2 mEq of potassium chloride (KCl)/100 mL at a maintenance rate of 52 mL/hour. After several hours, the nurse notices that the child has developed periorbital edema and that the urine output has dropped from 1 to 0.5 mL/kg per hour.

1. What is the most probable explanation for the development of the periorbital edema and the reduction in urine output?
a. Pneumonia causes a shift of fluid from the intravascular space to the interstitial spaces (e.g., wet lungs, periorbital edema). This shift of fluid results in a decrease in the circulating blood volume and a reduced urine output.
b. Increased PEEP causes an increase in thoracic pressure. The increased pressure inhibits venous return and causes retention of water in the dependent areas.
c. Mechanical ventilation causes an increase in insensible fluid loss, which results in a decreased circulating blood volume. Antidiuretic hormone (ADH) is secreted in response to the decreased circulating volume and stimulates the kidneys to retain water.
d. Increased PEEP and resulting decreased cardiac output stimulate ADH release. The ADH stimulates the kidneys to retain water.

After several more hours pass, the edema is increasing, and the urine output is 0.3 to 0.5 mL/kg per hour. J.'s breath sounds are "wet" on auscultation. Based on this assessment, the decision is made to attempt to diurese J. Lasix is ordered and given every 6 hours. The next morning's routine laboratory tests reveal the following electrolyte results:

Na$^+$: 135 mEq/L	Glu: 199 mg/dL
K$^+$: 2.7 mEq/L	BUN: 29 mg/dL
Cl$^-$: 104 mEq/L	Cr: 1.4 mg/dL
CO$_2$: 24 mEq/L	

The arterial blood gas determinations include hydrogen ion concentration (pH), partial pressures of oxygen (P$_{O_2}$) and carbon dioxide (P_{CO_2}), bicarbonate (HCO_3^-) level, and base excess (BE). The following values are the results for the initial determinations:

pH: 7.49 HCO_3^-: 24 mEq/L
P_{O_2}: 84 mmHg   BE: +1 mEq/L
P_{CO_2}: 40 mmHg

2. What is the probable cause of the alkalosis?
   a. Overventilation.
   b. Hypokalemia.
   c. Reduction in urine output resulting from ADH secretion.
   d. Aggressive diuresis.

3. What is the physiologic reason for the increased glucose level?
   a. Potassium and glucose have an inverse relationship.
   b. Hypokalemia and hyperglycemia are unrelated physiologic features.
   c. Hypokalemia impairs the release of insulin.
   d. Hypokalemia increases insulin secretion.

4. What clinical symptoms would the nurse expect J. to be exhibiting with a K^+ of 2.7 mEq/L?
   a. Flattened, inverted T waves on the electrocardiogram (ECG), muscle weakness, lethargy, and hyporeflexia.
   b. Peaked T waves on the ECG, irritability, and paralytic ileus.
   c. Flattened, inverted T waves and the presence of U waves on ECG, irritability, lethargy, and muscle weakness.
   d. Symptoms of hypokalemia are nonspecific, and it is difficult to establish a direct cause and effect relationship.

Based on the electrolyte determinations, the decision is made to administer a potassium bolus.

5. Which order is correct and why?
   a. Administer 7.5 mEq of KCl intravenously over 1 hour; the recommended maximum dose is 0.5 mEq/kg per hour. For any potassium concentration less than 3.0 mEq/L, a rapid correction within safety guidelines is preferred.
   b. Administer 7.5 mEq of KCl intravenously over 2 hours; the dosage is 0.5 to 1 mEq/kg per dose to infuse at 0.3 to 0.5 mEq/kg per hour. If the patient is not exhibiting symptoms directly related to the hypokalemia, a slower correction, which limits side effects, is preferred.

   c. Administer 15 mEq KCl orally. Oral replacement of potassium is preferred over intravenous replacement to prevent the side effects that may occur with intravenous administration.
   d. Administer 4.5 mEq potassium phosphate (KPO_4) over 1 hour. In cases of alkalosis, KPO_4 is preferred for the replacement of potassium.

Laboratory tests repeated 1 hour after the K^+ bolus is given show these results:

Na^+: 134 mEq/L   Glu: 135 mg/dL
K^+: 3.2 mEq/L   BUN: 29 mg/dL
Cl^-: 100 mEq/L   Cr: 1.4 mg/dL
CO_2: 23 mEq/L

The arterial blood gas results are

pH: 7.43 HCO_3^-: 23 mEq/L
P_{O_2}: 88 mmHg   BE: 0 mEq/L
P_{CO_2}: 41 mmHg

To treat the mild hypokalemia, the potassium in the maintenance fluids is changed from 2 to 3 mEq/100 mL.

Two days later, J. is successfully weaned from the ventilator, and the diuretics are discontinued. Twelve hours after the extubation, the nurse notices peaked T waves on the ECG. Laboratory values reveal the following:

Na^+: 131 mEq/L   Glu: 124 mg/dL
K^+: 5.8 mEq/L   BUN: 30 mg/dL
Cl^-: 98 mEq/L   Cr: 1.3 mg/dL
CO_2: 26 mEq/L

The arterial blood gas results are

pH: 7.35 HCO_3^-: 24 mEq/L
P_{O_2}: 94 mmHg   BE: −1 mEq/L
P_{CO_2}: 37 mmHg

6. What is the probable cause of the hyperkalemia?
   a. The potassium in the maintenance fluids was not readjusted after extubation, and the diuretics were discontinued.
   b. There is an inverse relationship between potassium and pH; therefore, the hyperkalemia is caused by the acidosis.
   c. The hyperkalemia is probably a result of hemolysis that occurs as a result of improper or difficult collection of the specimen. The result should be double-checked by repeating the laboratory tests.
   d. The fluid is redistributed from the intracellular to the extracellular space with resolution of the edema.

7. What is the best treatment of J.'s hyper-kalemia?
   a. Administer Kayexalate enema to re-duce the potassium rapidly without causing hypokalemia.
   b. Remove the potassium from the intra-venous fluids, and allow the body sys-tems to correct the potassium.
   c. Administer 100 mg/kg of calcium glu-conate intravenously to reduce the car-diac effects of the hyperkalemia.
   d. Administer 15 mEq of sodium bicar-bonate to correct the acidosis and force the K^+ to move back into the cells.

CASE 8-3

H. is a 7-year-old girl who was in good health until 2 days ago, when she was hit by a car while she was walking to school. She suffered a severe head injury and is comatose. H. is intubated and is being aggressively treated with therapies that include hyperventilation and administration of osmotic diuretics to combat the effects of increased intracranial pressure. During the initial assessment of H., tetany of her hands is noticed. Review of the morning laboratory results reveals an ionized calcium (Ca^{2+}) concentration of 3.5 mg/dL and a total serum calcium concen-tration of 10 mg/dL.

1. What is the most probable cause of H.'s hypocalcemia?
   a. Decreased intake of calcium.
   b. Multiple blood transfusions.
   c. Respiratory alkalosis caused by the hyperventilation.
   d. Administration of aminoglycosides for infection prophylaxis.

2. Should the hypocalcemia be treated?
   a. As clinical symptoms related to the hypocalcemia manifest, treatment should be started.
   b. Treatment is unnecessary, because the Ca^{2+} will return to a normal level as the pH is normalized.
   c. Because Ca^{2+} is the form of calcium used for metabolic functions, treat-ment is required to maintain the value in a normal range.
   d. Treatment should not be started, be-cause calcium therapy may exacerbate cellular injury.

The recommended dose for calcium chlo-ride ($CaCl_2$) is 10 to 20 mg/kg, and H. weighs 25 kg. The resident orders one 500-mg dose of calcium chloride delivered intravenously.

3. What precautions are taken when admin-istering a calcium chloride bolus?
   a. Dilute to a maximum concentration of 20 mg/mL, and administer at a rate no faster than 50 mg/minute; monitor for bradycardia and asystole; and do not infuse with other salt solutions.
   b. Administer into a central vein; dilute to a maximum concentration of 20 mg/mL, and administer over 1 hour; moni-tor for bradycardia and asystole; and do not infuse with other salt solutions.
   c. Administer into a central vein; di-lute to a maximum concentration of 100 mg/mL and administer over 1 hour; and monitor for bradycardia and asystole.
   d. Administer into a central vein; dilute to a maximum concentration of 20 mg/mL and administer over 1 hour; moni-tor for bradycardia and asystole; do not infuse with other salt solutions; and repeat the Ca^{2+} determination 1 hour after infusion.

While administering the calcium bolus, the nurse decides to assess H. for other potential electrolyte problems. She notices that H. is not receiving any nutritional support and that her intravenous solution is 10% dextrose in 0.2 NS with 2 mEq of KCl/100 mL at two-thirds maintenance rate. She has a suction-ing nasogastric (NG) tube that is draining at a rate of approximately 230 mL/24 hours, and she has hypoactive bowel sounds. Her parents state that she was in a good nutri-tional state before the accident. Two hours after completing the calcium bolus, the nurse notices that the tetany has not resolved. A repeated ionized calcium level is 3.7 mg/dL. After a second calcium bolus, the Ca^{2+} level is 3.8 mg/dL.

4. What is the probable rationale for the per-sistent hypocalcemia?
   a. Reduced protein administration causes a reduction in the total serum calcium level.
   b. Depleted calcium stored in bone and tissue is replaced before changes in Ca^{2+} are seen.
   c. Persistent hypocalcemia may be caused by hypomagnesemia.
   d. The calcium level cannot be corrected in a case of respiratory alkalosis.

A full review of the laboratory test results reveals the following:

Na$^+$: 129 mEq/L	Glu: 99 mg/dL
K$^+$: 4.0 mEq/L	BUN: 15 mg/dL
Cl$^-$: 98 mEq/L	Cr: 0.8 mg/dL
CO$_2$: 19 mEq/L	Ca^{2+}: 4.0 mg/dL
Mg^{2+}: 1.1 mEq/L	pH: 3.4

5. What factors may have contributed to the reduced magnesium (Mg^{2+}) level?
   a. Reduced intake, administration of diuretics, and alkalosis.
   b. Reduced intake, administration of diuretics, and loss of body fluid through NG suctioning.
   c. Administration of diuretics and loss of body fluid through NG suctioning.
   d. Reduced intake, administration of diuretics, alkalosis, and loss of body fluid through NG suctioning.

6. What is the best course of action for treating the hypomagnesemia?
   a. Aim treatment at the underlying cause of the hypomagnesemia, and begin parenteral nutrition, enteral nutrition, or both.
   b. Give a bolus dose of magnesium sulfate (MgSO$_4$) intravenously, place the NG tube to gravity, and begin parenteral nutrition, enteral nutrition, or both.
   c. Give a bolus dose of MgSO$_4$ intravenously and begin parenteral nutrition, enteral nutrition, or both.
   d. Give a bolus does of MgSO$_4$ intravenously and place the NG tube to gravity.

Two days later, H. remains comatose but is showing some improvement and is no longer being hyperventilated. She was begun on feedings through a nasoduodenal tube, but yesterday morning, she began having large amounts of diarrhea. The feedings were stopped, and hyperalimentation was begun. H. is receiving 15% dextrose in water with 2% amino acids. The laboratory results are

Na$^+$: 134 mEq/L	Glu: 126 mg/dL
K$^+$: 4.1 mEq/L	BUN: 21 mg/dL
Cl$^-$: 100 mEq/L	Cr: 1.0 mg/dL
CO$_2$: 24 mEq/L	Ca^{2+}: 4.6 mg/dL
Mg^{2+}: 1.6 mEq/L	pH: 2.4

7. What is the best course of action for treating the hypophosphatemia?
   a. Supplemental phosphate should be added to the enteral feedings for several days to increase the serum levels and replete the body stores.
   b. Administer a phosphate bolus intravenously until the level returns to normal.
   c. Resume the enteral feedings with a nutritionally complete formula, normalize the other electrolytes, and allow the phosphorus to self-correct.
   d. Increase the phosphate content of the hyperalimentation while determining and correcting the cause of the diarrhea.

8. What clinical symptoms are important to monitor for when caring for a comatose patient with actual or potential hypophosphatemia?
   a. Muscle weakness, irritability, hypoventilation, and reduced oxygen-carrying capacity.
   b. Decreased myocardial contractility, muscle weakness, decreased deep tendon reflexes, and bleeding.
   c. Bleeding and blood clotting abnormalities, tissue hypoxia, and immunosuppression.
   d. Muscle weakness, confusion, tissue hypoxia, cardiac arrhythmias, and immunosuppression.

ANSWERS ■ CASE 8-1

1. Answer (c). The most important initial assessment and treatment is aimed at ensuring the child has an adequate circulating blood volume. When signs of early shock are present, aggressive fluid resuscitation must be undertaken immediately to prevent a more profound circulatory collapse.

REFERENCE

Wetzel, R.C. (1991). Shock and fluid resuscitation. In D.G. Nichols, M. Yaster, D.G. Lappe, & J.R. Buck (Eds.). *Golden hour: The handbook of advanced pediatric life support* (p. 85). St. Louis: Mosby–Year Book.

2. Answer (b). The degree of dehydration is estimated in two ways: weight loss and the identification of physical findings. These findings are then applied to the criteria that are associated with one of the three classes of dehydration, and the child is categorized as being mildly, moderately, or severely dehydrated.

REFERENCE

Aoki, B.Y., & McCloskey, K. (1992). *Evaluation, stabilization, and transport of the critically ill child* (p. 136). St. Louis: Mosby–Year Book.

3. Answer (a). A 10% weight loss correlates with severe dehydration in children but with moderate dehydration in infants. Signs and symptoms that correlate with a moderate dehydration include a rapid, weak pulse; sunken fontanelle, normal blood pressure, lack of tears with dry mucous membranes; doughy skin turgor; cool extremities; small quantities of dark urine; lethargy; irritability in response to touch; and drowsiness when left alone.

REFERENCES

Brown, P.A., Blayney, F., Brown, C.A., & Evans, K.G. (1989). *Quick reference to pediatric intensive care nursing* (pp. 132–133). Rockville, MD: Aspen.
Samson, L.F., & Ouzts, K.M. (1996). Fluid and electrolyte regulation. In M.A.Q. Curley, J.B. Smith, & P.A. Moloney-Harmon (Eds.). *Critical care nursing of infants and children.* Philadelphia: W.B. Saunders.

4. Answer (b). Maturation of the renal system is not complete until adolescence. Infants and children under 2 years old have a tendency to produce more dilute urine because of immature and shorter loops in the nephron and because renal blood flow is primarily distributed in the renal medulla while the majority of the nephrons are located in the renal cortex.

REFERENCES

Andrews, M., & Mooney, K. (1990). Alteration of renal and urinary tract function in children. In K. McCance & S. Huether (Eds.). *Pathophysiology: The biologic basis for disease in adults and children* (pp. 1160–1171). St. Louis: Mosby–Year Book.

5. Answer (a). A.'s serum Na^+ level is 132 mEq/L, and she therefore meets the criteria for the diagnosis of isonatremic dehydration (i.e., normal serum Na^+). Isonatremic dehydration is also known as isotonic dehydration, and it occurs when there is a Na^+ loss equal to the fluid loss. Hyponatremic or hypotonic dehydration occurs when more Na^+ is lost than water, and hypernatremic or hypertonic dehydration occurs when more fluid is lost than Na^+.

REFERENCES

Brown, P.A., Blayney, F., Brown, C.A., & Evans, K.G. (1989). *Quick reference to pediatric intensive care nursing* (pp. 132–133). Rockville, MD: Aspen Publishers.
Samson, L.F., & Ouzts, K.M. (1996). Fluid and electrolyte regulation. In M.A.Q. Curley, J.B. Smith & P.A. Moloney-Harmon (Eds.). *Critical care nursing of infants and children.* Philadelphia: W.B. Saunders.

6. Answer (d). Fluid deficit is calculated by multiplying the actual weight (not the dehydrated weight) of the child by the percentage of dehydration. This provides the kilograms lost. Assuming that 1 g = 1 mL, multiplication of the kilogram loss by 1000 mL yields the total fluid loss: $11.8 \times 0.1 = 1.18$ kg loss $\times$ (1000 mL/1 kg) = 1180 mL total fluid loss.

REFERENCES

Aoki, B.Y., & McCloskey, K. (1992). *Evaluation, stabilization, and transport of the critically ill child* (p. 143). St. Louis: Mosby–Year Book.
Wetzel, R.C. (1991). Shock and fluid resuscitation. In D.G. Nichols, M. Yaster, D.G. Lappe, & J.R. Buck (Eds.). *Golden hour: The handbook of advanced pediatric life support* (p. 88). St. Louis: Mosby–Year Book.

7. Answer (c). Fluid loss is replaced as follows: *0 to 8 hours:* one half of the fluid loss over 8 hours plus the normal maintenance rate/hour; *9 to 24 hours:* one half of the fluid loss over 16 hours plus the normal maintenance rate per hour. A.'s calculated fluid loss is 1180 mL; one half of the fluid loss is 590 mL, and 590 mL/8 hours = 74 mL/hour. Maintenance fluids are calculated to be 1090 mL in 24 hours or 45 mL/hour. Replacement for *0 to 8 hours* is 74 + 45 = 119 mL/hour. Replacement for *9 to 24 hours* is as follows: 590 mL/16 hours = 37 mL/hour; 37 + 45 = 82 mL/hour.

REFERENCES

Wetzel, R.C. (1991). Shock and fluid resuscitation. In D.G. Nichols, M. Yaster, D.G. Lappe, & J.R. Buck (Eds.). *Golden hour: The handbook of advanced pediatric life support* (p. 88). St. Louis: Mosby–Year Book.

8. Answer (d). It is important to begin the rehydration as soon as possible. Because it is difficult to obtain intravenous access in a child with 10% dehydration, rehydration is begun with the existing intravenous line, making frequent assessments to ensure early identification of infiltration. After the child's hydration status improves, a second intravenous site should be started. In an effort to prolong the life of both intravenous sites, split the infusion equally between the two.

REFERENCE

Summerfield, A.L. (1991). Inserting intravenous catheters. In D.P. Smith (Ed.). *Comprehensive child and family nursing skills* (pp. 621–629). St. Louis: Mosby–Year Book.

9. Answer (a). Improvement in hydration

status is reflected early by the level of consciousness, heart rate, and urine output. If rehydration is successful, there will be an improvement in the level of consciousness. The child will become more alert and less irritable and lethargic. The heart rate will slow, and the production of urine will increase. Subsequently, as the total body water begins to be restored, there will be improvements in peripheral perfusion, mucous membrane moisture, skin turgor, and skin color. Because blood pressure changes occur only in severe dehydration, blood pressure is not a critical indicator of hydration status in stabilized patients.

REFERENCE

Barkin, R.M, & Rosen, P. (1990). *Emergency pediatrics, a guide to ambulatory care* (pp. 52–59). St. Louis: Mosby.

10. Answer (**a**). There are several nursing care priorities. The nurse should continue replacement therapy because replacement of the lost fluid is essential to recovery; monitor vital signs, which are the most sensitive indicator of response to therapy; and monitor intake and output, including insensible water loss. The nurse must ensure that the intake is exceeding the output, especially if the condition that caused the dehydration is still present. The nurse must assess the clinical status for fluid volume deficit or overload. It is important to ensure that the dissipating symptoms of dehydration are not replaced by symptoms of fluid excess (i.e., pulmonary edema). The nurse also must evaluate electrolyte results, which change more slowly than fluid status and therefore are generally monitored every 4 to 6 hours.

REFERENCE

Smith, D.P., & Breen, M. (1991). Monitoring hydration. In D.P. Smith (Ed.). *Comprehensive child and family nursing skills* (pp. 406–418). St. Louis: Mosby–Year Book.

ANSWERS ■ CASE 8-2

1. Answer (**d**). Increasing the PEEP causes an increase in the positive pressure in the thoracic cavity, which decreases cardiac output. The reduction in cardiac output is interpreted by the body to be a state of hypovolemia, and ADH is released in response. With the release of ADH, the kidneys are stimulated to conserve water, reducing the urine output and causing fluid retention.

REFERENCES

Bohn, D. (1993). Cardiopulmonary interactions. In P.R. Holbrook (Ed.). *Textbook of pediatric critical care* (pp. 475–477). Philadelphia: W.B. Saunders.
Samson, L.F., & Ouzts, K.M. (1996). Fluid and electrolyte regulation. In M.A.Q. Curley, J.B. Smith, & P.A. Moloney-Harmon (Eds.). *Critical care nursing of infants and children.* Philadelphia: W.B. Saunders.

2. Answer (**b**). Potassium and pH have an inverse relationship. As K+ decreases, pH increases, and vice versa. Because the HCO_3^- level of the patient is normal, it is clear that the alkalosis is not related to a primary acid-base disturbance but is a result of the hypokalemia.

REFERENCE

Paschall, J.A., & Melvin, T. (1993). Fluid and electrolyte therapy. In P.R. Holbrook (Ed.). *Textbook of pediatric critical care* (p. 690). Philadelphia: W.B. Saunders.
Samson, L.F., & Ouzts, K.M. (1996). Fluid and electrolyte regulation. In M.A.Q. Curley, J.B. Smith, & P.A. Moloney-Harmon (Eds.). *Critical care nursing of infants and children.* Philadelphia: W.B. Saunders.

3. Answer (**c**). Hypokalemia impairs the release of insulin. The alteration in insulin release causes a change in glucose hemostasis, which manifests as hyperglycemia.

REFERENCE

Clive, D., & Stoff, J. (1984). Renal syndromes associated with non-steroidal anti-inflammatory drugs. *New England Journal of Medicine,* 310, 563–572.

4. Answer (**d**). J.'s hypokalemia probably developed in response to the administration of diuretics and therefore occurred gradually over 24 hours. Symptoms of hypokalemia most commonly appear when a child suffers an acute potassium loss. Because only 24 hours have passed since the initiation of diuretic therapy, symptoms that take time to develop, such as abdominal distention and paralytic ileus, are not expected to be seen. Subtle changes in ECG patterns, such as flattened T waves and the presence of a U wave, are difficult to identify in children because of their faster heart rates. The most likely symptoms of hypokalemia include muscle weakness, irritability, lethargy, and nausea. However, in the clinical setting, it may be difficult to identify these symptoms as resulting from hypoka-

lemia. The symptoms may also be related to conditions such as pain, respiratory distress, and hunger.

REFERENCE

Brown, P.A., Blayney, F., Brown, C.A., & Evans, K.G. (1989). *Quick reference to pediatric intensive care nursing* (pp. 135–136). Rockville, MD: Aspen.
Samson, L.F., & Ouzts, K.M. (1996). Fluid and electrolyte regulation. In M.A.Q. Curley, J.B. Smith, & P.A. Moloney-Harmon (Eds.). *Critical care nursing of infants and children*. Philadelphia: W.B. Saunders.

5. Answer (**b**). Administer 7.5 mEq of KCl intravenously over 2 hours; the dosage range is 0.5 to 1 mEq/kg per dose to infuse at 0.3 to 0.5 mEq/kg per hour. If the patient is not exhibiting symptoms directly related to hypokalemia, a slower correction, which limits side effects, is preferred.

REFERENCE

Hamill, R.J., Robinson, L.M., Wexler, H.R., et al. (1991). Efficacy and safety of potassium infusion therapy in hypokalemic critically ill patients. *Critical Care Medicine,* 19 (5), 649.

6. Answer (**a**). The most probable cause of the hyperkalemia is maintenance fluids that were not readjusted after extubation and the diuretics were discontinued. The amount of potassium in the maintenance fluids was increased in response to the effect of mechanical ventilation and the use of diuretics. After those therapies are removed, the maintenance fluids must be readjusted accordingly.

REFERENCE

Samson, L.F., & Ouzts, K.M. (1996). Fluid and electrolyte regulation. In M.A.Q. Curley, J.B. Smith, & P.A. Moloney-Harmon (Eds.). *Critical care nursing of infants and children*. Philadelphia: W.B. Saunders.

7. Answer (**b**). The initial treatment of potassium levels less than 6.5 mEq/L is the removal of potassium from the fluids. If the potassium level does not decrease, more aggressive treatments aimed at reducing the serum potassium may be required.

REFERENCE

Paschall, J.A., & Melvin, T. (1993). Fluid and electrolyte therapy. In P.R. Holbrook (Ed.). *Textbook of pediatric critical care* (p. 692). Philadelphia: W.B. Saunders.

ANSWERS ■ CASE 8-3

1. Answer (**c**). Alkalosis increases the binding of calcium to protein and therefore decreases the Ca^{2+} level. Total serum calcium levels remain unchanged despite alkalosis. The ionized Ca^{2+} decreases by approximately 0.2 mg/dL, and the total serum calcium decreases by 0.12 mg/dL for each 0.1 increase in the pH.

REFERENCES

Chambers, J.K. (1987). Metabolic bone disorders: Imbalances of calcium and phosphorus. *Nursing Clinics of North America,* 22 (4), 861–874.
Paschall, J.A., & Melvin, T. (1993). Fluid and electrolyte therapy. In P.R. Holbrook (Ed.). *Textbook of pediatric critical care* (p. 693). Philadelphia: W.B. Saunders.

2. Answer (**a**). The tetany indicates that H. is beginning to display the clinical symptoms associated with hypocalcemia. Left untreated, she may begin to display more severe symptoms, such as decreased cardiac output and hypotension. Although the replacement of calcium may be associated with a loss of cell membrane integrity, the risks related to the hypocalcemia are the most immediate. Calcium replacement therapy is appropriate for a patient who demonstrates clinical and laboratory evidence of hypocalcemia. A patient who is hypocalcemic but not demonstrating symptoms of hypocalcemia may not require immediate intervention.

REFERENCES

Paschall, J.A., & Melvin, T. (1993). Fluid and electrolyte therapy. In P.R. Holbrook (Ed.). *Textbook of pediatric critical care* (p. 694). Philadelphia: W.B. Saunders.

3. Answer (**b**). Many precautions should be taken when administering calcium salts. Because the extravasation of calcium chloride may cause severe necrosis and tissue sloughing, calcium is best administered into a central line. In a cardiac arrest situation, calcium chloride may be given undiluted at a maximum concentration of 100 mg/mL, infused at a rate of 50 to 100 mg/mL. However, to minimize the potential side effects of calcium administration outside the arrest, it is best to dilute the calcium chloride to a maximum concentration of 20 mg/mL and administer over 1 hour. During the administration, the child must be monitored for negative cardiac effects, most notably bradycardia and asystole. A precipitate may be formed when calcium is administered with bicarbonates, phosphates, and sulfates, depending on the concentration,

and calcium must not be infused into the lines used for those solutions.

REFERENCES

Samson, L.F., & Ouzts, K.M. (1996). Fluid and electrolyte regulation. In M.A.Q. Curley, J.B. Smith, & P.A. Moloney-Harmon (Eds.). *Critical care nursing of infants and children.* Philadelphia: W.B. Saunders.

Taketomo, C. (1994). *Pediatric dosing handbook & formulary* (pp. 140–141). Los Angeles: Division of Pharmacy, Children's Hospital, Los Angeles.

4. Answer (c). The persistence of hypocalcemia and hypokalemia is an indication of hypomagnesemia. The relationship between the levels of calcium and magnesium is generally directly proportional, and when there is a reduction in one level, the other is also decreased. Confirmation of hypomagnesemia should be made by laboratory analysis. The signs and symptoms of hypomagnesemia are similar to those seen with hypocalcemia and hypokalemia, and one condition cannot be differentiated from the other without laboratory analysis.

REFERENCES

Samson, L.F., & Ouzts, K.M. (1996). Fluid and electrolyte regulation. In M.A.Q. Curley, J.B. Smith, & P.A. Moloney-Harmon (Eds.). *Critical care nursing of infants and children.* Philadelphia: W.B. Saunders.

Workman, M.L. (1992). Magnesium and phosphorus: The neglected electrolytes. *AACN Clinical Issues in Critical Care Nursing, 3* (3), 655–663.

5. Answer (d). Hypomagnesemia is caused by any or all of the following circumstances. *Insufficient intake:* malnutrition; prolonged NG suctioning; and large losses of body fluids. *Diuretic therapy:* administration of diuretics increases the excretion of magnesium from the kidneys; diuretics that are potassium-wasting are also magnesium wasting. *Alkalosis:* The shift in pH causes extracellular magnesium to move into the intracellular space, producing a transient but potentially clinically significant hypomagnesemia.

REFERENCES

Ryzen, E., Wagners, P.W., & Singer, F.R. (1985). Magnesium deficiency in a medical ICU. *Critical Care Medicine, 13* (1), 19–21.

Workman, M.L. (1992). Magnesium and phosphorus: The neglected electrolytes. *AACN Clinical Issues in Critical Care Nursing, 3* (3), 655–663.

6. Answer (b). Priorities for the treatment of electrolyte disturbances are determined by the clinical presentation. In H.'s case, with the persistent tetany, the priority treatment consists of three steps: replace the magnesium by administering a $MgSO_4$ bolus to increase the level to a normal range and therefore alleviate the clinical symptoms; place the NG tube to gravity to reduce the body fluid losses that contribute to hypomagnesemia; and begin nutritional support to provide sufficient intake of magnesium.

REFERENCES

Graves, L. (1990). Disorders of calcium, phosphorus, and magnesium. *Critical Care Nursing Quarterly, 14* (3), 231–236.

Workman, M.L. (1992). Magnesium and phosphorus: The neglected electrolytes. *AACN Clinical Issues in Critical Care Nursing, 3* (3), 655–663.

7. Answer (d). The correction of hypophosphatemia is best done slowly through enteral feedings. However, until the diarrhea is slowed or stopped, administering replacement through the enteral route probably will compound the problem. In H.'s case, the best course of action is to increase the phosphate content of the hyperalimentation while determining and correcting the cause of the diarrhea. After the diarrhea is under control, enteral feedings should begin. The adverse effects of phosphate administration (e.g., hypocalcemia, hypotension, extravasation injury) limit the use of a phosphate bolus except in cases of acute symptoms or if the serum level falls below 2 mg/dL.

REFERENCES

Kingston, M., & Badawi Al-Siba', I. (1985). Treatment of severe hypophosphatemia. *Critical Care Medicine, 13* (1), 16–18.

Samson, L.F., & Ouzts, K.M. (1996). Fluid and electrolyte regulation. In M.A.Q. Curley, J.B. Smith, & P.A. Moloney-Harmon (Eds.). *Critical care nursing of infants and children.* Philadelphia: W.B. Saunders.

8. Answer (c). The symptoms of hypophosphatemia (e.g., weakness, irritability, confusion, seizures) are often difficult to differentiate from other electrolyte disturbances. In the critically ill patient, many of the clinical symptoms, such as decreased myocardial contractility and hypoventilation due to muscle weakness, may be caused by a variety of conditions and are therefore difficult to attribute to hypophosphatemia. The symptoms unique to hypophosphatemia are related to the effect on the metabolic activity of platelets, erythrocytes, and leukocytes.

Platelets demonstrate a decreased ability to aggregate and to initiate the clotting cascade. Erythrocytes have a reduced ability to bind and release oxygen, resulting in tissue hypoxia. Leukocytes demonstrate reduced phagocytic activity, resulting in immunosuppression despite normal leukocyte counts.

REFERENCE

Workman, M.L. (1992). Magnesium and phosphorus: The neglected electrolytes. *AACN Clinical Issues in Critical Care Nursing,* 3 (3), 655–663.

CHAPTER 9

Renal Disorders

BEVERLY J. D'ANGIO, RN,C, MS

CASE 9-1

K., a 3-week-old, 3.4-kg infant, is admitted from the health department. K.'s mother noticed puffiness around the baby's eyes several days ago and states she is having to change K.'s diapers less frequently than when she first brought her home from the hospital. K. is admitted to the intensive care unit with a diagnosis of possible renal failure.

1. The immature kidney of an infant is less capable of concentrating urine to conserve water than the adult kidney. Several factors contribute to this phenomenon, including
   a. Increased excretion of sodium (Na^+).
   b. Short length of the loop of Henle.
   c. High glomerular filtration rate.
   d. Patent ductus arteriosus.

2. Simple chemical testing of urine is performed with multiple dipsticks by the nurse. To adequately interpret values seen on a dipstick of a patient in possible renal failure, the nurse must know that
   a. Normal 24-hour protein excretion is 10 to 20 mg.
   b. Persistent proteinuria usually initiates renal disease.
   c. Persistent proteinuria indicates renal trauma.
   d. Persistent proteinuria is a normal finding in infants.

3. Two key indicators of intrinsic renal failure are
   a. Increased blood pressure and decreased respiratory rate.
   b. Proteinuria and hematuria.
   c. Increased serum Na^+ and edema.
   d. Polyuria.

On physical examination, K. has significant periorbital edema and 2+ pedal edema, indicating fluid overload.

4. How can the nurse explain K.'s specific gravity (SG) value of 1.028 with accompanying signs and symptoms of fluid overload?
   a. SG of 1.028 is a normal finding with fluid overload.
   b. The laboratory made an error.
   c. SG is not a reliable indicator of kidney function in the infant.
   d. SG in an infant is usually elevated because of increased phosphorus excretion.

5. Critically ill infants or children have a tendency to retain fluids because of
   a. Increased antidiuretic hormone secretion.
   b. Decreased aldosterone.
   c. Hypertension.
   d. Hypotension.

The physician orders a fluid challenge of 60 mL (15 mL/kg) of normal saline solution followed by mannitol.

6. The rationale for ordering a fluid challenge is to
   a. Accurately measure the glomerular filtration rate.
   b. Restore the circulating blood volume.
   c. Decrease the SG.
   d. Stimulate cardiac stretch receptors in an effort to increase cardiac output.

7. Before administering a fluid challenge to an oliguric patient, the nurse should evaluate the
   a. Blood urea nitrogen (BUN) and creatinine.
   b. Glomerular filtration rate.
   c. Cause of the oliguria.
   d. Status of hypovolemia.

8. Osmotic agents, such as mannitol and glucose, have an immediate effect on the patient, as evidenced by
   a. Decreased urine output.
   b. Decreased intravascular volume.
   c. Increased intravascular volume.
   d. Decreased glomerular filtration rate and increased urine volume.

9. Mannitol is contraindicated in a 2700-g premature infant with a patent ductus arteriosus because
   a. Mannitol increases the risk of intravascular hemorrhage.
   b. Mannitol is never administered to infants weighing less than 3 kg.
   c. Acute renal failure in a premature infant with a patent ductus arteriosus will resolve without treatment.
   d. Mannitol may cause hyperkalemia.

10. Diuril is contraindicated in a patient with which of the following laboratory values?
    a. Serum potassium (K^+) less than 3.0 mEq/L.
    b. Serum K^+ greater than 6.0 mEq/L.
    c. Total serum calcium greater than 9.2 mg/dL.
    d. Total serum calcium less than 8.0 mg/dL.

11. Furosemide (Lasix) is a widely used diuretic. In which of the following patients is furosemide administration contraindicated?
    a. A 10-year-old girl with acute renal failure (ARF).
    b. A patient in early renal failure on a dopamine drip.
    c. A 2-day-old, weak neonate.
    d. A patient with a serum K^+ concentration of 5.0 mEq/L and serum Na^+ concentration of 140 mEq/L.

K. is diagnosed with ARF due to ischemia related to renal thrombosis.

12. Renal failure is frequently categorized as prerenal, renal, and post-renal failure. Prerenal failure means that events have compromised renal perfusion before glomerular filtration. In prerenal failure, oliguria is the body's compensatory mechanism to
    a. Increase the glomerular filtration rate.
    b. Conserve bicarbonate to alter the acid-base balance.
    c. Restore the intravascular volume to increase tissue perfusion.
    d. Keep the patent ductus arteriosus open.

13. An important indicator of K.'s degree of renal damage is the
    a. Persistence of a patent ductus arteriosus.
    b. Glomerular filtration rate.
    c. Duration of ischemia.
    d. Degree of metabolic alkalosis.

14. Oliguric acute tubular necrosis may occur after an ischemic event. Which of the following laboratory values are likely to be seen for a patient with oliguric acute tubular necrosis?
    a. SG of 1.035 and a serum K^+ concentration of 2.0 mEq/L.
    b. Microscopic hematuria.
    c. Increased BUN and decreased creatinine levels.
    d. Increased BUN, increased creatinine level, and decreased urine osmolality.

15. Potential complications during the oliguric phase of acute tubular necrosis are
    a. K^+ concentration of 4.0 mEq/L.
    b. Serum osmolality of 260 mOsm/L.
    c. Congestive heart failure.
    d. Urine output of 1 mL/kg per hour.

Serum concentrations are determined for K.'s sodium (Na^+), potassium (K^+), phosphorus and phosphates (P), calcium (Ca^{2+}), magnesium (Mg^{2+}), and osmolality (Osm), and her hemoglobin (Hgb), hematocrit (Hct), platelet (Plat) count, and leukocyte count (WBC) are also determined:

Na^+: 133 mEq/L	Osm: 300 mOsm/L
K^+: 4.0 mEq/L	Hgb: 24 g/dL
P: 8.0 mg/dL	Hct: 45%
Total serum Ca^{2+}: 6.2 mg/dL	WBC: 20,000/mm³
Mg^{2+}: 6.0 mEq/L	Plat: 300,000/mm³

16. Accurate monitoring and documentation of intake and output is essential in the care of the critically ill infant. Daily weights, vital signs, and laboratory values are also critical values to be moni-

tored by the nurse. An early sign of decreased tissue perfusion includes unexplained metabolic acidosis. Late symptoms of distress include
   a. Hyperactivity.
   b. Decreased urine output and lethargy.
   c. Bounding peripheral pulses.
   d. Increased blood pressure.

17. Based on K.'s laboratory values, which of the following will the nurse monitor for?
   a. Increased urine output.
   b. Hypercarbia.
   c. Peaked T waves.
   d. Seizures.

18. How can K.'s hemoglobin and hematocrit values be explained?
   a. Gestational age.
   b. Decreased cardiac output.
   c. Furosemide therapy.
   d. Result of a fluid challenge.

19. Which of the following may be the result of severe Na^+ imbalance?
   a. Intracranial pressure of 24 mmHg.
   b. SG of 1.012.
   c. Systolic blood pressure of 80 mmHg.
   d. Serum K^+ concentration of 5.0 mEq/L.

CASE 9-2

J.'s mother took him to the local pediatrician and said, "He just lies around all the time and looks very pale to me." J., a 5-year-old boy, was treated by the pediatrician 3 weeks before this visit for an episode of nausea, vomiting, and diarrhea that lasted 8 days.

1. Based on the history and his physical appearance, what would be an important diagnostic test?
   a. Urinalysis.
   b. Prothrombin time and partial thromboplastin time.
   c. Blood culture.
   d. Complete blood count.

J. is sent to the local tertiary care center for a complete workup. Hemolytic uremic syndrome (HUS) is diagnosed the next day. He develops significant hepatosplenomegaly.

2. Classic signs and symptoms of HUS are
   a. Chronic renal failure, oliguria, and pernicious anemia.
   b. Chronic renal failure, leukopenia, and hemolytic anemia.

   c. Thrombocytopenia, hemolytic anemia, and ARF.
   d. Acute renal failure, positive Coombs' test result, and anemia.

3. In HUS, anemia results from
   a. Bleeding into the kidney.
   b. Decreased vitamin K metabolism.
   c. Destruction of damaged red blood cells (RBCs).
   d. Hepatosplenomegaly.

4. Why is hepatosplenomegaly a factor in HUS?
   a. The cause is unknown.
   b. HUS virus attacks the splenic microvasculature.
   c. The spleen works overtime to clear damaged RBCs from the circulation.
   d. Kidneys of ARF patients emit a toxin that attacks the liver and spleen.

Despite conservative treatment with packed RBC transfusions, intravenous fluids, and diuretics, J.'s condition worsens. He develops serious electrolyte imbalances.

5. Hyperkalemia may be a life-threatening complication of HUS because
   a. Immature kidneys cannot concentrate urine.
   b. Kidneys are responsible for 90% of K^+ excretion.
   c. Dopamine receptors are rendered inactive in ARF.
   d. Hyperkalemia may cause seizures.

6. Indications of hyponatremia in the patient with HUS include
   a. Hypokalemia.
   b. Hypocalcemia.
   c. Cerebral edema and seizures.
   d. Cardiac arrhythmias.

7. An appropriate treatment for hypocalcemia is
   a. Dopamine.
   b. Lasix.
   c. Aluminum hydroxide.
   d. Potassium bolus.

8. What laboratory values are expected with HUS?
   a. K^+ concentration of 6.0 mEq/L, increased BUN, and increased creatinine level.
   b. K^+ concentration of 2.0 mEq/L, increased BUN, and increased creatinine level.

c. K$^+$ concentration of 6.0 mEq/L, decreased BUN, and decreased creatinine level.

d. K$^+$ concentration of 2.0 mEq/L, decreased BUN, and decreased creatinine level.

J.'s condition worsens and the decision is made to begin hemodialysis. A temporary large, double-lumen central venous line is placed in the right subclavian vein.

9. Hemodialysis is preferred for treating J.'s condition rather than peritoneal dialysis because
   a. Severe electrolyte imbalance is not corrected with peritoneal dialysis.
   b. Hemodialysis is more efficient and faster at removing nitrogenous wastes and restoring fluid and acid-base balance.
   c. Peritoneal dialysis is contraindicated for the patient with a history of bloody diarrhea.
   d. Peritoneal dialysis is contraindicated in the patient less than 6 years old.

10. Heparin is administered during hemodialysis to
    a. Prevent hyperkalemia.
    b. Prevent clot formation.
    c. Treat hypovolemia.
    d. Treat hypervolemia.

J.'s laboratory values, including a determination of creatine (Cr), are

K$^+$: 6.3 mEq/L	BUN: 54 mg/dL
Cr: 8.1 mg/dL	Hgb: 6.8 g/dL
Plat: 148,000/mm^3	

The arterial blood gas determinations include hydrogen ion concentration (pH), partial pressures of oxygen (Po_2) and carbon dioxide (Pco_2), bicarbonate (HCO$_3^-$) level, and base excess (BE). The following values are the results for the initial determinations:

pH: 7.20	HCO$_3^-$: 19 mEq/L
Po_2: 93.5 mmHg	BE: 17 mEq/L
Pco_2: 30 mmHg	

11. After reviewing the laboratory values, the nurse knows J. is
    a. In metabolic acidosis.
    b. In respiratory acidosis.
    c. At risk for intracranial bleeding.
    d. At risk for liver failure.

12. As with peritoneal dialysis, the content and concentration of the hemodialysis dialysate controls fluid and solute movement across a semipermeable membrane. Considering J.'s current laboratory values and arterial blood gas values, the nurse expects the dialysate to be
    a. Low in K$^+$ and high in HCO$_3^-$.
    b. Low in K$^+$ and high in protein.
    c. High in K$^+$ and low in HCO$_3^-$.
    d. High in K$^+$ and low in glucose.

13. During hemodialysis, J. becomes irritable and confused and complains of a headache. The nurse recognizes these as signs and symptoms of cerebral edema, possibly attributed to
    a. Too much K$^+$ in the dialysate.
    b. An untoward reaction to heparinization.
    c. Hypervolemia.
    d. Solutes being too rapidly removed from the intravascular space.

CASE 9-3

N. is a 4-year-old girl diagnosed with Wilms' tumor who underwent a bilateral nephrectomy 1 month ago. N. has been managed successfully on peritoneal dialysis.

1. Principles of peritoneal dialysis include
   a. Osmolarity and dilution.
   b. Hemodynamics and glomerular filtration rate.
   c. Osmosis and diffusion.
   d. Osmolarity and diffusion.

2. Peritoneal dialysis is more efficient in smaller pediatric patients, because they
   a. Have immature kidneys.
   b. Have high cardiac outputs.
   c. Have a larger ratio of peritoneal space to body mass.
   d. Have low blood pressures.

3. Based on a knowledge of renal replacement, which of the following patients would be the most likely candidate for hemodialysis?
   a. A patient with decreased urine output and a high SG.
   b. A chronically ventilated patient with potential renal complications.
   c. An intensive care unit patient who is hemodynamically unstable.
   d. An ARF patient 2 days after exploratory laparotomy who also has possible renal complications.

N. is exhibiting signs and symptoms of fluid overload. The nephrologist wishes to remove as much fluid as quickly and safely as possible to prevent N. from developing congestive heart failure.

4. Which of the following dialysate concentrations would the nurse expect the nephrologist to order?
   a. A 2.5% dialysate with 20 mEq of potassium chloride (KCl)/L.
   b. A 2.5% dialysate with 40 mEq of KCl/L.
   c. A 4.25% dialysate with 20 mEq of KCl/L.
   d. A 2.5% dialysate with 1000 U of heparin/L and 40 mEq of KCl/L.

5. Which of the following patient conditions may cause transient hyperglycemia in a peritoneal dialysis patient?
   a. Pancreatitis.
   b. Mechanical ventilation.
   c. Congestive heart failure.
   d. Hypokalemia.

6. Reliable indications of uremia are
   a. Nausea, vomiting, and azotemia.
   b. Elevated BUN and decreased creatinine levels.
   c. Elevated creatinine and decreased BUN levels.
   d. High cardiac output and a PR interval of 0.2 seconds.

N. is admitted to the intensive care unit in septic shock. Her treatment includes the following: mechanical ventilation, vecuronium drip, arterial blood gas determinations every 4 hours, and dopamine administered at 10 μg/kg per minute.

7. The arterial blood gas results are significant because, based on knowledge of the kidney,
   a. Respiratory alkalosis is a prognostic factor in renal failure.
   b. Base deficit is an indication of the severity of renal failure.
   c. Acid-base balance is regulated by the kidneys, lungs, and chemical buffering systems.
   d. Erythropoietin is secreted by the kidney.

8. If a neonate's arterial blood gas values show a pH of 7.28 and HCO_3^- level of 18 mEq/L, the nurse knows that
   a. The values are normal.
   b. The patient is in respiratory acidosis.
   c. The patient has ARF.
   d. HUS is suspected.

ANSWERS ■ CASE 9-1

1. Answer (**b**). Infant kidneys are less efficient at concentrating urine because of immature tubular function, a short loop of Henle, decreased Na^+ excretion, and a low glomerular filtration rate.

REFERENCE
Madder, S.M., & Milberger, P.M. (1996). Renal critical care problems. In M.A.Q. Curley, J.B. Smith, & P.A. Moloney-Harmon (Eds.). *Critical care nursing of infants and children*. Philadelphia: W.B. Saunders.

2. Answer (**b**). Proteinuria is an abnormal finding on a urine dipstick and indicates renal disease. Hematuria occurs in cases of glomerulonephritis and renal trauma. Normal 24-hour protein excretion is less than 150 mg.

REFERENCES
Jackle, M., & Rasmussen, C. (1980). *Renal problems: A critical care nursing focus* (p. 58). London: Prentice-Hall.
Madder, S.M., & Milberger, P.M. (1996). Renal critical care problems. In M.A.Q. Curley, J.B. Smith, & P.A. Moloney-Harmon (Eds.). *Critical care nursing of infants and children*. Philadelphia: W.B. Saunders.

3. Answer (**b**). Proteinuria and hematuria are classic signs and symptoms of intrinsic renal failure. Polyuria, increased blood pressure, serum Na^+, edema, and a decreased respiratory rate may have other causes.

REFERENCES
Jackle, M., & Rasmussen, C. (1980). *Renal problems: A critical care nursing focus* (p. 108). London: Prentice-Hall.
Madder, S.M., & Milberger, P.M. (1996). Renal critical care problems. In M.A.Q. Curley, J.B. Smith, & P.A. Moloney-Harmon (Eds.). *Critical care nursing of infants and children*. Philadelphia: W.B. Saunders.

4. Answer (**c**). Because the immature kidney is unable to concentrate urine, the SG is not diagnostic. SG of 1.028 in a child or adult indicates dehydration, not fluid overload.

REFERENCE
Madder, S.M., & Milberger, P.M. (1996). Renal critical care problems. In M.A.Q. Curley, J.B. Smith, & P.A. Moloney-Harmon (Eds.). *Critical care nursing of infants and children*. Philadelphia: W.B. Saunders.

5. Answer (**a**). Antidiuretic hormone and aldosterone hormone secretion are increased during an infant's critical illness. Hypertension and hypotension do not have an effect on fluid retention.

REFERENCES

Jackle, M., & Rasmussen, C. (1980). *Renal problems: A critical care nursing focus* (p. 123). London: Prentice-Hall.

Kennedy, J. (1992). Renal disorders. In M.F. Hazinski (Ed.). *Nursing care of the critically ill child* (2nd ed., p. 649). St. Louis: Mosby–Year Book.

6. Answer (**b**). In the absence of hypervolemia, a 10 to 20 mL/kg fluid challenge helps to restore intravascular volume, which ensures adequate cardiac output. Stimulating the cardiac stretch receptors does not increase cardiac output. A fluid challenge followed by diuretics decreases the SG.

REFERENCE

Madder, S.M., & Milberger, P.M. (1996). Renal critical care problems. In M.A.Q. Curley, J.B. Smith, & P.A. Moloney-Harmon (Eds.). *Critical care nursing of infants and children*. Philadelphia: W.B. Saunders.

7. Answer (**d**). Administering a fluid challenge to a patient who is not in a state of hypovolemia may seriously compromise cardiac and respiratory function. Therefore, accurate assessment of hypovolemia is critical. The BUN and creatinine levels and the glomerular filtration rate may contribute to the cause of the ARF, but the deciding factor is the intravascular volemic state.

REFERENCE

Madder, S.M., & Milberger, P.M. (1996). Renal critical care problems. In M.A.Q. Curley, J.B. Smith, & P.A. Moloney-Harmon (Eds.). *Critical care nursing of infants and children*. Philadelphia: W.B. Saunders.

8. Answer (**c**). Osmotic agents (when filtered through the glomerulus) pull additional free water into the filtrate. This action slows sodium and water reabsorption in the proximal tubule and results in an increased glomerular filtration rate and urine volume. A temporary increase in intravascular volume may result.

REFERENCE

Kennedy, J. (1992). Renal disorders. In M.F. Hazinski (Ed.). *Nursing care of the critically ill child.* (2nd ed., p. 650). St. Louis: Mosby–Year Book.

9. Answer (**a**). Mannitol has a significant effect on fluid shifts and may precipitate intravascular hemorrhage. Age alone is not a contraindication, and ARF does not resolve without treatment.

REFERENCE

Madder, S.M., & Milberger, P.M. (1996). Renal critical care problems. In M.A.Q. Curley, J.B. Smith, & P.A. Moloney-Harmon (Eds.). *Critical care nursing of infants and children*. Philadelphia: W.B. Saunders.

10. Answer (**a**). Diuril is not a potassium-sparing diuretic and may worsen a hypokalemic state. A diuretic of choice would be spironolactone (Aldactone).

REFERENCE

Kennedy, J. (1992). Renal disorders. In M.F. Hazinski (Ed.). *Nursing care of the critically ill child.* (2nd ed., pp. 650–651). St. Louis: Mosby–Year Book.

11. Answer (**c**). The primary diuretic effect of furosemide is inhibition of chloride reabsorption in the ascending limb of the loop of Henle, and it may be involved in the persistence of a patent ductus arteriosus in a 2-day-old neonate. Furosemide can help decrease serum potassium and sodium levels and is a valuable medication in treating ARF.

REFERENCE

Madder, S.M., & Milberger, P.M. (1996). Renal critical care problems. In M.A.Q. Curley, J.B. Smith, & P.A. Moloney-Harmon (Eds.). *Critical care nursing of infants and children*. Philadelphia: W.B. Saunders.

12. Answer (**c**). Oliguria helps the body conserve water in an effort to restore intravascular volume.

REFERENCE

Madder, S.M., & Milberger, P.M. (1996). Renal critical care problems. In M.A.Q. Curley, J.B. Smith, & P.A. Moloney-Harmon (Eds.). *Critical care nursing of infants and children*. Philadelphia: W.B. Saunders.

13. Answer (**c**). The duration of ischemia is the primary indicator of the extent of renal damage.

REFERENCE

Madder, S.M., & Milberger, P.M. (1996). Renal critical care problems. In M.A.Q. Curley, J.B. Smith, & P.A. Moloney-Harmon (Eds.). *Critical care nursing of infants and children*. Philadelphia: W.B. Saunders.

14. Answer (**d**). During oliguria, the serum BUN and creatinine levels rise, the urine SG is less than 1.018, urine osmolality falls, and the patient develops hyperkalemia because of tubular dysfunction.

REFERENCE

Madder, S.M., & Milberger, P.M. (1996). Renal critical care problems. In M.A.Q. Curley, J.B. Smith, & P.A. Moloney-Harmon (Eds.). *Critical care nursing of infants and children*. Philadelphia: W.B. Saunders.

15. Answer (**c**). Electrolyte imbalances, acid-base disturbances, congestive heart failure, pulmonary edema, or all of these factors are potential complications during the oliguric phase because of tubular dysfunction and the inability to concentrate urine. Urine output of 1 mL/kg per hour is a normal finding in an infant.

REFERENCE
Madder, S.M., & Milberger, P.M. (1996). Renal critical care problems. In M.A.Q. Curley, J.B. Smith, & P.A. Moloney-Harmon (Eds.). *Critical care nursing of infants and children*. Philadelphia: W.B. Saunders.

16. Answer (**b**). Late signs of distress include decreased urine output, weak peripheral pulses, cool extremities, lethargy, hypotension, and congestive heart failure.

REFERENCE
Madder, S.M., & Milberger, P.M. (1996). Renal critical care problems. In M.A.Q. Curley, J.B. Smith, & P.A. Moloney-Harmon (Eds.). *Critical care nursing of infants and children*. Philadelphia: W.B. Saunders.

17. Answer (**d**). Neurologic sequelae of hypocalcemia include seizures, muscle cramps, and tetany. Hypokalemia or hyperkalemia affects cardiac function.

REFERENCES
Jackle, M., & Rasmussen, C. (1980). *Renal problems: A critical care nursing focus* (p. 85). London: Prentice-Hall.
Kennedy, J. (1992). Renal disorders. In M.F. Hazinski (Ed.). *Nursing care of the critically ill child*. (2nd ed., p. 213). St. Louis: Mosby–Year Book.

18. Answer (**a**). The normal hemoglobin concentration for an infant is 10 to 15 g/dL, and the normal hematocrit is 30% to 40%.

REFERENCE
Pagana, K.D., & Pagana, T.J. (1986). *Pocket nurse guide to laboratory and diagnostic tests* (p. 450). St. Louis: Mosby–Year Book.

19. Answer (**a**). Hyponatremia may cause cerebral edema, increased intracranial pressure, or seizures because of changes in osmolality. Hyperkalemia may cause cardiac arrhythmias. The SG of 1.012 is low normal, and systolic blood pressure of 80 mmHg is not indicative of a sodium problem.

REFERENCE
Madder, S.M., & Milberger, P.M. (1996). Renal critical care problems. In M.A.Q. Curley, J.B. Smith, & P.A.

Moloney-Harmon (Eds.). *Critical care nursing of infants and children*. Philadelphia: W.B. Saunders.

ANSWERS ■ CASE 9-2

1. Answer (**d**). In a patient with HUS, as RBCs pass through vessels lined with fibrin deposits, they become fragmented and are easily seen on a peripheral complete blood count smear. Platelet function is altered by the increased use of platelets, but the prothrombin time and partial thromboplastin time are within normal limits.

REFERENCES
Jackle, M., & Rasmussen, C. (1980). *Renal problems: A critical care nursing focus* (p. 187). London: Prentice-Hall.
Madder, S.M., & Milberger, P.M. (1996). Renal critical care problems. In M.A.Q. Curley, J.B. Smith, & P.A. Moloney-Harmon (Eds.). *Critical care nursing of infants and children*. Philadelphia: W.B. Saunders.

2. Answer (**c**). The primary site of injury in a patient with HUS is the endothelial lining of small arteries and arterioles, especially in the kidney. This process results in the intravascular deposition of platelets and fibrin, resulting in partial or complete occlusion of small arterioles and capillaries in the kidney. As erythrocytes and platelets travel through these occluded vessels, they are fragmented. The result is functional thrombocytopenia and hemolytic anemia. The cells of the renal endothelium tend to swell and detach from the basement membrane, reducing renal blood flow and the glomerular filtration rate. The resulting ARF can be reversed in as little as 5 to 7 days with prompt treatment.

REFERENCE
Kennedy, J. (1992). Renal disorders. In M.F. Hazinski (Ed.). *Nursing care of the critically ill child* (2nd ed., p. 699). St. Louis: Mosby–Year Book.

3. Answer (**c**). The renal microvasculature becomes occluded with fibrin deposits and damages RBCs as they travel through. Even though the RBC count may not be decreased by a significant amount, the RBCs are damaged and nonfunctional. Hepatosplenomegaly results from the clearance of damaged RBCs.

REFERENCE
Kennedy, J. (1992). Renal disorders. In M.F. Hazinski (Ed.). *Nursing care of the critically ill child* (2nd ed., p. 699). St. Louis: Mosby–Year Book.

4. Answer (**c**). RBCs are damaged as they travel through vessels occluded with fibrin deposits. The liver and spleen work overtime in an effort to clear the damaged RBCs from circulation. The virus suspected of causing HUS attacks the microvasculature of the kidney.

REFERENCE

Kennedy, J. (1992). Renal disorders. In M.F. Hazinski (Ed.). *Nursing care of the critically ill child* (2nd ed., p. 699). St. Louis: Mosby–Year Book.

5. Answer (**b**). Kidneys are the primary source of potassium excretion, and any alteration in kidney function alters potassium clearance or reabsorption. Dopamine receptors are not inactive in patients with ARF, and the concentration of urine is not a factor in hyperkalemia. Hyponatremia and hypocalcemia may cause seizures.

REFERENCE

Madder, S.M., & Milberger, P.M. (1996). Renal critical care problems. In M.A.Q. Curley, J.B. Smith, & P.A. Moloney-Harmon (Eds.). *Critical care nursing of infants and children.* Philadelphia: W.B. Saunders.

6. Answer (**c**). Cerebral edema, seizures, and coma result from hyponatremia. Hypocalcemia accompanies hyperphosphatemia, and hyperkalemia or hypokalemia result in cardiac arrhythmias.

REFERENCE

Jackle, M. & Rasmussen, C. (1980). *Renal problems: A critical care nursing focus* (p. 103). London: Prentice-Hall.

7. Answer (**c**). Aluminum hydroxide and calcium inhibit the reabsorption of phosphorus in the gastrointestinal tract and reduce the serum level. Treating hyperphosphatemia treats the hypocalcemia.

REFERENCE

Madder, S.M., & Milberger, P.M. (1996). Renal critical care problems. In M.A.Q. Curley, J.B. Smith, & P.A. Moloney-Harmon (Eds.). *Critical care nursing of infants and children.* Philadelphia: W.B. Saunders.

8. Answer (**a**). Because of the renal failure, potassium excretion is altered, resulting in hyperkalemia. Increased BUN and creatinine levels are indications of ARF.

REFERENCE

Kennedy, J. (1992). Renal disorders. In M.F. Hazinski (Ed.). *Nursing care of the critically ill child.* (2nd ed., p. 700). St. Louis: Mosby–Year Book.

9. Answer (**b**). Hemodialysis is the fastest and most efficient artificial method of removing nitrogenous wastes from the body and of restoring fluids. Peritoneal dialysis can correct an electrolyte imbalance, but it does so slower than hemodialysis. Peritoneal dialysis catheters may be placed safely in patients with abdominal difficulties and can significantly control fluid balance; it is not contraindicated in patients with bloody diarrhea or in young children.

REFERENCE

Kennedy, J. (1992). Renal disorders. In M.F. Hazinski (Ed.). *Nursing care of the critically ill child* (2nd ed., pp. 686–687). St. Louis: Mosby–Year Book.

10. Answer (**b**). Clot formation may be a life-threatening complication of hemodialysis. Regional or systemic heparinization prevents clot formation.

REFERENCE

Madder, S.M., & Milberger, P.M. (1996). Renal critical care problems. In M.A.Q. Curley, J.B. Smith, & P.A. Moloney-Harmon (Eds.). *Critical care nursing of infants and children.* Philadelphia: W.B. Saunders.

11. Answer (**a**). Metabolic acidosis is reflected by a decrease in pH, increase in P_{CO_2}, and a base excess of a minus value. The normal platelet count is 100,000 to $400,000/mm^3$, and intravascular hemorrhage is not a new-onset complication for a 5-year-old child.

REFERENCE

Jackle, M. & Rasmussen, C. (1980). *Renal problems: A critical care nursing focus* (p. 165). London: Prentice-Hall.

Kennedy, J. (1992). Renal disorders. In M.F. Hazinski (Ed.). *Nursing care of the critically ill child* (2nd ed., p. 405). St. Louis: Mosby–Year Book.

12. Answer (**a**). The dialysate is low in K+ and high in HCO_3^- in an effort to correct the patient's hyperkalemia and acidosis.

REFERENCE

Madder, S.M., & Milberger, P.M. (1996). Renal critical care problems. In M.A.Q. Curley, J.B. Smith, & P.A. Moloney-Harmon (Eds.). *Critical care nursing of infants and children.* Philadelphia: W.B. Saunders.

13. Answer (**d**). The acceptable rate of solute clearance is affected by how the child tolerates hemodialysis. As fluid is removed during hemodialysis, disequilibrium between intravascular and intracellular spaces may develop, leading to severe fluid shifts and cerebral edema. Hyperkalemia affects cardiac function.

REFERENCE

Madder, S.M., & Milberger, P.M. (1996). Renal critical care problems. In M.A.Q. Curley, J.B. Smith, & P.A. Moloney-Harmon (Eds.). *Critical care nursing of infants and children*. Philadelphia: W.B. Saunders.

ANSWERS ■ CASE 9-3

1. Answer (**c**). The patient's peritoneum serves as a semipermeable membrane to allow movement of solutes by diffusion and water by osmosis.

REFERENCE

Jackle, M., & Rasmussen, C. (1980). *Renal problems: A critical care nursing focus* (p. 207). London: Prentice-Hall.

2. Answer (**c**). Peritoneal dialysis can be affected by the concentration of dialysate, dwell time, and surface area. The smaller the patient, the larger the ratio of peritoneal space to body mass; peritoneal dialysis therefore is more efficient in smaller pediatric patients. Cardiac output and blood pressure have no effect on the relative efficiency of peritoneal dialysis.

REFERENCE

Madder, S.M., & Milberger, P.M. (1996). Renal critical care problems. In M.A.Q. Curley, J.B. Smith, & P.A. Moloney-Harmon (Eds.). *Critical care nursing of infants and children*. Philadelphia: W.B. Saunders.

3. Answer (**c**). There are no absolute contraindications to peritoneal dialysis. However, patients with peritonitis, peritoneal adhesions, or diaphragmatic defects and those healing from recent abdominal surgery are not ideal candidates for peritoneal dialysis. Patients with potential renal complications are not treated aggressively with hemodialysis. Decreased urine output and increased SG may be corrected with less invasive procedures. Peritoneal dialysis is a safe and reliable method to treat the critically ill patient who is hemodynamically unstable.

REFERENCE

Jackle, M., & Rasmussen, C. (1980). *Renal problems: A critical care nursing focus* (p. 254). London: Prentice-Hall.

4. Answer (**c**). The higher the concentration of glucose in the dialysate, the faster the water moves from the intravascular space into the peritoneal fluid. The KCl concentration is not a factor.

5. Answer (**a**). During peritoneal dialysis, glucose may move from the peritoneal to the intravenous space, resulting in hyperglycemia. This is usually temporary, persisting until the pancreas is able to increase insulin production.

REFERENCE

Madder, S.M., & Milberger, P.M. (1996). Renal critical care problems. In M.A.Q. Curley, J.B. Smith, & P.A. Moloney-Harmon (Eds.). *Critical care nursing of infants and children*. Philadelphia: W.B. Saunders.

6. Answer (**a**). Uremia (i.e., urine in the blood) causes the clinical features of nausea, vomiting, confusion, and disorientation. Azotemia refers to a high concentration of nitrogenous wastes in blood. Elevated BUN and creatinine levels alone are not indicative of uremia.

REFERENCE

Jackle, M., & Rasmussen, C. (1980). *Renal problems: A critical care nursing focus* (p. 99). London: Prentice-Hall.

7. Answer (**c**). The kidney selectively secretes or absorbs hydrogen and bicarbonate ions to bring the serum pH within normal range. Along with the lungs and chemical buffering system, the kidneys play a large part in acid-base balance. Erythropoietin is secreted by the kidney, but it does not affect arterial blood gas values.

REFERENCE

Madder, S.M., & Milberger, P.M. (1996). Renal critical care problems. In M.A.Q. Curley, J.B. Smith, & P.A. Moloney-Harmon (Eds.). *Critical care nursing of infants and children*. Philadelphia: W.B. Saunders.

8. Answer (**a**). Renal regulation of acid-base balance in the immature kidney is different from that in older infants and children. Serum pH and HCO_3^- levels are lower because of the low renal threshold for HCO_3^-. This is not necessarily an indication of acidosis.

REFERENCE

Madder, S.M., & Milberger, P.M. (1996). Renal critical care problems. In M.A.Q. Curley, J.B. Smith, & P.A. Moloney-Harmon (Eds.). *Critical care nursing of infants and children*. Philadelphia: W.B. Saunders.

CHAPTER *10*

Gastrointestinal Disorders

JODY A. HOLLAND, RN, MN

CASE 10-1

S., a 7-month-old boy, was diagnosed with hepatoblastoma 4 months ago. He has been hospitalized for a liver biopsy, radiation therapy, Hickman central line placement, and chemotherapy. S. undergoes a second laparotomy for partial excision of the tumor mass and a visceral angiogram for chemoembolization of the residual mass. He returns to the pediatric intensive care unit (PICU) postoperatively.

1. On admission to the PICU, what baseline laboratory tests are obtained?
   a. Complete blood count and electrolytes.
   b. Hemoglobin and hematocrit.
   c. Transaminase and alkaline phosphatase.
   d. Blood cultures and bleeding time.

2. Additional orders include daily determinations of the bilirubin level, albumin concentration, and prothrombin time. The rationale for monitoring these laboratory values is to
   a. Define liver function.
   b. Predict bleeding diathesis.
   c. Determine readiness for enteral feedings.
   d. Ascertain the presence of infection.

   S.'s admitting laboratory tests found these levels of alkaline phosphatase (Alk), direct (Bil_D) and total (Bil_T) bilirubin, lactate dehydrogenase (LDH), serum glutamic-oxaloacetic transaminase (SGOT), albumin (Alb), total protein (Prot), and glucose (Glu):

Alk: 39 U/L	SGOT: 35 U/L
Bil_D: 0.4 mg/dL	Alb: 4.1 g/dL
Bil_T: 1.6 mg/dL	Prot: 5.2 g/dL
LDH: 425 U/L	Glu: 50 mg/dL

   S.'s admitting orders include starting an intravenous solution of glucose.

3. The rationale for this is that
   a. Patients with liver failure are kept off oral intake, because eating interferes with ventilation.
   b. Gluconeogenesis is no longer completed because of liver failure.
   c. Appetite stimulation is greatly decreased because of hepatic encephalopathy.
   d. Decreased bile production compromises digestion and absorption.

   Clinical examination reveals a heart rate of 165 beats per minute (bpm), respiratory rate of 65 breaths per minute, bilateral rhonchi, use of accessory muscles, and nasal flaring. The arterial blood gas determinations include the hydrogen ion concentration (pH), oxygen saturation (Sao_2), and partial pressures of oxygen (Po_2) and carbon dioxide (Pco_2):

pH: 7.35	Pco_2: 42 mmHg
Sao_2: 70%	Po_2: 54 mmHg

   Supplemental O_2 is provided.

4. Respiratory failure with liver failure probably is caused by
   a. Fluid overload.
   b. Pulmonary bleeding.
   c. Cerebral ischemia.
   d. Overwhelming sepsis.

5. S.'s level of consciousness decreases, he does not recognize his parents, and he re-

sponds minimally to painful stimuli. Initial care should be directed toward
a. Intubation and hyperventilation.
b. Volume expansion and infusions of an inotropic agent.
c. Hypertonic glucose infusions and administration of histamine blockers.
d. Diuretics and colonic gavage to decrease ammonia absorption.

S.'s neurological status deteriorates further. A Camino catheter is inserted for intracranial pressure monitoring.

S.'s parents are anxious and ask what they can do.

6. Which of the following would help the parents?
a. Instruct them of the intracranial pressure values and ask them to let the nurse know when it goes up.
b. Acknowledge that there is little they can do at this time.
c. Encourage them to touch and stroke their child.
d. Have them speak to a social worker.

The conventional therapies of hyperventilation, mannitol administration, and increasing serum osmolarity have been ineffective in controlling the intracranial pressure. Barbiturate-induced coma is initiated.

7. This treatment
a. Reduces cerebral metabolism.
b. Increases cerebral metabolism.
c. Shifts intracellular sodium to the extracellular space.
d. Decreases the cerebral perfusion pressure.

Ammonia levels have decreased from 110 to 75 μg/dL.

8. Surveillance of ammonia levels is valuable for patients with hepatic failure, because ammonia levels are
a. A predictor of gastrointestinal bleeding.
b. A nonspecific indicator of gastrointestinal function.
c. Responsible for fluid shifts from the intracellular space to the extracellular space.
d. An indicator of the amount of ammonia detoxified by the liver.

The nurse caring for S. is concerned about the development of stress gastritis. She knows that gastritis in patients with hepatic failure can be reduced by maintaining the gastric pH above 4.5.

9. Interventions that can accomplish this goal include
a. Vitamin K.
b. H_2-receptor antagonists plus antacids.
c. Prophylactic heparin.
d. Lactulose.

CASE 10-2

M. is a 3-year-old girl who was transferred from a rural hospital to the intensive care unit. She was in a motor vehicle accident 3 days ago and has been on mechanical ventilation because of an unresolved pneumothorax. On M.'s admission, the nurse notices flecks of blood in the nasogastric aspirate, which a nurse from the referring hospital states was not evident before. The gastric aspirate tests positive for blood.

1. Based on this information, the plan of care includes observation and management of
a. Adult respiratory distress syndrome.
b. Stress ulcers.
c. Intracranial pressure.
d. Renal replacement therapy.

2. The most likely cause of the condition in question 1 is
a. Sepsis.
b. Intracranial hypertension.
c. Ischemia-anoxia.
d. Abdominal trauma.

3. The diagnostic procedure of choice to evaluate the extent of the stress ulcers is
a. Abdominal computed tomography.
b. Evaluation of gastric pH.
c. Serial prothrombin times.
d. Endoscopy.

4. Interventions for treatment of stress ulcers should include
a. Maintenance of an alkaline gastric pH.
b. Initiation of ice water lavage.
c. Calculation of maintenance and deficit fluid requirements.
d. Monitoring peak, mean, and end-positive pressures.

5. The physician orders administration of antacids and an H_2-histamine blocker, cimetidine. The desired effect of cimetidine in the treatment of stress ulcers is to
a. Decrease gastric motility.
b. Increase gastric pH.
c. Prevent gastric reflux.
d. Enhance food absorption.

CASE 10-3

R., an 8-year-old girl who suffered blunt abdominal trauma from a soccer injury, is being transferred to the PICU from the general pediatric unit. She has been in the hospital for 24 hours without significant problems, but 2 hours ago, R. started to experience mild discomfort in her epigastric region, and the discomfort has increased in severity since then. R. rates her pain as 5 on a pain scale of 1 to 10. She is admitted to the PICU to assess the possibility of pancreatitis.

1. Acute pancreatitis can best be defined as
   a. Infection of the head of the pancreas.
   b. An autodigestive process.
   c. An overproduction of bile.
   d. Ischemia to the pancreas.

2. One of the most frequent causes of pancreatitis in children is
   a. Alcoholism.
   b. Gallstones.
   c. Blunt abdominal trauma.
   d. Vascular disease.

3. The nurse observes for a positive Cullen's sign in R., which is indicative of
   a. Impending disseminated intravascular coagulopathy.
   b. Hemorrhagic pancreatitis.
   c. Necrotic bowel process.
   d. Sepsis.

Laboratory tests reveal an amylase level of 325 Somogyi units/dL and a glucose concentration of 562 md/dL.

4. Hyperglycemia is caused by
   a. Dehydration leading to hyperconcentration of glucose.
   b. Fat necrosis.
   c. The starvation response.
   d. Hypersecretion of glycogen.

It has been 2 days since R. was transferred to the PICU, and her condition during that time has deteriorated. She has required oxygen by nasal cannula at 3 L/min and now has a central venous pressure line. Her condition is consistent with hypovolemia due to third spacing. Assessment reveals a heart rate of 170 bpm, respiratory rate of 53 breaths per minute, a central venous pressure of 5 mmHg, crackles in both lung fields, extremities that are cool to the touch, ascites, and a urine specific gravity greater than 1.028.

5. Third spacing in the patient with pancreatitis results from
   a. Release of pancreatic enzymes.
   b. Hemorrhagic process in the small bowel.
   c. Bowel necrosis.
   d. Azotemia.

6. Administration of fluids is anticipated. R. weighs 18 kg. The initial fluid bolus is
   a. 180 mL.
   b. 1000 mL.
   c. 500 mL.
   d. 360 mL.

7. R. is put on "pancreatic rest," which consists of no oral intake. The rationale for this is to
   a. Produce an ileus.
   b. Stop the release of cholecystokinin.
   c. Prevent bowel obstruction.
   d. Prevent bowel perforation.

8. R.'s pain is being controlled with meperidine. Opioids are contraindicated because
   a. They would blunt the signs of neurologic decompensation.
   b. They increase spasms in the sphincter of Oddi.
   c. The pain of pancreatitis is treated more effectively with antacids.
   d. Opioids alter the signs of duodenal perforation.

9. R. is ready to be transferred back to the ward. She is to receive 5% dextrose in 0.45% normal saline with 20 mEq/L of KCl at a maintenance rate. Based on her weight of 18 kg, what hourly rate is reported to the receiving nurse?
   a. 100 mL/hour.
   b. 18 mL/hour.
   c. 56 mL/hour.
   d. 150 mL/hour.

ANSWERS ■ CASE 10-1

1. Answer (c). Liver function tests are usually drawn at the time of admission and include transaminases and alkaline phosphatase. Transaminases increase with altered hepatocellular membrane integrity. Alkaline phosphatase of liver origin increases in response to extrahepatic or intrahepatic obstruction to bile flow.

REFERENCE
Rogers, M. (1992). *Handbook of pediatric intensive care* (2nd ed.). Baltimore: Williams & Wilkins.

2. Answer (**a**). Neither transaminases nor alkaline phosphatase define liver function. Liver function can be best determined by monitoring the levels of serum bilirubin and albumin and the prothrombin time, all of which are influenced by hepatocyte metabolism and thus reflect function.

REFERENCE

Rogers, M. (1992). *Handbook of pediatric intensive care* (2nd ed.). Baltimore: Williams & Wilkins.

3. Answer (**b**). The liver is essential to the process of carbohydrate metabolism. With hepatic failure, the liver is unable to store glycogen or generate new glucose. Hypoglycemia becomes a problem. Because glucose is the major nutrient for the brain, hypoglycemia further compromises cerebral function.

REFERENCES

Belknap, W.M. (1990). Acute hepatic failure. In D.L. Levine and F. Morriss (Eds.). *Essential aspects of pediatric intensive care* (pp. 137–143). St. Louis: Quality Medical Publishing.

Jakabowski, D.S., Harmon, T., Peck, S., & Stellar, J. (1996). Gastrointestinal critical care problems in infants and children. In M.A.Q. Curley, J.B. Smith, & P.A. Moloney-Harmon (Eds.). *Critical care nursing of infants and children* (pp. 724–755). Philadelphia: W.B. Saunders.

4. Answer (**a**). Fluid overload from the antidiuretic-like activity seen in patients with liver failure and intrapulmonary shunting due to the release of vasoactive products in liver failure may be responsible for the hypoxia seen in 40% to 60% of patients with hepatic failure.

REFERENCE

Rogers, M. (1992). *Handbook of pediatric intensive care* (2nd ed.). Baltimore: Williams & Wilkins.

5. Answer (**a**). Intubation is indicated for the development of respiratory failure. Intubation also facilitates hyperventilation if it is required to decrease intracranial pressure.

REFERENCE

Halpin, T.J. (1990). Acute hepatic failure. In J.L. Blumer (Ed.). *A practical guide to pediatric intensive care* (3rd ed., pp. 135–138). St. Louis: Mosby–Year Book.

6. Answer (**c**). Mitchell and colleagues (1985) conducted a study that examined the effects of touch on children with intracranial hypertension. They found that, because touch never increased the intracranial pressure to a life-threatening level, the fear of doing harm by gentle touch was not well founded. They suggested that nurses increase the amount of nonprocedural touch and encourage parents to touch their children.

REFERENCE

Mitchell, P.H., Habeem-Little, B., Johnson, F., et al. (1985). Critically ill children: The importance of touch in a high-technology environment. *Nursing Administration Quarterly, 9* (3), 38–46.

7. Answer (**a**). The use of barbiturates to produce a protective coma is controversial, because it is difficult to judge whether a good outcome is produced as the result of therapy. The concept underlying the use of barbiturates in brain injury is that cerebral metabolism is reduced, which may protect the brain. However, arterial hypotension and hemodynamic instability occur with barbiturate coma, and barbiturates may aggravate hepatic encephalopathy.

REFERENCES

Jakabowski, D.S., Harmon, T., Peck, S., & Stellar, J. (1996). Gastrointestinal critical care problems in infants and children. In M.A.Q. Curley, J.B. Smith, & P.A. Moloney-Harmon (Eds.). *Critical care nursing of infants and children* (pp. 724–755). Philadelphia: W.B. Saunders.

Rogers, M. (1992). *Handbook of pediatric intensive care* (2nd ed.). Baltimore: Williams & Wilkins.

8. Answer (**d**). Ammonia is absorbed by the blood into the portal vein and is detoxified by the liver. Blood ammonia levels can assist the nurse in evaluating the severity of coma and determining whether the patient is responding to treatment.

REFERENCE

Grant, M., & McFarland, M. (1982). *Nursing implications of laboratory tests* (pp. 216–218). New York: John Wiley & Sons.

9. Answer (**b**). Stress gastritis in patients with hepatic failure can be prevented by maintaining the gastric pH above 4.5. This level has been associated with a decrease in severe bleeding and mortality. Maintaining the gastric pH above 4.5 can be accomplished by H_2-receptor antagonists, antacids, or both and gentle nasogastric suction.

REFERENCE

Rogers, M. (1992). *Handbook of pediatric intensive care* (2nd ed.). Baltimore: Williams & Wilkins.

ANSWERS ■ CASE 10-2

1. Answer (b). Stress ulcers frequently occur in children who have experienced burns, severe head trauma, major surgical procedures, sepsis, multiple trauma, and respiratory failure.

REFERENCE

Jakabowski, D.S, Harmon, T., Peck, S., & Stellar, J. (1996). Gastrointestinal critical care problems in infants and children. In M.A.Q. Curley, J.B. Smith, & P.A. Moloney-Harmon (Eds.). *Critical care nursing of infants and children* (pp. 724–755). Philadelphia: W.B. Saunders.

2. Answer (c). Stress ulcers occur when the integrity of the mucosal cell membrane of the gastric mucosa is impaired. Mucosal ischemia due to impaired blood flow increases the membrane's susceptibility to damage by acid.

REFERENCE

Rogers, M. (1992). *Handbook of pediatric intensive care* (2nd ed.). Baltimore: Williams & Wilkins.

3. Answer (d). Endoscopy is often performed to locate, evaluate, and definitively treat the exact source if bleeding persists after lavage and antacid therapy.

REFERENCE

Hotter, A. (1990). The pathophysiology of multi-system organ failure in the trauma patient. *AACN Clinical Issues in Critical Care Nursing*, 1 (3), 465–476.

4. Answer (a). Maintaining an alkaline gastric environment through the administration of an antacid is indicated to prevent bleeding. Attention to nutrition early in the course of the illness also may play a role in the prevention of stress bleeding.

REFERENCE

Thelan, L., Davie, J., & Urden, L. (1990). *Textbook of critical care nursing: Diagnosis and management* (p. 694). St. Louis: Mosby–Year Book.

5. Answer (b). Cimetidine, a histamine H_2-receptor antagonist, predictably inhibits histamine-stimulated acid secretion.

REFERENCE

Chernow, B. *Essentials of critical care pharmacology* (2nd. ed., p. 384). Baltimore: Williams & Wilkins.

ANSWERS ■ CASE 10-3

1. Answer (b). Pancreatitis, which may be acute or chronic, is an autodigestive process that results from the release and activation of proteolytic enzymes in the pancreas or from the reflux of enzymes into the pancreas because of an obstruction. These digestive enzymes are normally inactive while in the pancreas and become active only in the small intestine. During pancreatitis, the enzymes are activated within the pancreas and begin the process of digestion before reaching the small intestine.

REFERENCES

Jakabowski, D.S., Harmon, T., Peck, S., & Stellar, J. (1996). Gastrointestinal critical care problems in infants and children. In M.A.Q. Curley, J.B. Smith, & P.A. Moloney-Harmon (Eds.). *Critical care nursing of infants and children* (pp. 724–755). Philadelphia: W.B. Saunders.
Thelan, L., Davie, J., & Urden, L. (1990). *Textbook of critical care nursing: Diagnosis and management* (pp. 695–696). St. Louis: Mosby–Year Book.

2. Answer (c). There are multiple causes of acute pancreatitis in children. One of the most frequent causes is blunt abdominal trauma.

REFERENCE

Jakabowski, D.S., Harmon, T., Peck, S., & Stellar, J. (1996). Gastrointestinal critical care problems in infants and children. In M.A.Q. Curley, J.B. Smith, & P.A. Moloney-Harmon (Eds.). *Critical care nursing of infants and children* (pp. 724–755). Philadelphia: W.B. Saunders.

3. Answer (b). In severe cases of hemorrhagic pancreatitis, the Gray-Turner sign (i.e., bluish discoloration of the flanks) or Cullen sign (i.e., bluish discoloration of the periumbilical area) may be seen.

REFERENCE

Walker, A., Durie, P., Hamilton, R., Walker-Smith, J., & Watkins, J. (1991). *Pediatric gastrointestinal disease: Pathophysiology, diagnosis, management* (p. 1218). Philadelphia: B.C. Decker.

4. Answer (d). Hyperglycemia often occurs early in the course of pancreatitis, because damaged pancreatic alpha cells release glucagon.

REFERENCE

Barnard, J.F., & Hazinski, M.F. (1992). Pediatric gastrointestinal disorders. In M.F. Hazinski (Ed.). *Nursing care of the critically ill child* (2nd ed., pp. 715–801). St. Louis: Mosby–Year Book.

5. Answer (a). Large amounts of fluid can be lost from the intravascular space into the peritoneal and pleural cavities because of the release of pancreatic enzymes, which can increase capillary permeability. The pancreatic enzymes may change pulmonary and peripheral capillary permeability, resulting in respiratory failure, peripheral edema, and the third spacing of fluid, leading to cardiovascular failure.

REFERENCE

Barnard, J.F., & Hazinski, M.F. (1992). Pediatric gastrointestinal disorders. In M.F. Hazinski (Ed.). *Nursing care of the critically ill child* (2nd ed., pp. 715–801). St. Louis: Mosby–Year Book.

6. Answer (**d**). Bolus fluid resuscitation therapy consists of 20 mL/kg of isotonic crystalloid solution administered as rapidly as possible (<20 minutes) immediately after intravenous or intraosseous access is obtained.

REFERENCE

Chaimedes, L., & Hazinski, M.F. (1994). *Pediatric advanced life support*. Dallas: American Heart Association.

7. Answer (**b**). Pancreatic rest, which usually entails keeping the patient off oral intake, is an effective therapy for the patient with pancreatitis. It is important to keep fat and protein out of the proximal bowel, because they cause the release of cholecystokinin, which leads to pancreatic enzyme release. This is extremely destructive to an already inflamed pancreas.

REFERENCE

Rogers, E.L., & Perman. J.A. (1992). Gastrointestinal and hepatic failure in the pediatric intensive care unit. In M. Rogers (Ed.). *Textbook of pediatric intensive care* (2nd ed., Vol. 2, pp. 1133–1158). Baltimore: Williams & Wilkins.

8. Answer (**b**). Pain relief is achieved with meperidine rather than opiates, because meperidine causes less spasm of the sphincter of Oddi.

REFERENCE

Thelan, D., Davie, J., & Urden, L. (1990). *Textbook of critical care nursing: Diagnosis and management* (p. 696). St. Louis: Mosby–Year Book.

9. Answer (**c**). The following recommendations are used to calculate daily fluid requirements:

4 mL/kg per hour for the first 10 kg of body weight, or 100 mL/kg per day

2 mL/kg per hour for the second 10 kg of body weight, or 50 mL/kg per day

1 mL/kg per hour for each additional 1 kg of body weight, or 20 mL/kg per day

R. weighs 18 kg, and the answer is calculated by this equation:

$$(4 \text{ mL/kg/hour} \times 10 \text{ kg}) + (2 \text{ mL/kg/hour} \times 8 \text{ kg}) = 40 + 16 = 56 \text{ mL/hour}.$$

REFERENCE

Johnson, K. (1993). Harriett Lane Handbook (13th ed., pp. 164–165). St. Louis: Mosby–Year Book.

CHAPTER *11*

Immunologic Disorders

JOYCE BANSBACH-BAILEY, RN, MSN

CASE 11-1

K. is an 8-month-old girl who was diagnosed at 1 month of age with congenital acute lymphocytic leukemia. K. received induction chemotherapy but relapsed 3 months later with central nervous system involvement. Another course of chemotherapy was begun that included intrathecal methotrexate and daily prednisone. Concurrently, a workup for a bone marrow transplantation was done, and a donor search was initiated. One month later, a bone marrow aspiration showed fewer than 5% blasts, and a related donor was identified who matched four of six human leukocyte antigen (HLA) types.

K. is being admitted into the transplant unit of the hospital, where she will undergo a conditioning regimen of high-dose cytosine arabinoside (ARA-C) and cyclophosphamide (Cytoxan) plus total body irradiation (TBI).

The primary nurse meets with K. and her parents for the initial assessment and education about K.'s treatment plan. K.'s physical assessment shows a 1.4-kg weight gain in the last 6 weeks and soft, spongy skin turgor.

1. This presentation reflects
   a. K.'s disease course.
   b. T cell proliferation.
   c. An increase in antidiuretic hormone.
   d. Extended steroid use.

2. Because K. will be undergoing chemotherapy and TBI, K.'s parents should be instructed about which of the following pre- and post-transplantation diagnostic tests for growth and development evaluation?

   a. Endocrinologic, pulmonary function, psychomotor, vision, and hearing tests.
   b. Endocrinologic and psychological tests.
   c. Renal and psychomotor tests.
   d. Endocrinologic, pulmonary function, and psychomotor tests.

3. K. will be undergoing an allogeneic transplantation. Because graft-versus-host disease (GVHD) is a common complication, which organs are expected to be primary targets initially?
   a. Skin, kidneys, and gut.
   b. Skin, kidneys, and liver.
   c. Skin, liver, and gut.
   d. Liver, gut, and kidneys.

4. Prophylactic drugs and other agents that may be used to prevent or lessen the effects of GVHD include
   a. T cell–depleted bone marrow, polyvalent intravenous immunoglobulin (IVIG), methotrexate, and antithymocyte globulin (ATG).
   b. T cell–depleted bone marrow, methotrexate, and ATG.
   c. Methotrexate, IVIG, and ATG.
   d. ATG, IVIG, and granulocyte colony-stimulating factor (G-CSF).

5. K. has a central line surgically placed, and her conditioning regimen is begun. As part of her conditioning regimen, she is placed in a totally protected environment. The components of this environment are
   a. Gut and skin decontamination, a laminar flow isolation room, sterile

supplies, and specialized nursing procedures.

    b. Gut and skin decontamination, good handwashing only for those entering the room, and sterile supplies.

    c. Low-microbial diet, removal of unwanted cell populations, specialized nursing procedures, and bathing.

    d. Low-microbial diet, restriction of all visitors, sterile supplies, and removal of unwanted cell populations.

6. Considering that K. is at high risk for infection, the nurse knows that the most appropriate interventions to decrease K.'s endogenous sources of infection include

    a. Antiviral prophylaxis, vaginal decontamination, nystatin mouthwashes, and antimicrobial baths.

    b. Antiviral prophylaxis, nystatin mouthwashes, and antimicrobial baths

    c. Nystatin mouthwashes, antimicrobial baths, and vaginal decontamination.

    d. Baths with antimicrobials.

K. will be placed in a private room with high-efficiency particulate air (HEPA) filtration, be placed in reverse isolation, and have gut decontamination.

7. The nurse discusses with K.'s family that the most important intervention for preventing transmission of infectious organisms is

    a. Adherence to reverse isolation.

    b. Strict handwashing.

    c. Continual HEPA filtration.

    d. Obtaining negative cultures after gut decontamination.

8. To prevent GVHD, K. is started on cyclosporine. The effects of cyclosporine are to

    a. Inhibit interleukin-2 production, which impairs helper and cytotoxic T cell activation and replication while sparing B lymphocytes.

    b. Suppress production of interleuken-4, which promotes production of helper T cells.

    c. Inhibit the production of complement cluster designation 8 (CD8) to suppress cytotoxic T cells and natural killer cells.

    d. Suppress mature T cell activation.

On day 5 before transplantation, K.'s white blood cell (WBC) count, red blood cell (RBC)

count, hemoglobin (Hbg) level, hematocrit (Hct), platelet (Plat) count, polymorphonuclear neutrophil (PMN) count, and immature neutrophil (Band) count are determined by a complete blood count (CBC). The results of the CBC analysis are

$$WBC: 1900/mm^3 \quad Plat: 18,000/mm^3$$
$$RBC: 2,320,000/ \quad PMN: 40\%$$
$$mm^3$$
$$Hct: 19.4\% \quad Band: 15\%$$
$$Hgb: 7.2 \text{ g/dL}$$

9. Based on these results, the nurse expects the following intervention:

    a. Packed RBCs and platelets.

    b. Irradiated packed RBCs and platelets.

    c. Cytomegalovirus (CMV)-negative, irradiated, packed RBCs and platelets.

    d. Platelets and a repeat CBC.

10. K.'s absolute neutrophil count is

    a. $105/mm^3$.

    b. $760/mm^3$.

    c. $1045/mm^3$.

    d. $1900/mm^3$.

11. Cytoxan is part of K.'s conditioning regimen. A major toxic effect of Cytoxan is hemorrhagic cystitis. Which of the following interventions may be implemented to maintain renal function?

    a. Encourage and increase oral fluids, maintain intake and output, and anchor the urinary catheter.

    b. Maintain strict intake and output and begin fluid restriction.

    c. Start intravenous fluids.

    d. Encourage and increase oral fluids, maintain intake and output, and start intravenous fluids.

12. On day 4 before transplantation, the nurse finds redness and swelling inside K.'s mouth. K. has been taking little food or fluids. Interventions to maintain K.'s nutritional status are

    a. Hyperalimentation, antiemetics, narcotic analgesics, and consultation with a child psychiatrist.

    b. Hyperalimentation, enteral feedings, antiemetics, and consultation with a child psychiatrist.

    c. Enteral feedings, antiemetics, and consultation with a dietitian.

    d. Hyperalimentation or enteral feedings, antiemetics, narcotic analgesics, and consultation with a dietitian.

13. Factors to be considered in K.'s hematopoietic recovery include
    a. Age, nutritional status, renal and hepatic functions, bone marrow functioning, and absence of infection.
    b. Age, nutritional status, disease state, absence of infection, and the chemotherapeutic agents previously received.
    c. Pretransplantation clinical status, family support, previous therapies, age, and cardiac function.
    d. Age, nutritional status, hepatic and renal function, family support, and the number of infections.

14. Bacteremia is a common complication in patients before and soon after transplantation. Common causative bacterial pathogens include all but
    a. *Staphylococcus epidermidis* and CMV.
    b. *Staphylococcus epidermidis, Klebsiella,* and *Pseudomonas.*
    c. *Klebsiella, Aspergillus,* and *Escherichia coli.*
    d. *Pseudomonas, Aspergillus,* and *Enterobacter.*

On day 2 after K.'s bone marrow infusion, she develops a temperature of 39.5°C.

15. What interventions should the nurse anticipate?
    a. Start antibiotics and obtain blood cultures.
    b. Obtain culture samples, including one from the central line, and start antibiotics.
    c. Start antibiotics only.
    d. Start antibiotics, obtain culture samples, and discontinue and culture a central line sample.

16. The nurse recognizes that normal inflammatory symptoms may not be present in immunosuppressed patients because of
    a. Neutropenia, preventing an immune response.
    b. Suppression of T cells.
    c. Delayed cell-mediated response.
    d. Hypoproduction of immunoglobulin G (IgG).

K. receives her bone marrow infusion, and on day 12 after transplantation, the nurse finds K. irritable and crying. The child has slight maculopapular rashes on the bottom of her feet. In a 3-hour period, K. has two large, watery, green stools. K.'s liver enzymes are slightly elevated.

17. The nurse recognizes that this may be indicative of
    a. Septicemia.
    b. Veno-occlusive disease.
    c. Neutropenia.
    d. GVHD.

K. is started on high-dose steroids. On day 15 after transplantation, K.'s stools have decreased, and the rash has resolved. K. has an absolute neutrophil count of 620 cells/mm³, and she is beginning to take small bites and small amounts of fluid orally. K. is receiving G-CSF.

18. The purpose of G-CSF is to
    a. Stimulate granulocytes, macrophages, and eosinophils.
    b. Stimulate proliferation and maturation of erythroid precursors.
    c. Stimulate granulocyte colonies.
    d. Stimulate macrophage precursors and colonies.

On day 20 after transplantation, K.'s absolute neutrophil count is 1540/mm³, and K. is orally taking 50% of her daily caloric requirement. A discharge conference with K.'s parents and the multidisciplinary team is scheduled. K.'s drug therapy at home will include cyclosporine, ganciclovir, trimethoprim-sulfamethoxazole (Bactrim), and IVIG.

19. This regimen helps to decrease the following post-transplantation risks:
    a. Chronic GVHD and CMV, *Aspergillus,* and herpesvirus infections.
    b. Chronic GVHD, CMV and *Aspergillus* infections, and restrictive lung disease.
    c. Acute GVHD, CMV infection, and pneumococcal sepsis.
    d. Chronic GVHD, CMV and herpesvirus infections, and pneumococcal sepsis.

20. Because K. will continue to be immunosuppressed after discharge, K.'s parents need to know that she must avoid
    a. Crowds, visitors, and those with a cold or fever.
    b. Crowds, visitors, those with a cold or fever, and those exposed to communicable diseases.
    c. Crowds, some visitors, those with a cold or fever, animals, and those exposed to communicable diseases.
    d. Crowds, those exposed to communi-

cable diseases, and those with a cold or fever.

21. K. will be receiving IVIG at home. The mode of action of IVIG is to
    a. Inhibit viral replication.
    b. Increase suppressor T cell activity.
    c. Inhibit cytotoxic T cell proliferation.
    d. Promote helper T cell proliferation.

CASE 11-2

Four-year-old S. is being admitted to the pediatric intensive care unit (PICU) with closed head injuries and possible abdominal injuries after a motor vehicle accident in which she was inadequately restrained. In the emergency room, S.'s modified Glasgow Coma scale score was 8. A computed tomography (CT) scan of the head shows a contralateral contusion, and a CT scan of the abdomen shows no abnormality. Roentgenography has ruled out cervical or other spinal injuries.

S. arrives in the PICU sedated and intubated. An intracranial pressure (ICP) monitor is placed, and the initial pressure reading is 14 to 17 mmHg. The PICU nurse's assessment of S. finds multiple superficial scalp and facial lacerations. S.'s Glasgow Coma scale score is 9, and the ICP value is 16 to 18 mmHg. Abdominal assessment reveals a soft, nontender abdomen with hypoactive bowel sounds. Breath sounds are clear, with a respiratory rate of 32. The apical heart rate is 120, and the cardiac monitor shows sinus tachycardia. The blood pressure is 90/50 mmHg, and her temperature is 37.4°C. A central line is placed; mannitol, steroids, and ranitidine are begun. Arterial blood gases, electrolytes, CBC, serum osmolality, urinalysis, and osmolality determinations are ordered. A nasogastric tube and urinary catheter are placed.

1. What age-related immunologic considerations should the nurse be aware of?
   a. Decreased immunity to bacteria, immature T cell function, and limited chemotactic activity.
   b. Inadequate endogenous antibody, immature granulocyte function, and limited opsonic activity.
   c. Increased immunity to common viruses and bacteria and immature B cell function.
   d. Decreased immunity to common viruses, immature development of T cell function, and inadequate endogenous antibody.

2. Which clinical features demonstrate respiratory tract host defenses compromised by intubation?
   a. Depressed cough reflex, decreased lymphatic flow, and increased secretions.
   b. Depressed cough reflex, atelectasis, and increased secretions.
   c. Depressed cough reflex, decreased cilia activity, and increased secretions.
   d. Depressed cough reflex, increased cilia activity, and increased secretions.

3. The nurse initiates which interventions to support S.'s respiratory defenses while preventing intracranial hypertension?
   a. Suctioning every 2 hours, turning on a regular schedule, and aggressive pulmonary toilet.
   b. Suctioning as needed, with frequent assessment of respiratory status and chest physical therapy every 4 hours.
   c. Suctioning and chest physical therapy every 2 hours, with the head of the bed elevated 30 degrees.
   d. Maintaining the head of the bed at 30 degrees, straight-head alignment, frequent assessment of respiratory status, and suctioning as needed.

S. maintains a stable ICP, and nasogastric tube feedings are begun. The nurse notices fine, scattered rales bilaterally, and she observes that the oxygen saturation of arterial blood (SaO_2) has dropped from 99% to 93% during the last 20 minutes. S.'s temperature has risen from 37.3 to 38.2°C. The intake and output balance is positive at 130 mL. Laboratory values include a creatinine (Cr) concentration of 0.4 mg/dL and blood urea nitrogen (BUN) level of 18 mg/dL.

4. What interventions should the nurse anticipate?
   a. Obtain a chest x-ray, determine arterial blood gases, increase the fraction of inspired oxygen (FIO_2), and administer diuretics.
   b. Obtain a chest x-ray, determine arterial blood gases, increase the FIO_2, and obtain sputum for culture and sensitivity testing.

c. Obtain a chest x-ray, determine arterial blood gases, increase the F_{IO_2}, obtain sputum for culture and sensitivity testing, and administer diuretics.
d. Obtain a chest x-ray, determine arterial blood gases and electrolyte levels, increase intravenous fluids, and obtain sputum for culture and sensitivity testing.

S.'s Sao_2 returns to 98%. The arterial blood gas determinations include the hydrogen ion concentration (pH), partial pressures of oxygen (Po_2) and carbon dioxide (Pco_2), and bicarbonate (HCO_3^-) level:

Po_2: 83 mmHg   pH: 7.36
Pco_2: 33 mmHg HCO_3^-: 23 mEq/L

Her chest x-ray shows fluffy infiltrates. S. is initially diagnosed with nosocomial pneumonia.

5. Predisposing risk factors for the development of nosocomial pneumonia in S. include
   a. Age, depressed level of consciousness, and central line placement.
   b. Depressed level of consciousness, intracranial monitoring, and large-volume aspiration.
   c. Depressed consciousness, mechanical ventilation, and frequent suctioning.
   d. Depressed consciousness, intracranial monitoring, mechanical ventilation, and H_2 blockers.

6. The primary bacterial organisms identified in nosocomial pneumonias are
   a. Gram-positive enteric bacilli.
   b. Gram-negative enteric bacilli.
   c. Gram-positive cocci.
   d. Gram-negative cocci.

7. Initial treatment of nosocomial pneumonia includes which classification(s) of antibiotics?
   a. Aminoglycoside and third-generation cephalosporin.
   b. Aminoglycoside only.
   c. Penicillin.
   d. First-generation cephalosporin.

8. S.'s nosocomial pneumonia probably resulted from
   a. Nasopharyngeal colonization.
   b. Colonization through direct contact.
   c. Gastric colonization, oropharyngeal colonization, or both.
   d. Colonization from immunosuppression.

The nurse reviews S.'s daily CBC and electrolyte results and finds the following:

Na^+: 137 mEq/L	Cr: 0.3 mg/dL
K^+: 3.3 mEq/L	Hgb: 8.7 g/dL
Cl^-: 100 mEq/L	Hct: 30%
CO_2: 23 mEq/L	RBC: 3,200,000/mm^3
Ca^{2+}: 9 mEq/L	WBC: 16,500/mm^3
Glu: 92 mg/dL	Plat: 170,000/mm^3
BUN: 12 mg/dL	

9. What interventions can be expected based on these laboratory values?
   a. Administration of whole blood and a potassium chloride (KCl) bolus.
   b. Administration of packed RBCs and addition of KCl to the intravenous fluids.
   c. Administration of packed RBCs and KCl piggyback.
   d. Increase of intravenous fluids and administration of packed RBCs and platelets.

On day 5 of hospitalization, S.'s ICP readings have been stable, and her monitor is removed. The arterial blood gas results for the morning are

Po_2: 92 mmHg   pH: 7.40
Pco_2: 34 mmHg HCO_3^-: 24 mEq/L

Weaning from the ventilator is begun.
   The nurse notices that S.'s urine is slightly cloudy and has a small amount of sediment. S. has had a low-grade temperature for the last 2 days. The nurse suspects the S. may have a urinary tract infection (UTI).

10. What intervention(s) should the nurse take?
    a. Obtain a urinalysis and culture and sensitivity testing.
    b. Irrigate the catheter and replace it if needed.
    c. Manipulate the catheter to ensure patency.
    d. Increase intravenous fluids and maintain accurate intake and output.

11. The bacterial pathogens most likely responsible for S.'s UTI are
    a. Gram-negative bacilli.
    b. Gram-positive cocci.
    c. Gram-positive bacilli.
    d. Gram-negative cocci.

12. The antibiotic classes most effective for

treatment of pediatric nosocomial UTI include

a. Cephalosporins, aminoglycosides, quinolones, and penicillins.
b. Cephalosporins, quinolones, and β-lactamase inhibitors.
c. Aminoglycosides, β-lactamase inhibitors, and quinolones.
d. Cephalosporins, aminoglycosides, and β-lactamase inhibitors.

On day 7 of S.'s hospitalization, she is successfully weaned from the ventilator and extubated. Her neurologic status is stable, with a Glasgow Coma scale score of 14, but she continues to be intermittently confused. S.'s nasogastric tube is discontinued, and she is started on a liquid diet. Plans are begun for transfer to the step-down unit.

CASE 11-3

J. is a 5-month-old boy who was referred from the community health center to the community hospital's emergency room. Information from the community health center indicates that J.'s mother brought him to the clinic because he was taking only small amounts of formula and he had increased diarrhea for the last 2 days. Clinic notes indicate that J.'s mother may be infected with the human immunodeficiency virus (HIV).

On assessment, the nurse finds J. underweight, with poor skin turgor and whitish patches in his mouth. His respiratory rate is 42 breaths per minute, pulse is 136, and temperature is 38.5°C. J. is alert but irritable. A CBC, urinalysis, electrolyte determination, chest x-ray, blood cultures, stool culture, and culture for HIV are ordered. After blood samples are drawn for testing, intravenous fluids and antibiotics are started. J. is admitted to the floor. A few days later, the results of HIV testing return positive. J. is begun on zidovudine.

1. The type of HIV testing in infants and newborns is important, because some HIV tests result in
   a. A false-positive result because of passive maternal IgG antibody transfer.
   b. A false-negative result because of passive maternal IgG antibody transfer.
   c. A false-positive result because of passive maternal IgM antibody transfer.
   d. A false-positive result because of passive maternal antigen transfer.

2. The pathology of immunocompromise by the HIV virus reflects
   a. Viral cytotoxicity of suppressor T cells.
   b. Viral cytotoxicity of helper T cells.
   c. Autoimmune response to host antigens.
   d. Autoimmune response to cytotoxic T cells.

3. One of the primary symptoms of HIV-infected children that J. presents with is
   a. Diarrhea.
   b. CMV pneumonia.
   c. Failure to thrive.
   d. Oral candidiasis.

4. Zidovudine acts primarily by
   a. Inhibiting attachment of HIV virions to complement cluster designation 4 (CD4).
   b. Providing a virostatic effect against retroviruses.
   c. Stimulating production of helper T cells, which interact with macrophages.
   d. Inhibiting replication of viral DNA.

The next day, J.'s respiratory rate increases to 44, with increased respiratory effort and decreased breath sounds bilaterally. The SaO_2 drops to 82% to 84%. An immediate chest x-ray and arterial blood gas determination are ordered. Oxygen is begun to keep the SaO_2 above 95%. The chest x-ray shows bilateral infiltrates, and the arterial blood gas results are

PO_2: 75 mmHg   pH: 7.33
PCO_2: 46 mmHg HCO_3^-: 22 mEq/L

J. is transferred to the PICU, where bronchoscopy with lavage is done. J.'s respiratory status continues to deteriorate, and he is intubated and mechanically ventilated with positive end-expiratory pressure.

5. Interventions to decrease nosocomial infections and prevent further respiratory compromise include
   a. Maintaining an alkaline stomach pH.
   b. Pulmonary toileting using aseptic technique.
   c. Suctioning every hour.
   d. Limiting mobility.

Pneumocystis carinii is cultured from J.'s bronchoalveolar washings. J. is started on steroids and trimethoprim-sulfamethoxazole. After several days, J.'s respiratory status improves, and he is weaned from the ventilator. As his respiratory function becomes stronger, J. is transferred to the floor, and discharge planning is begun.

ANSWERS ■ CASE 11-1

1. Answer (**d**). Extended or long-term steroid use increases appetite and fluid retention, resulting in weight gain, fluid retention, and a cushingoid appearance.

REFERENCES

Brown, J.K., & Hagan, C.M. (1990). Chemotherapy. In S.L. Groenwald, M.H. Frogge, M. Goodman, et al. (Eds.). *Cancer nursing* (pp. 230–283). Boston: Jones & Bartlett Publishers.

Lyons, M. (1993). Immunosuppressive therapy after cardiac transplantation: Teaching pediatric patients and their families. *Critical Care Nurse,* 13 (1), 39–45.

2. Answer (**c**). Late effects of chemotherapy and TBI may affect many body systems, but TBI used in conditioning regimens causes abnormalities and slowing of growth rates. K.'s parents should be counseled about the endocrinologic and psychomotor testing that is completed before and after transplantation.

REFERENCES

Moore, I.M., & Ruccione, K. (1990). Late effects of cancer treatment. In S.L. Groenwald (Ed.). *Cancer nursing* (pp. 669–685). Boston: Jones & Bartlett Publishers.

Ostroff, J.S., & Lesko, L.M. (1991). Psychosexual adjustment and fertility issues. In M.B. Whedon (Ed.). *Bone marrow transplantation* (pp. 312–333). Boston: Jones & Bartlett Publishers.

3. Answer (**c**). The epithelium of the skin, gastrointestinal tract and hepatic biliary ducts, and lymphoid system are immediate targets. The reason for this targeting is unknown.

REFERENCE

Caudell, K.A. (1991). Graft-versus-host disease. In M.B. Whedon (Ed.) *Bone marrow transplantation* (pp. 160–181). Boston: Jones & Bartlett Publishers.

4. Answer (**b**). All of the drugs except IVIG can be used individually or in combinations to prevent GVHD. IVIG is used to provide immunoglobulin protection for immunosuppressed patients.

REFERENCES

Caudell, K.A. (1991). Graft-versus-host disease. In M.B. Whedon (Ed.). *Bone marrow transplantation* (pp. 160–181). Boston: Jones & Bartlett Publishers.

NIH Consensus Conference. (1990). Intravenous immunoglobulin: Prevention and treatment of disease. *Journal of the American Medical Association,* 264 (124), 3189–3193.

5. Answer (**a**). The goal of the totally protected environment is to eradicate the normal microbial flora and to prevent colonization by new microorganisms from the hospital environment. This type of environment includes several components. *Gut and skin decontamination* reduces endogenous normal flora that may serve as a source on infection. Gut decontamination is accomplished by a sterile or low-microbial diet and by administration of oral nonabsorbable antibiotics and an antifungal agent. Skin decontamination is achieved with a daily bath with an antimicrobial solution and application of antibiotic solutions and creams to body surfaces, where microbes may exist. A *laminar flow isolation room* makes the air in the room essentially microbe free. *Sterile supplies* augment the protected environment. *Specialized nursing procedures* help to maintain the environment, because this type of environment requires a strict protocol of care. An allied component of these procedures is minimizing the stress of this environment on the child and family. Because data show that this type of environment does not improve long-term survival, most bone marrow transplantation centers use the totally protected environment for selected groups of patients.

REFERENCES

Frederick, B., & Hanigan, M.J. (1993). Bone marrow transplantation. In G.V. Foley, D. Fochtman, & K.H. Mooney (Eds.). *Nursing care of the child with cancer* (pp. 130–177). Philadelphia: W.B. Saunders.

Mooney, B.R., Reeves, S.A., & Larson, E. (1993). Infection control and bone marrow transplantation. *American Journal of Infection Control,* 21 (6), 131–138.

Poe, S.S., Larson, E., McGuire, D., et al. (1994). A national survey of infection prevention practices on bone marrow transplant units. *Oncology Nursing Forum,* 21 (10), 1687–1694.

6. Answer (**b**). Antiviral prophylaxis prevents reactivation of herpes simplex virus and decreases the incidence and severity of CMV. Nystatin is used to prevent or decrease the incidence and severity of candidiasis. Baths with antimicrobials decrease the amount of normal skin flora that may become infectious in a neutropenic state. Vaginal decontamination may be used for menarcheal women, but it is not appropriate for children unless there is a history of vaginal infections.

REFERENCES

Caudell, K.A., & Whedon, M.B. (1991). Hematopoietic complications. In M.B. Whedon (Ed.). *Bone marrow* transplantation (pp. 135–159). Boston: Jones & Bartlett Publishers.

Poe, S.S., Larson, E., McGuire, D., et al. (1994). A national survey of infection prevention practices on bone marrow transplant units. *Oncology Nursing Forum,* 21 (10), 1687–1694.

7. Answer (**b**). Handwashing is the single most effective intervention for preventing infection.

REFERENCE

Poe, S.S., Larson, E., McGuire, D., et al. (1994). A national survey of infection prevention practices on bone marrow transplant units. *Oncology Nursing Forum,* 21 (10), 1687–1694.

8. Answer (**a**). Cyclosporine inhibits production of interleukin-2, which suppresses cytotoxic and helper T cells while sparing B lymphocytes.

REFERENCES

Lyons, M. (1993). Immunosuppressive therapy after cardiac transplantation: Teaching pediatric patients and their families. *Critical Care Nurse,* 13 (1), 39–45.
Payne, J.L. (1992). Immune modification and complications of immunosuppression. *Critical Care Nursing Clinics of North America,* 4 (1), 43–57.

9. Answer (**c**). Maintenance of the hemoglobin and platelet levels is critical for engraftment support and immune system recovery. RBCs are irradiated to inactivate contaminating lymphocytes that may cause GVHD. CMV-negative blood products are administered to decrease the risk of CMV infections.

REFERENCE

Caudell, K.A., & Whedon, M.B. (1991). Hematopoietic complications. In M.B. Whedon (Ed.). *Bone marrow transplantation* (pp. 135–159). Boston: Jones & Bartlett Publishers.

10. Answer (**c**). The absolute neutrophil count is found by multiplying the total WBC count (1900 cells/mm^3) by the percentage of PMNs (40%) plus the percentage of bands (15%), or a total of 55%: 1900 cells/mm^3 × 0.55 = 1045 cells/mm^3.

REFERENCE

Klemm, P.R., & Hubbard, S.M. (1990). Infection. In S.L. Groenwald, M.H. Frogge, M. Goodman, et al. (Eds.). *Cancer nursing* (pp. 442–466). Boston: Jones and Bartlett Publishers.

11. Answer (**d**). Oral fluids and intravenous hydration increase diuresis. Maintenance of strict intake and output assists in managing fluid therapy to maintain adequate output. Placement of a catheter is unnecessary unless there is urinary retention.

REFERENCE

Whedon, M.B. (1991). Allogeneic bone marrow transplantation: Clinical indications, treatment process, and outcomes. In M.B. Whedon (Ed.). *Bone marrow transplantation* (pp. 20–48). Boston: Jones & Bartlett Publishers.

12. Answer (**d**). Nutritional support may be provided by hyperalimentation or enteral feedings. Antiemetics assist in relieving nausea and vomiting and therefore support continued nutritional intake. Analgesics relieve the pain associated with mucositis. A dietary consultation and calorie count are needed to assess daily nutritional requirements and adjust total parenteral nutrition, enteral feedings, or both.

REFERENCE

Buchsel, P.C. (1990). Bone marrow transplantation. In S.L. Groenwald, M.H. Frogge, M. Goodman, et al. (Eds.). *Cancer nursing* (pp. 307–337). Boston: Jones and Bartlett Publishers.

13. Answer (**a**). All of the listed factors correlate with hematopoietic recovery.

REFERENCE

Caudell, K.A., & Whedon, M.B. (1991). Hematopoietic complications. In M.B. Whedon (Ed.). *Bone marrow transplantation* (pp. 135–159). Boston: Jones & Bartlett Publishers.

14. Answer (**b**). The primary causative organisms are bacterial and are commonly an infectious problem during the neutropenic period. CMV is a viral agent. *Aspergillus* is a fungal organism that causes aspergillosis, a condition immunosuppressed patients are at risk for during their prolonged periods of granulocytopenia.

REFERENCE

Press, O.W., Schaller, R.T., & Thomas, E.D. (1987). Bone marrow transplant complications. In L.H. Toledo-Pereyra (Ed.). *Complications of organ transplantation* (pp. 399–426). New York: Marcel Dekker.

15. Answer (**b**). Infections in neutropenic patients can be life threatening and should be treated aggressively. Samples for cultures are obtained, including those from any invasive lines. Because fever may be nonspecific, pulling the central line is not appropriate until culture results are obtained.

REFERENCE

Caudell, K.A., & Whedon, M.B. (1991). Hematopoietic complications. In M.B. Whedon (Ed.). *Bone marrow transplantation* (pp. 135–159). Boston: Jones & Bartlett Publishers.

16. Answer (**a**). Neutropenia prevents normal expression of typical signs of infection. Subsequently, redness, pus formation, and an elevated WBC count are absent or present atypically.

REFERENCES

Buchsel, P.C. (1990). Bone marrow transplantation. In S.L. Groenwald, M.H. Frogge, M. Goodman, et al. (Eds.). *Cancer nursing* (pp. 307–337). Boston: Jones and Bartlett Publishers.
Caudell, K.A., & Whedon, M.B. (1991). Hematopoietic complications. In M.B. Whedon (Ed.). *Bone marrow transplantation* (pp. 135–159). Boston: Jones & Bartlett Publishers.

17. Answer (**d**). A maculopapular rash on the trunk, soles, palms, and ears accompanied by watery stools and elevated levels of liver enzymes are cardinal signs of GVHD. Elevated levels of liver enzymes and an elevated alkaline phosphatase concentration are also early symptoms of veno-occlusive disease, but they are usually accompanied by hepatomegaly, right upper quadrant pain, and jaundice.

REFERENCES

Buchsel, P.C. (1990). Bone marrow transplantation. In S.L. Groenwald, M.H. Frogge, M. Goodman, et al. (Eds.). *Cancer nursing* (pp. 307–337). Boston: Jones & Bartlett Publishers.
Press, O.W., Schaller, R.T., & Thomas, E.D. (1987). Bone marrow transplant complications. In L.H. Toledo-Pereyra (Ed.). *Complications of organ transplantation* (pp. 399–426). New York: Marcel Dekker.

18. Answer (**c**). Growth factors are needed to stimulate proliferation of progenitor cells and activity of mature cells. Different growth factors act more specifically on certain cell types. G-CSF stimulates granulocyte colonies, granulocyte-macrophage CSF stimulates granulocyte-macrophage and eosinophil colonies, macrophage CSF stimulates macrophage precursors and colonies. Erythropoietin increases RBC production through stimulation and maturation of erythroid precursors.

REFERENCE

Ommann, A.J. (1990). Biologic and immunomodulating factors in the treatment of pediatric-acquired immunodeficiency syndrome. *Pediatric Infectious Disease Journal*, 9 (12), 894–904.

19. Answer (**d**). Cyclosporine is used to control GVHD. Ganciclovir is prophylaxis for CMV. Acyclovir prevents reactivation of a herpesvirus infection. Trimethoprim-sulfamethoxazole provides protection from pneumococcal pneumonia. IVIG provides exogenous humoral antibody support while the patient is immunosuppressed. There is no prophylaxis for aspergillosis. Steroids are most often used in conjunction with cyclosporine for acute GVHD.

REFERENCES

Mooney, B.R., Reeves, S.A., & Larson, E. (1993). Infection control and bone marrow transplantation. *American Journal of Infection Control*, 21 (6), 131–138.
Mudge-Grout, C.L. (1994). Immunoglobulin therapy. In S. Schrefer (Ed.). *Immunologic disorders* (pp. 314–348). St. Louis: Mosby–Year Book.

20. Answer (**c**). Because K.'s immune system will take 6 to 12 months to recover, special precautions should be taken to decrease K.'s exposure to potentially infectious organisms. Visitors should be allowed, but the number should be limited. Anyone with a cold or fever or those who have been exposed to any communicable disease should be avoided. Pets and animals should also be avoided during this time.

REFERENCES

Bone Marrow Transplant Unit of All Children's Hospital (1992). *Discharge teaching tool*. St. Petersburg, FL: All Children's Hospital.
Buchsel, P.C. (1991). Ambulatory care: Before and after BMT. In M.B. Whedon (Ed.). *Bone marrow transplantation* (pp. 296–311). Boston: Jones & Bartlett Publishers.

21. Answer (**b**). IVIG has been found to increase T cell activity, decreasing the incidence and severity of CMV infections, interstitial pneumonia, and bacterial infections.

REFERENCES

Rechewi, G., & Mandel, M. (1993). Principles of autoimmunity in pediatric practice. In Z. Spirer, C.M. Roifman, & D. Branski (Eds.). *Pediatric immunology* (pp. 28–47). Farmington, CT: S. Karger.
Poe, S.S., Larson, E., McGuire, D., et al. (1994). A national survey of infection prevention practices on bone marrow transplant units. *Oncology Nursing Forum*, 21 (10), 1687–1694.

ANSWERS ■ CASE 11-2

1. Answer (**d**). In early childhood, the child has had limited exposure to organisms. If the child has not been previously exposed to the organism, it is not seen as foreign, and an immune response is not mounted against it. T cell function and endogenous antibody production is not yet fully developed.

REFERENCES

Hazinski, M.F. (1992). Children are different. In M.F. Hazinski (Ed.). *Nursing care of the critically ill child* (pp. 1–17). St. Louis: Mosby–Year Book.

Rosenthal, C.H., & Allen, M. (1996). In M.A.Q. Curley, J.B. Smith, & P.A. Moloney-Harmon (Eds.). *Critical care nursing of infants and children*. Philadelphia: W.B. Saunders.

2. Answer (**c**). The endotracheal tube prevents normal cough reflexes while also decreasing cilia activity. The endotracheal tube also becomes an irritant to the respiratory tract, which increases mucus production. Mucus carries phagocytized cells that are expelled through cilia activity and coughing. Because these defenses are altered by intubation, the secretions pool and become instead a reservoir for bacterial growth.

REFERENCE

Stacy, K.M. (1994). Pulmonary disorders. In L.A. Thelan, J.K. Davie, L.D. Urden, & M.E. Laugh (Eds.). *Critical care nursing* (pp. 413–435). St. Louis: Mosby–Year Book.

3. Answer (**d**). S.'s airway should be kept clear for optimal oxygenation, but because intracranial hypertension must be prevented, suctioning should be done only as needed. Frequent respiratory assessment can identify when suctioning is needed. Keeping the head of the bed at 30 degrees, with straight alignment of the patient, assists in preventing intracranial hypertension and assists with good diaphragmatic expansion.

REFERENCES

Cox, S.A. (1994). Pediatric trauma: Special patients/special needs. *Critical Care Nursing Quarterly,* 17 (2), 51–61.

Johnson, K.L. (1994). Trauma. In L.A. Thelan, J.K. Davie, L.D. Urden, & M.E. Laugh (Eds.). *Critical care nursing* (pp. 729–765). St. Louis: Mosby–Year Book.

4. Answer (**b**). A chest x-ray, arterial blood gas determinations, and sputum culture assist in determining the definitive diagnosis and further treatment course. The FIO_2 should be increased until the underlying reason for decompensation has been diagnosed. Changes in SaO_2 and the presence of rales and increased temperature indicate possible respiratory infection. S.'s fluid balance should be carefully monitored, but at this point, she does not require diuretics and can instead depend on normal renal functioning.

REFERENCE

Few, B. (1996). Pulmonary critical care problems. In M.A.Q. Curley, J.B. Smith, & P.A. Moloney-Harmon (Eds.). *Critical care nursing of infants and children* (pp. 619–655). Philadelphia: W.B. Saunders.

5. Answer (**d**). Predisposing factors include depressed consciousness, intracranial monitoring, mechanical ventilation, frequent ventilator circuit changes, large-volume aspiration, chest surgery, chronic lung disease, and advanced age (≥70 years). H_2 blockers create an alkaline environment in the upper gastrointestinal tract that allows colonization from the lower gastrointestinal tract. Subsequent aspiration or reflux predisposes the patient to pneumonia.

REFERENCE

McRaney, S., & Rapp, R. (1993). Antibiotic agents in critical care. *Critical Care Nursing Clinics of North America,* 5 (2), 313–323.

6. Answer (**b**). The primary bacterial pathogens found in more than one half of nosocomial pneumonia cases are gram-negative enteric bacilli.

REFERENCE

McRaney, S., & Rapp, R. (1993). Antibiotic agents in critical care. *Critical Care Nursing Clinics of North America,* 5 (2), 313–323.

7. Answer (**a**). Empiric therapy is started while awaiting the culture and sensitivity reports to cover aerobic gram-negative bacilli. Combination therapy is used to prevent resistance.

REFERENCE

McRaney, S., & Rapp, R. (1993). Antibiotic agents in critical care. *Critical Care Nursing Clinics of North America,* 5 (2), 313–323.

8. Answer (**c**). Gastric acidity is a normal defense of the gastrointestinal tract. When the pH of the stomach becomes more alkaline, as during nasogastric suctioning, the risk of colonization from the lower gastrointestinal tract is increased. Mechanically ventilated patients are at risk for oropharyngeal colonization from humidified oxygen and tubing.

REFERENCE

McRaney, S., & Rapp, R. (1993). Antibiotic agents in critical care. *Critical Care Nursing Clinics of North America, 5* (2), 313–323.

9. Answer (**b**). Because S.'s potassium is not seriously below normal, additional potassium can be added to the intravenous fluids. Packed RBCs are given to increase hemoglobin while limiting additional volume administration. Bolus potassium administration should be avoided, because it may produce arrhythmias or cardiac arrest.

REFERENCES

Hazinski, M.F. (1992). Cardiovascular disorders. In M.F. Hazinski (Ed.). *Nursing care of the critically ill child* (pp. 117–194). St. Louis: Mosby–Year Book.
Luban, N. (1992). Basics of transfusion medicine. In B.P. Fuhrman & J.J. Zimmerman (Eds.). *Pediatric critical care* (pp. 829–840). St. Louis: Mosby–Year Book.

10. Answer (**a**). Catheterization is a risk factor for the colonization of bacterial pathogens. A urinalysis with culture and sensitivity testing can definitively diagnose the causative organism of the UTI. Because the catheter is draining properly without clots, the closed system should not be opened for irrigation. Accurate intake and output should be maintained, but increasing the intravenous fluids at this time is not indicated.

REFERENCE

Skippen, P., Cox, P., Langley, J., et al. (1992). Nosocomial infections in the PICU: Epidemiology and control. In B.P. Fuhrman & J.J. Zimmerman (Eds.). *Pediatric critical care* (pp. 965–988). St. Louis: Mosby–Year Book.

11. Answer (**a**). The gram-negative bacilli most commonly identified in UTI infections are *E. coli, Pseudomonas, Enterobacter,* and *Klebsiella.*

REFERENCE

McRaney, S., & Rapp, R. (1993). Antibiotic agents in critical care. *Critical Care Nursing Clinics of North America, 5* (2), 313–323.

12. Answer (**d**). Culture and sensitivity reports provide the definitive diagnostic tool to determine specific antibiotic treatment. The antibiotic groups most effective in treating pediatric patients'

UTIs from gram-negative bacilli through single or combination therapy include cephalosporins, β-lactamase inhibitors, aminoglycosides, and extended-spectrum penicillins. Quinolones are often used in adult populations but are contraindicated in pediatric patients because of possible arthropathy.

REFERENCE

Schell, K.H. (1993). Current trends in antimicrobial therapy for the critically ill patient. *Critical Care Nursing Quarterly, 15* (4), 23–32.

ANSWERS ■ CASE 11-3

1. Answer (**a**). HIV culture testing is necessary in children younger than 18 months of age, because passive transfer of maternal IgG antibody renders standard HIV antibody tests falsely positive.

REFERENCES

Church, J.A. (1993). Clinical aspects of HIV infection in children. *Pediatric Annals, 22* (7), 417–427.
Francis, B. (1994). The incidence of HIV/AIDS in children and their care needs. *Nursing Times, 90* (26), 47–49.

2. Answer (**b**). The HIV virus attaches itself to CD4 on the surface of helper T cells and with virus-specific reverse transcriptase enters the target cell's cytoplasm.

REFERENCES

Church, J.A. (1993). Clinical aspects of HIV infection in children. *Pediatric Annals, 22* (7), 417–427.
Czarniecki, L., & Dillman, P. (1992). Pediatric HIV/AIDS. *Critical Care Nursing Clinics of North America, 4* (3), 447–456.

3. Answer (**c**). HIV-infected children may have a history of bacterial or opportunistic infections, but instead of manifesting other symptoms, they may present with failure to thrive. Failure to thrive is universally seen in HIV-infected children.

REFERENCES

Landor, M., & Rubinstein, A. (1993). Human immunodeficiency virus infection in children. In Z. Spirer, C.M. Roifman, & D. Branski (Eds.). *Pediatric immunology* (pp. 102–130). Farmington: S. Karger.
Czarniecki, L., & Dillman, P. (1992). Pediatric HIV/AIDS. *Critical Care Nursing Clinics of North America, 4* (3), 447–456.

4. Answer (**b**). Zidovudine inhibits replication of retroviruses by interfering with viral RNA-directed DNA polymerase.

REFERENCE

American Hospital Formulary Service (1994). *AHFS drug information* (pp. 438–448). Bethesda, MD: American Society of Hospital Pharmacists.

5. Answer (**b**). Proper technique in pulmonary toileting removes secretions and improves alveolar oxygenation while preventing transmission of infectious organisms. Alkaline gut pH encourages colonization from the lower gastrointestinal tract, and immobility increases the risk of pneumonia. Hourly suctioning may be necessary but is probably overzealous.

REFERENCES

Czarniecki, L., & Dillman, P. (1992). Pediatric HIV/ AIDS. *Critical Care Nursing Clinics of North America, 4* (3), 447–456.

Church, J.A. (1993). Clinical aspects of HIV infection in children. *Pediatric Annals, 22* (7), 417–427.

CHAPTER *12*

Oncologic Disorders

LINDA OAKES, RN, MSN, CCRN

CASE 12-1

J., a 4-year-old boy, has been admitted to the intensive care unit (ICU) for possible dialysis. He has a probable diagnosis of acute lymphoblastic leukemia. The results of an aspirate of J.'s bone marrow reported by his referring physician indicate that 89% of his cells are blasts (i.e., immature blood cells). On admission to the ICU, his temperature is 36.6°C, heart rate is 109 beats per minute (bpm), respiratory rate is 24 breaths per minute, and blood pressure is 116/70 mmHg. The physical examination reveals that J. is a well-nourished, pale, and mildly ill–appearing child. The nurse notices that he has anterior cervical adenopathy and scattered ecchymoses across his trunk. Auscultation of his lung sounds reveals diminished breath sounds on the right side. The nurse also observes that he has hepatosplenomegaly and is grunting with respirations. His history is negative for hematuria, bleeding, fevers, headaches, or neurologic problems. The chest x-ray film reveals that J. has a mediastinal mass and a large right pleural effusion.

In the emergency room, he has been unable to urinate for more than 6 hours, and after a urinary catheter is placed in J. in the ICU, 30 mL of urine is obtained. His laboratory results from the emergency room analysis include a white blood cell (WBC) count of 220,000/mm³, a hemoglobin concentration of 9.2 g/dL, and a platelet count of 59,000/mm³. The results of his blood chemistry tests are compared with normal values in Table 12–1.

1. J. is exhibiting clinical features caused by tumor lysis syndrome, which is associated with
   a. Slow-growing tumors.
   b. Cancers resistant to chemotherapy and radiation therapy.
   c. Coagulation defects at the time of diagnosis.
   d. Products of cell degradation collected in the renal tubules from fast-growing tumors.

2. Reviewing his laboratory results, the nurse notices hyperuricemia, hyperkalemia, hyperphosphatemia, and hypocalcemia. These findings are related to the tumor lysis syndrome because
   a. The intracellular potassium, phosphates, and purines are being released into the blood as the large number of cells die.
   b. Hepatosplenomegaly causes a variety of these imbalances, including those seen in J.
   c. The blast cells kill the healthy cells, which release urate, potassium, and phosphorus.
   d. These imbalances are commonly seen in children with cancer.

3. J.'s electrocardiographic pattern shows increasingly elevated T waves. This abnormality is associated with
   a. Hypocalcemia.
   b. Hyperkalemia.
   c. Hyponatremia.
   d. Hypercalcemia.

J. continues to be anuric, begins to become more lethargic, and exhibits increasing respiratory effort.

TABLE 12-1. Results of J.'s Blood Chemistry Analysis Compared With Normal Values

	J.'s Value	Normal Value
Sodium (Na$^+$)	127 mmol/L	137–145 mmol/L
Potassium (K$^+$)	5.7 mmol/L	3.4–4.8 mmol/L
Chloride (Cl$^-$)	92 mmol/L	98–107 mmol/L
Blood urea nitrogen (BUN)	40 mg/dL	7–21 mg/dL
Creatinine (Cr)	3.9 mg/dL	0.1–0.7 mg/dL
Calcium (Ca^{2+})	0.98 mmol/L	1.2–1.44 mmol/L
Phosphorus (P)	11 mg/dL	3.3–5.6 mg/dL
Uric acid (UA)	16.5 mg/dL	2.0–5.1 mg/dL

4. The nurse should begin to prepare for the following medical intervention:
   a. Insulin and glucose administration.
   b. Kayexalate.
   c. Hemodialysis.
   d. Peritoneal dialysis.

J. undergoes dialysis for 6 hours, after which his electrolytes are as follows:

   K$^+$: 3.5 mmol/L   BUN: 20 mg/dL
   UA: 8.1 mg/dL   Cr: 2.0 mg/dL
   P: 5.0 mg/dL

His respiratory status has improved, and he is no longer grunting. His urine output is 0.5 mL/kg per hour.

5. The goal of treatment for J. at this point would be to
   a. Maintain renal blood flow and glomerular filtration in the kidney while preventing fluid overload.
   b. Initiate measures to restrict fluid volume to minimal needs.
   c. Provide care during this period in the outpatient setting as much as possible.
   d. Restart hemodialysis as soon as possible.

J. is started on 5% dextrose in 0.25 normal saline with 30 mEq of bicarbonate at a rate of 175 mL/hour. Two hours later, J. has a urine output of 1 mL/kg per hour. Additional tests indicate his urine pH is 5.5.

6. Considering the laboratory results, what is the first priority for medical management?
   a. Prepare for measures to decrease the pH of J.'s urine as part of the medical plan.
   b. Hydrate J., and increase the pH of his urine.
   c. Inform J. and his parents that it will be necessary to restrict his oral intake to 1000 mL/day.

   d. Prepare J. and his family for a probable thoracotomy to remove the mediastinal mass.

Laboratory studies are ordered at 4-hour intervals, and J.'s intake and output are carefully measured. His urine output is maintained at a rate of 3.5 mL/kg per hour. His urine pH is tested every hour. A bone marrow aspirate performed the next morning confirms the diagnosis of acute lymphocytic leukemia; 100% of the marrow is replaced by leukemic blasts. Remission-induction chemotherapy is initiated after obtaining consent for treatment from his parents.

7. The physician orders allopurinol to be given orally three times daily. J. is asleep, and his mother asks that the first dose be held until he awakens. The most appropriate action is to
   a. Honor the mother's request, indicating in the medical record why the dose was held for a few hours.
   b. Call the physician to ask for his concurrence with holding the medication until J. awakens.
   c. Explain to her that it is important for J. to start this medication, because it will decrease the uric acid concentration in his blood.
   d. Decrease his intravenous fluid rate during this period to decrease urine output.

8. A nursing intervention for normalization of J.'s fluid and electrolyte status is to
   a. Notify the physician of any neuromuscular irritability such as tetany or muscle cramps.
   b. Ensure that the physician adds potassium to J.'s intravenous fluid if the child's serum potassium starts to decrease below 3.2 mg/dL.

c. Hold the ordered aluminum hydroxide if J. tells the nurse that he does not have any gas pains.

d. Ensure that calcium supplements are ordered in case his calcium level further decreases.

Over the next 5 days J.'s electrolytes, BUN, and creatinine levels slowly normalize. However, antibiotics are ordered because J. develops a fever.

9. The dosing of potentially nephrotoxic antibiotics is
   a. Irrelevant because his laboratory values have normalized.
   b. Important to avoid further damage to normal functioning kidneys.
   c. Easily guided by the patient's serum BUN and creatinine.
   d. Imperative because his kidneys have already undergone a significant insult and may have compromised function.

10. A primary nursing intervention associated with caring for children receiving cancer treatment is to
    a. Provide reverse isolation for all patients.
    b. Notify the physician of any incidence of fever.
    c. Provide mouth care regimen medications as needed.
    d. Obtain his temperature rectally at least once during each shift.

11. Discharge teaching topics related to J.'s risk for infection include
    a. Prevention of exposures to persons with varicella zoster.
    b. Avoidance of all children until his chemotherapy is complete.
    c. Compliance with taking the trimethoprim-sulfamethoxazole when he is neutropenic.
    d. Information that handwashing is unnecessary for family members except if they are ill.

CASE 12-2

R., a 15-year-old boy, has been admitted to the ICU for mild respiratory distress, particularly on exertion. The chest x-ray film obtained in the emergency room reveals a large mediastinal mass that is narrowing the tracheal diameter. R. is alert and oriented. Jugular venous distention and enlargement of one of his axillary lymph nodes is noticed on physical examination. The nurse can hear mild stridor on chest auscultation. His mother reports that he has had respiratory symptoms for the past month.

1. Based on the physical examination and the x-ray findings, what would be the nurse's first impression regarding R.'s diagnosis?
   a. Foreign body obstruction.
   b. Pneumonia.
   c. Superior vena cava syndrome.
   d. Pneumothorax.

2. What is the first priority in R.'s care?
   a. Maintaining adequate ventilation.
   b. Providing venous access.
   c. Sedating to relieve anxiety.
   d. Administering diuretics to relieve the heart failure.

3. The diagnostic workup of a mediastinal mass includes
   a. An emergency thoracotomy under general anesthesia.
   b. Bronchoscopy with sedation to keep the patient minimally distressed.
   c. A needle biopsy of the mass (if superficial tissue is available) or bone marrow aspirate with local anesthesia only.
   d. Cardiac catheterization as soon as the airway can be stabilized.

A peripheral lymph node biopsy is performed with local anesthesia.

4. The immediate intervention if R.'s respiratory distress suddenly worsens is
   a. Immediate tracheostomy.
   b. Immediate intubation without sedation.
   c. Referral to a pulmonologist.
   d. Emergency irradiation or chemotherapy.

5. A post-irradiation nursing intervention for R. is
   a. Observing for worsening of his respiratory status after radiation therapy.
   b. Positioning him supine, with the head of the bed at less than a 20-degree elevation.
   c. Avoiding supplemental oxygen.
   d. Removing the simulation marks from the patient's skin.

Radiation treatments continued to be given twice each day. The pathology report on the lymph node biopsy indicated that R. has Hodgkin's lymphoma.

After four radiation treatments, R.'s respiratory distress decreased. Chemotherapy was initiated for long-term control of his disease. Further improvement of his clinical status occurred, and he was released from the hospital 10 days after admission.

CASE 12-3

M., a 10-year-old girl, is brought to the emergency room by her parents, who are concerned about her complaints of "weak arms and legs" during the past 24 hours. On admission, her temperature is 37°C, heart rate is 120 bpm, respiratory rate is 28 breaths per minute, and blood pressure is 116/92 mmHg. Further assessment reveals a very distended bladder. Her parents report that she has been complaining of shoulder and back pain, which has been treated with acetaminophen.

The emergency room physician requests a neurologic consultation for further evaluation. The neurologist is concerned that M. may have a neurologic defect within the spinal canal.

1. Which diagnostic tool would be the best to confirm the diagnosis?
   a. Magnetic resonance image (MRI).
   b. Lumbar puncture.
   c. Spinal films.
   d. Bone scan.

The MRI reveals epidural masses from the cervical to lumbar spine, beginning as high as C-4.

2. Based on this history, what does the nurse suspect is occurring at this time?
   a. Spinal meningitis and a bladder infection.
   b. Spinal cord compression from tumor invasion of the epidural space.
   c. Neurologic toxicity from the chemotherapy.
   d. Hysterical reaction to past experiences with lumbar punctures.

3. What should be included in the nurse's assessment for this patient?
   a. Preparation of the family for permanent disability.
   b. An immediate physical therapy consultation.
   c. Psychological interventions.
   d. Questions relating to bowel and bladder functions.

Other symptoms related to this diagnosis include paresthesia and back pain aggravated by coughing or sneezing.

4. This condition requires prompt assessment because
   a. The syndrome will become more painful.
   b. Brain damage could result if it is not treated quickly.
   c. Early intervention is critical in preventing permanent damage.
   d. The spinal cord tumor will metastasize to other tissues.

M. is demonstrating increasing respiratory distress after her sedation for the MRI. A blood sample is drawn for arterial blood gas determinations.

5. With the concern about hypoventilation due to compromise of diaphragmatic and intercostal muscle function, the nurse would expect to find the following abnormalities on the arterial blood gas results:
   a. Low P_{O_2} and low P_{CO_2}.
   b. High P_{O_2} and low P_{CO_2}.
   c. Low P_{O_2} and high P_{CO_2}.
   d. Normal P_{O_2} and normal P_{CO_2}.

M. is admitted to the ICU for more complete respiratory and neurologic monitoring.

6. In addition to capnography, other parameters to follow would be
   a. Forced vital capacity measured with a bedside spirometer.
   b. Capillary or arterial blood gases.
   c. Serial chest expansions to trend diaphragmatic expansion.
   d. Alterations in mental status secondary to hypercapnia.

7. The treatment of choice at this time is
   a. Surgery scheduled for the next day.
   b. Irradiation or chemotherapy to begin immediately.
   c. A bone scan.
   d. Complete bed rest in a supine position.

8. Independent nursing actions should include
   a. Limitation of fluid intake to prevent incontinence.
   b. Avoidance of movement of affected limbs, such as range of motion exercises.
   c. Assessment for pressure sores, contracture, and muscle atrophy.
   d. No further need for assessment of respiratory failure.

After 72 hours in the ICU and eight radiation treatments, the nurse notices that M.'s leg strength and movement are improving, and she is transferred to the floor. She later undergoes a thoracotomy, which reveals she has Ewing's sarcoma.

ANSWERS ■ CASE 12-1

1. Answer (**d**). Tumor lysis syndrome refers to a group of metabolic effects associated with rapidly growing tumors, such as leukemia cells that are highly sensitive to destruction by chemotherapy. Debris from the lysed cells must be excreted by the kidneys, or the debris accumulates. The excretion rate through the renal tubules is even more critical if the tumor cells are numerous (i.e., high tumor burden). Symptoms of tumor lysis syndrome are flank pain, lethargy, nausea, vomiting, oliguria, hematuria, pruritus, tetany, and altered level of consciousness. In this patient, the laboratory values are abnormal, most notably the BUN and creatine levels. These findings indicate that renal function has been impaired and that the kidneys cannot excrete metabolic byproducts at an appropriate rate.

REFERENCES
Akers, P.A. (1990). Tumor lysis syndrome. *Dimensions in Oncology Nursing,* 4 (4), 10–13.
Kozlowski, L.J. (1996). Oncology. In M.A.Q. Curley, J.B. Smith, & P.A. Moloney-Harmon (Eds.). *Critical care nursing of infants and children* (pp. 756–776). Philadelphia: W.B. Saunders.

2. Answer (**a**). Leukemia cells have an abundance of potassium, phosphorus, and purines. In patients such as J. with high white cell counts, the abundant white cells are rapidly dividing and dying. As these cells die, their membranes rupture and release the cellular contents into the bloodstream, leading to hyperkalemia and hyperphosphatemia. There is a reciprocal balance between phosphorus and calcium, and as phosphorus increases in the intravascular compartment, calcium is deposited in soft tissues, leading to hypocalcemia. As the purines released from the leukemia cells are metabolized, uric acid, an end product of this metabolism, accumulates in the bloodstream. This process occurs before chemotherapy is given, but chemotherapeutic agents accelerate the process by destroying the leukemic cells. The chemotherapeutic drugs are most effective against rapidly dividing cells. These imbalances in J. are associated only with a large number of tumor cells. Hepatosplenomegaly is not related to these imbalances.

REFERENCES
Nace, C.S., & Nace, G.S. (1985). Acute tumor lysis syndrome: Pathophysiology and nursing management. *Critical Care Nurse,* 5 (3), 26–34.
Patterson, K.L., & Klopovich, P. (1987). Metabolic emergencies in pediatric oncology: The acute tumor lysis syndrome. *Journal of Association of Pediatric Oncology Nurses,* 4 (3), 19–24.

3. Answer (**b**). Electrocardiographic abnormalities that may occur with hyperkalemia are elevated T waves and prolonged PR and QRS intervals. These abnormalities are not associated with the other electrolyte imbalances.

REFERENCE
Patterson, K.L., & Klopovich, P. (1987). Metabolic emergencies in pediatric oncology: The acute tumor lysis syndrome. *Journal of Association of Pediatric Oncology Nurses,* 4 (3), 19–24.

4. Answer (**c**). Because of J.'s life-threatening potassium levels and his hyperuricemia, emergent hemodialysis is necessary. Other treatment strategies such as peritoneal dialysis or the administration of Kayexalate or insulin and glucose would not be appropriate, because they would not be able to lower the serum potassium quickly enough.

REFERENCES
Kozlowski, L.J. (1996). Oncology. In M.A.Q. Curley, J.B. Smith, & P.A. Moloney-Harmon (Eds.). *Critical care nursing of infants and children* (pp. 756–776). Philadelphia: W.B. Saunders.
Patterson, K.L., & Klopovich, P. (1987). Metabolic emergencies in pediatric oncology: The acute tumor lysis syndrome. *Journal of Association of Pediatric Oncology Nurses,* 4 (3), 19–24.

5. Answer (**a**). Vigorous hydration is essential for promoting a rapid renal tubular flow rate to prevent accumulation of uric acid and phosphorus in the kidneys. Monitoring the balance between the intake and output and the patient's weight is critical to prevent fluid overload. The nurse should assess for other signs of hypervolemia, such as distended neck veins, edema, and rales. This assess-

ment should be done by a nurse familiar with oncologic emergencies and at a frequency that usually requires admission to the ICU to detect acute changes in the fluid and electrolyte balance. Dialysis is employed only if hydration fails to prevent life-threatening electrolyte imbalances. Restarting dialysis would reroute blood flow away from the kidney and potentially increase the risk of metabolite accumulation by decreasing glomerular filtration.

REFERENCES

Allegretta, G.J., Weisman, S.J., & Altman, A.J. (1985). Oncologic emergencies I: Metabolic and space-occupying consequences of cancer and cancer treatment. *Pediatric Clinics of North America, 32* (3), 601–607.

Kozlowski, L.J. (1996). Oncology. In M.A.Q. Curley, J.B. Smith, & P.A. Moloney-Harmon (Eds.). *Critical care nursing of infants and children* (pp. 756–776). Philadelphia: W.B. Saunders.

6. Answer (**b**). The first priority for managing patients with actual or potential tumor lysis syndrome is to prevent renal failure and serious electrolyte imbalances. To be excreted by the kidney, uric acid must be soluble in urine. Uric acid becomes less soluble as the urine pH decreases, resulting in higher serum uric acid levels. Because his serum uric acid levels are high, therapies are initiated to encourage the solubility of the uric acid in the urine, which promotes excretion by the kidneys. One method is to increase his urine pH to between 6 and 7 by administering sodium bicarbonate intravenously. Another alternative is the use of acetazolamide, a mild diuretic, that increases the bicarbonate excretion in the urine, alkalizing the urine. These interventions should be initiated before the institution of chemotherapy, which increases cell lysis. However, if the pH reaches 7.5, the bicarbonate should be withheld, because hypoxanthine or calcium phosphate stones may occur in the kidneys when serum pH is alkalinized to that degree. Hydration is often accomplished by intravenous fluids such as 5% dextrose in 0.45% normal saline at a rate of 3 L/m^2 per 24 hours. The urine output should be monitored closely to prevent fluid overload.

REFERENCES

Akers, P.A. (1990). Tumor lysis syndrome. *Dimensions in Oncology Nursing, 4* (4), 10–13.

Stucky, L. (1993). Acute tumor lysis syndrome: Assessment and nursing interventions. *Oncology Nursing Forum, 20* (1), 49–56.

7. Answer (**c**). To normalize the patient's uric acid, allopurinol is given at regular intervals and before chemotherapy is initiated. This medication is given to decrease the formation of uric acid by inhibiting the enzyme, xanthine oxidase. High levels of uric acid in the blood will lead to formation of uric acid crystals in the distal tubules and collecting ducts of the kidney. Uric acid crystals can obstruct urine flow and lead to nephropathy and the need for dialysis.

REFERENCES

Hunter, J.C. (1992). Nursing care of patients with structural oncological emergencies. In J.C. Clark & R.F. McGee (Eds.). *Core curriculum for oncology nursing* (2nd ed., p. 177). Philadelphia: W.B. Saunders.

Stucky, L. (1993). Acute tumor lysis syndrome: Assessment and nursing interventions. *Oncology Nursing Forum, 20* (1), 49–56.

8. Answer (**a**). Neuromuscular irritability such as tetany, muscle cramps, and carpopedal spasm may indicate hypocalcemia, which is one of the electrolyte imbalances associated with tumor lysis syndrome. This fall in the serum calcium level is a result of the rise in the phosphate level occurring as the cells lyse. The best method to reduce this process is to give oral phosphate-binding antacids. Aluminum hydroxide gels, such as Amphojel, are given on a regular basis every 4 to 6 hours. The aluminum binds the phosphate to form an insoluble substance that is excreted by the bowel. In the context of hyperphosphatemia, treatment with calcium supplements is withheld unless the patient is significantly symptomatic. This treatment could promote further calcium-phosphorus precipitation in the body. Because chemotherapy and subsequent lysis of the cells will probably elevate the potassium level, correction of the serum potassium levels is not recommended at this time. An important nursing consideration is to ensure that potassium is not added to any of J.'s intravenous fluids to avoid hyperkalemia.

REFERENCES

Kozlowski, L.J. (1996). Oncology. In M.A.Q. Curley, J.B. Smith, & P.A. Moloney-Harmon (Eds.). *Critical care nursing of infants and children* (pp. 756–776). Philadelphia: W.B. Saunders.

Lange, B., D'Angio, G., Ross, A.J., O'Neill, J.A., & Packer, R.J. (1993). Oncologic emergencies. In P.A. Pizzo and D.G. Poplack (Eds.). *Principles and practice of pediatric oncology* (2nd ed., pp. 966–967). Philadelphia: J.B. Lippincott.

Nace, C.S., & Nace, G.S. (1985). Acute tumor lysis syndrome: Pathophysiology and nursing management. *Critical Care Nurse,* 5 (3), 26–34.

9. **Answer (d).** Normal serum creatinine and BUN levels do not necessarily reflect the glomerular filtration rate. Normal serum values only indicate that there is adequate renal function to clear wastes accumulated from the stresses occurring at that time. However, an infection or a nephrotoxic drug used to treat the infection may lead to renal failure, because the kidneys must handle the additional metabolic waste.

REFERENCE

Feld, L.G., Springate, J.E., & Fildes, R.D. (1986). Acute renal failure. Part I. Pathology and diagnosis. *Journal of Pediatrics,* 109 (3), 401–408.

10. **Answer (b).** Fever (>38.3°C or 101°F) may be the only sign of infection. In the presence of neutropenia, persons may not exhibit signs and symptoms of an inflammatory response, such as pain, edema, and erythema. Scrupulous mouth care (at least four times each day) can reduce the incidence of secondary systemic infections. Cancer treatments affect rapidly growing cells, including those of the gastrointestinal system. Damage to the gastrointestinal mucosa may allow anaerobic organisms to enter the bloodstream. Further damage to rectal mucosa from taking rectal temperatures or administering medications by this route should be avoided. The rate of infection can also be reduced by placing the child in a private room with the door closed and by maintaining a strict handwashing regimen. Reverse isolation techniques are unnecessary.

REFERENCES

Clark, J.C., McGee, R.F., & Preston, R. (1992). Nursing management of responses to the cancer experience. In J.C. Clark & R.F. McGee (Eds.). *Core curriculum for oncology nursing* (2nd ed., pp. 111–112). Philadelphia: W.B. Saunders.

Griffin, J.P. (1986). *Hematology and immunology: Concepts for nursing.* Norwalk, CT: Appleton-Century-Crofts.

Panzarella, C., & Duncan, J. (1993). Nursing management of physical care needs. In G.V. Foley, D. Fochman, & K.H. Mooney (Eds.). *Nursing care of the child with cancer* (2nd ed., pp. 346–347). Philadelphia: W.B. Saunders.

11. **Answer (a).** Herpes infections are usually more severe in children undergoing cancer treatment. Varicella zoster (i.e., chickenpox) is particularly threatening because of the altered cell-mediated response to this viral agent in children with immunosuppression due to chemotherapy. Dissemination of varicella zoster to the liver, lung, and central nervous system produces significant morbidity and mortality. Handwashing by all those who come in contact with immunocompromised persons remains the best preventative measure for infections. For normal social development, J. can safely play with well children when he is not neutropenic. The prevention of *Pneumocystis carinii* infections is best provided by administering oral trimethoprim-sulfamethoxazole twice each day for 3 consecutive days each week for 3 to 6 months after chemotherapy has been completed. Infection-related deaths are still the major cause of death in children with cancer.

REFERENCES

Clark, J.C., McGee, R.F., & Preston, R. (1992). Nursing management of responses to the cancer experience. In J.C. Clark & R.F. McGee (Eds.). *Core curriculum for oncology nursing* (2nd ed., pp. 106–108). Philadelphia: W.B. Saunders.

Kozlowski, L.J. (1996). Oncology. In M.A.Q. Curley, J.B. Smith, & P.A. Moloney-Harmon (Eds.). *Critical care nursing of infants and children* (pp. 756–776). Philadelphia: W.B. Saunders.

Weintraub, M.H. (1993). Nursing management of the child or adolescent with infection. In G.V. Foley, D. Fochman, & K.H. Mooney (Eds.). *Nursing care of the child with cancer* (2nd ed., pp. 372–382). Philadelphia: W.B. Saunders.

ANSWERS ■ CASE 12-2

1. **Answer (c).** Superior vena cava syndrome is a set of symptoms resulting from compression of the structures in the superior mediastinum by a large mass in the vena cava or next to the vena cava in the mediastinal space. In R., the mass is extrinsic to the vena cava. Faro (1987) qualifies this in the diagnostic term "superior mediastinal syndrome." The mass obstructs blood returned by the superior vena cava and air passing through the lower airways, resulting in a medical emergency. This obstruction results in venous hypertension in the upper vessels. Such masses in children are most frequently associated

with Hodgkin's or non-Hodgkin's lymphomas. The urgency in treating this syndrome is related to the rapidity and degree of the obstruction, the location of the mass, and whether the circulation is aided by collateral vessels.

REFERENCES

Faro, V. (1987). Superior vena cava syndrome. *Journal of Association of Pediatric Oncology Nurses,* 4 (3), 32–35.

Sheppard, K.C. (1986). Care of the patient with superior vena cava syndrome. *Heart & Lung,* 15 (6), 636–641.

2. Answer (**a**). Alleviating respiratory distress and maximizing airway size are critical. Edema of the airway occurs from obstruction of venous drainage, leading to life-threatening signs of inspiratory stridor and respiratory distress. Cardiovascular symptoms such as jugular vein distention result from decreased venous drainage from the head, upper thorax, and upper extremities. However, treatment for this symptom is not a priority, because heart failure is not R.'s diagnosis.

REFERENCES

Baker, G.L., & Barnes, H.J. (1992). Superior vena cava syndrome: Etiology, diagnosis, and treatment. *American Journal of Critical Care,* 1 (1), 54–64.

Morse, L.K., Heery, M.L., & Flynn, K.T. (1985). Early detection to avert the crisis of superior vena cava syndrome. *Cancer Nursing,* 8 (4), 228–232.

3. Answer (**c**). It is ideal to obtain a tissue diagnosis before initiating treatment of the mediastinal mass. A sample may be obtained by a biopsy of superficial tissue or aspiration of fluid. Only local anesthesia can be provided for pain in patients with mediastinal masses. Even sedative medications probably will lead to airway collapse with the degree of airway compromise that R. exhibits, and he cannot tolerate general anesthesia. Airway collapse results in an area of obstruction lower than the area that can be assisted by placement of an endotracheal tube. Immediate surgery is not an option because of a high risk of hemorrhage in the area of vascular engorgement. Further risk to the patient will result if mechanical ventilation is required during surgery, because the positive pressure from the ventilator will further impede venous return of blood to the heart.

REFERENCES

Faro, V. (1987). Superior vena cava syndrome. *Journal of Association of Pediatric Oncology Nurses,* 4 (3), 32–35.

Sheppard, K.C. (1986). Care of the patient with superior vena cava syndrome. *Heart & Lung,* 15 (6), 636–641.

4. Answer (**d**). If tissue cannot be obtained for the diagnosis or diagnostic testing is not complete and respiratory distress occurs, treatment must begin without a definitive diagnosis. Although treatment may alter the tissue that would be involved in future biopsies, it must begin with the goal of trying to avoid the need for mechanical ventilation. Traditionally, the treatment has been radiation therapy. It may be possible to spare a part of the mass from the radiation to provide less altered tissue for future diagnosis. Chemotherapy may be used if irradiation does not provide relief or if the lesion is thought not to be radiosensitive. Immediate tracheostomy or intubation without sedation will increase the risk for airway collapse because of stressing the patient and potentially traumatizing and increasing edema in the area.

REFERENCES

Baker, G.L., & Barnes, H.J. (1992). Superior vena cava syndrome: Etiology, diagnosis, and treatment. *American Journal of Critical Care,* 1 (1), 54–64.

Lange, B., D'Angio, G., Ross, A.J., O'Neill, J.A., & Packer, R.J. (1993). Oncologic emergencies. In P.A. Pizzo & D.G. Poplack (Eds.). *Principles and practice of pediatric oncology* (2nd ed., pp. 951–953). Philadelphia: J.B. Lippincott.

5. Answer (**a**). After radiation treatments, the respiratory symptoms may worsen as a result of radiation-induced edema. Steroids may be given to decrease the inflammatory reaction. The patient should avoid lying supine to minimize respiratory distress. A semi-Fowler position is best to improve gas exchange and promote gravity drainage of the upper body. Supplemental oxygen may improve tissue perfusion. Simulation marks must remain on the skin until all radiation treatments are complete to provide effective treatments.

REFERENCES

Allegretta, G.J., Weisman, S.J., & Altman, A.J. (1985). Oncologic emergencies I: Metabolic and space-occupying consequences of cancer and cancer treatment. *Pediatric Clinics of North America,* 32 (3), 601–607.

Baker, G.L., & Barnes, H.J. (1992). Superior vena cava syndrome: Etiology, diagnosis, and treatment. *American Journal of Critical Care,* 1 (1), 54–64.

Lange, B., D'Angio, G., Ross, A.J., O'Neill, J.A., & Packer, R.J. (1993). Oncologic emergencies. In P.A. Pizzo & D.G. Poplack (Eds.). *Principles and practice of pediatric oncology* (pp. 799–804). Philadelphia: J.B. Lippincott.

Sheppard, K.C. (1986). Care of the patient with superior vena cava syndrome. *Heart & Lung,* 15 (6), 636–641.

ANSWERS ■ CASE 12-3

1. Answer (a). An MRI is the most useful tool. Other methods of diagnosing an epidural mass are a computed tomography scan or myelogram. A lumbar puncture may lead to cord herniation and worsening of symptoms and outcome. Spinal films cannot rule out compression.

REFERENCES

Hunter, J.C. (1992). Nursing care of patients with structural oncological emergencies. In J.C. Clark & R.F. McGee (Eds.). *Core curriculum for oncology nursing* (2nd ed., p. 159). Philadelphia: W.B. Saunders.

Pack, B., & Maria, B.L. (1987). Neurological emergencies in pediatric oncology. *Journal of Association of Pediatric Oncology Nurses,* 4 (3), 12–14.

Panzarella, C., & Duncan, J. (1993). Nursing management of physical care needs. In G.V. Foley, D. Fochman, & K.H. Mooney (Eds.). *Nursing care of the child with cancer* (2nd ed., pp. 336–337). Philadelphia: W.B. Saunders.

2. Answer (b). The symptoms of pain, neurologic deficits, and bladder dysfunction occur as the result of tumor invasion of the epidural space and subsequent compression of the spinal cord from metastasis or direct extension of the tumor. Metastatic tumor in the spinal epidural space is the most common cause of this condition in a patient with the history of cancer.

REFERENCES

Cairncross, J.G., & Posner, J.B. (1981). Neurological complications of systemic cancer. In J.W. Yarbro & R.S. Bornstein (Eds.). *Oncologic emergencies* (pp. 82–83). New York: Grune & Sutton.

Kozlowski, L.J. (1996). Oncology. In M.A.Q. Curley, J.B. Smith, & P.A. Moloney-Harmon (Eds.). *Critical care nursing of infants and children* (pp. 756–776). Philadelphia: W.B. Saunders.

Pack, B., & Maria, B.L. (1987). Neurological emergencies in pediatric oncology. *Journal of Association of Pediatric Oncology Nurses,* 4 (3), 12–14.

3. Answer (d). Changes in bowel and bladder dysfunction, including loss of control or severe constipation, may indicate spinal cord compression. Physical therapy, although useful after the diagnosis is made, is not an effective treatment at this time.

REFERENCES

Pack, B., & Maria, B.L. (1987). Neurological emergencies in pediatric oncology. *Journal of Association of Pediatric Oncology Nurses,* 4 (3), 12–14.

Panzarella, C., & Duncan, J. (1993). Nursing management of physical care needs. In G.V. Foley, D. Fochman, & K.H. Mooney (Eds.). *Nursing care of the child with cancer* (2nd ed., pp. 336–337). Philadelphia: Saunders.

4. Answer (c). A delay in diagnosis and treatment can lead to severe neurologic morbidity. If paraplegia occurs, treatment must begin within a few hours or full neurologic function may be lost. Motor dysfunction precedes sensory losses.

REFERENCES

Kozlowski, L.J. (1996). Oncology. In M.A.Q. Curley, J.B. Smith, & P.A. Moloney-Harmon (Eds.). *Critical care nursing of infants and children* (pp. 756–776). Philadelphia: W.B. Saunders.

Lewis, D.W., Packer, R.J., Raney, B., Rak, I.W., Belasco, J., & Lange, B. (1986). Incidence, presentation, and outcome of spinal cord disease in children with systemic cancer. *Pediatrics,* 78 (3), 438–443.

Pack, B., & Maria, B.L. (1987). Neurological emergencies in pediatric oncology. *Journal of Association of Pediatric Oncology Nurses,* 4 (3), 12–14.

5. Answer (c). Because of compression of the phrenic nerve, ventilation is being affected, leading to M.'s decreased ability to exhale CO_2. With further compromise of ventilation, hypoxia follows. A low P_{O_2} due to hypoventilation is always accompanied by an elevated P_{CO_2}.

REFERENCE

Martin, L. (1987). Oxygen transfer. In L. Martin (Ed.). *Pulmonary physiology in clinical practice* (pp. 88–111). St. Louis: Mosby.

6. Answer (a). These parameters offer increased sensitivity of deteriorating muscle strength over arterial or capillary blood gases. A forced vital capacity is the best method for accuracy. If not available, a negative inspiratory flow and peak expiratory flow may be used. Blood gases remain stable until a critical amount of strength is lost, and then they acutely worsen. Lung volumes seen on the chest x-ray film do not correlate well with actual minute ventilation. Altered mental status is an extremely late finding with severe hypoventilation and is inappropriate to use as a screening test for ventilatory status.

REFERENCES

Hund, E.F., Borel, C.O., Cornblath, D.R., Hanley, D.F., & McKhann, G.M. (1993). Intensive management and treatment of severe Guillain-Barré syndrome. *Critical Care Medicine,* 21 (3), 433–466.

Ropper, A.H., & Kehne, S.M. (1985). Guillain-Barré syndrome: Management of respiratory failure. *Neurology,* 35, 1662–1665.

7. Answer (**b**). After the diagnosis has been confirmed, treatment must begin immediately because the condition may rapidly progress over the next few hours. After paraplegia occurs, the likelihood of successful reversal of symptoms and deficits is lessened. Because most cancer cells are sensitive to radiation therapy and chemotherapy and there is no evidence of spinal instability, irradiation is the treatment of choice. Surgical decompression is indicated if irradiation is not effective and clinical deterioration continues. Chemotherapy is used if the tumor recurs at the site that received radiation therapy.

REFERENCES

Cairncross, J.G., & Posner, J.B. (1981). Neurological complications of systemic cancer. In J.W. Yarbro & R.S. Bornstein (Eds.). *Oncologic emergencies* (pp. 82–83). New York: Grune & Sutton.
Hunter, J.C. (1992). Nursing care of patients with structural oncological emergencies. In J.C. Clark & R.F. McGee (Eds.). *Core curriculum for oncology nursing* (2nd ed., p. 159). Philadelphia: W.B. Saunders.

8. Answer (**c**). Skin care measures are crucial, because the syndrome puts the child at risk for skin breakdown from the loss of physical mobility and the loss of sensation of pressure. Range of motion exercises are necessary until motor function is restored.

REFERENCES

Hunter, J.C. (1992). Nursing care of patients with structural oncological emergencies. In J.C. Clark & R.F. McGee (Eds.). *Core curriculum for oncology nursing* (2nd ed., p. 159). Philadelphia: W.B. Saunders.
Kozlowski, L.J. (1996). Oncology. In M.A.Q. Curley, J.B. Smith, & P.A. Moloney-Harmon (Eds.). *Critical care nursing of infants and children* (pp. 756–776). Philadelphia: W.B. Saunders.

ACKNOWLEDGMENT

I wish to acknowledge the careful review of and contributions to this chapter by Sam Zuckerman, M.D.

CHAPTER *13*

Endocrine Disorders

KATHLEEN MILLER, ARNP, MSN, PhD
BONNIE LYSY-NESTLER, RN, BSN, CCRN

CASE 13-1

C., a 12-year-old boy, is brought to the emergency room by his parents. They state, "For the last week, he has had a cold; he plays out in the snow as often as he can. At the beginning of the week, he was drinking nonstop and seemed to be eating even more than usual, and now all he wants to do is sleep." On admission, C. demonstrates lethargic behavior, complains about blurry vision, has abdominal pain, and has fruity breath. His heart rate is 130 beats per minute (bpm), blood pressure is 80/50 mmHg, respiratory rate is 20 breaths per minute, and temperature is 102.1°F. Laboratory tests are ordered.

1. The subjective and objective findings on admission indicate
   a. Diabetes insipidus (DI).
   b. Cushing's disease.
   c. Diabetic ketoacidosis (DKA).
   d. Syndrome of inappropriate antidiuretic hormone (SIADH).

Levels are determined for sodium (Na^+), potassium (K^+), chloride (Cl^-), bicarbonate (HCO_3^-), osmolality (Osm), glucose (Glu), blood urea nitrogen (BUN), creatine (Cr), hemoglobin (Hgb), hematocrit (Hct), and white blood cell (WBC) count. The initial laboratory tests reveal the following results:

Na^+: 128 mEq/L	Glu: 600 mg/dL
K^+: 5.0 mEq/L	BUN: 33 mg/dL
Cl^-: 100 mEq/L	Cr: 0.8 mg/dL

HCO_3^-: 15 mEq/L		Hgb: 18 g/dL	
Osm: 320 mOsm/kg		Hct: 55%	
WBC: 15,000/mm³			

2. Based on admission findings and the laboratory values, the initial treatment is
   a. 5-mL/kg boluses of Ringer's lactate.
   b. Boluses of Humulin R insulin every hour.
   c. Insulin infusion of Humulin N.
   d. 10–20 mL/kg boluses of 0.9% normal saline.

During the initial treatment, the nurse observes that C. is more stuporous and having Kussmaul respirations. The nurse requests an arterial blood gas determination.

3. Based on his condition, the nurse anticipates that the arterial blood gas values will reveal
   a. Respiratory acidosis.
   b. Metabolic acidosis.
   c. Metabolic alkalosis.
   d. Respiratory alkalosis.

C. is in a state of dehydration and catabolism from a metabolic derangement.

4. One of the components that lead to an osmotic diuresis and a metabolic derangement is
   a. Serum hypoglycemia.
   b. Serum hypercalcemia.
   c. Lactic acidosis.
   d. Serum hyperkalemia.

5. The initial treatment for C.'s decompensation is

a. Endotracheal intubation.
b. Sodium bicarbonate ($NaHCO_3$) infusion.
c. Insulin infusion of Humulin R.
d. An electrocardiogram.

6. The primary reason a 5% glucose solution is added to the treatment as blood glucose levels fall is to
   a. Slow osmotic diuresis.
   b. Avoid depleting glycogen stores.
   c. Maintain serum osmolality.
   d. Prevent the development of hypoglycemia.

7. Serum potassium levels decrease during the management of DKA as
   a. Serum alkalosis begins.
   b. Calcium levels rise.
   c. Serum sodium levels rise.
   d. Insulin moves glucose into the cells.

8. The body finds alternative ways of making glucose by the
   a. Inhibition of catecholamine.
   b. Hepatic breakdown of glycogen stores.
   c. Acceleration of protein synthesis.
   d. Inhibition of glycogenolysis.

At this point in treatment, C.'s laboratory values have shifted. The serum osmolality has dropped, and C. is becoming increasingly combative and unresponsive to verbal stimuli and pain. The nurse caring for C. suspects that cerebral swelling may be occurring.

9. Cerebral edema in DKA is a potential complication related to
   a. Rapid increase in serum osmolality.
   b. Rapid increase in glucose levels.
   c. Rapid increase in serum sodium levels.
   d. Rapid increase in serum potassium levels.

10. The cerebral edema should be treated with
   a. Boluses of Humulin R insulin.
   b. Insertion of an intraventricular catheter.
   c. Restriction of fluid to one half to two thirds of maintenance levels.
   d. Increase in the insulin drip to 2 U per hour.

C.'s diagnosis and treatment are discussed with him and his parents. C. appears to be a withdrawn, emotionally labile child.

11. Strong coping abilities and a stable social environment are important factors in the management of C.'s condition because
   a. Stress in the environment increases the release of catecholamine.
   b. A calm environment facilitates glycogenolysis.
   c. A calm environment increases the manufacturing of insulin.
   d. A stressful environment escalates gluconeogenesis.

CASE 13-2

M., a 15-year-old girl, underwent surgical excision of a pituitary tumor and is admitted to the pediatric intensive care unit (PICU) from the recovery room.

1. During her postoperative course, M. is closely monitored for the effects of alterations in pituitary function. The most common metabolic dysfunction that could occur as a result of surgical trauma to the pituitary gland is
   a. DI.
   b. Diabetes mellitus.
   c. Thyrotoxicosis.
   d. Primary adrenal insufficiency.

2. Hormone regulation in the body is controlled primarily by
   a. A negative feedback loop between the target organ and the gland that initiated the stimulus for hormone production.
   b. A positive feedback loop between the target organ and the gland that initiated the stimulus for hormone production.
   c. The release of regulatory catecholamines in response to stress.
   d. The release of counter-regulatory substances into the bloodstream.

On postoperative day 3, M. becomes excessively thirsty and constantly requests water. Her urine output has been nearly 2000 mL during the past 6 hours, with an intake of 850 mL. Her blood pressure is 140/74 mmHg, pulse is 74, and respiratory rate is 22 breaths per minute. The following values come back from the morning laboratory tests:

Serum	Urine
Na^+: 155 mEq/L	Na^+: 14 mEq/L
K^+: 3.7 mEq/L	Osm: 65 mOsm/kg
Cl^-: 114 mEq/L	Sp. grv: 1.004
HCO_3^-: 23 mEq/L	
Osm: 312 mOsm/kg	

3. Based on the preceding information, which condition is likely to be developing?
   a. SIADH.
   b. Type I diabetes mellitus.
   c. Anterior pituitary stimulation.
   d. DI.

4. An acceptable treatment of choice for this condition is
   a. A 300-mL/hour bolus of 5% dextrose in water.
   b. Desmopressin acetate (DDAVP).
   c. Diuretics.
   d. Fluid restriction.

5. Appropriate treatment for this condition produces
   a. Decreased serum osmolality, increased urine osmolality, and increased specific gravity of urine.
   b. Decreased urine output with no change in specific gravity or osmolality.
   c. Excessive sodium losses in the urine and a decreased feeling of thirst.
   d. Increased serum osmolality, decreased urine osmolality, and increased specific gravity of urine.

CASE 13-3

A 3-month-old infant is brought to the emergency room by his 18-year-old mother. She states that the baby "is hungry all the time and takes 10 bottles of formula each day. He wants to drink all the time and is constantly wet." Based on the data obtained, DI is considered as a possible cause.

1. One method of differentiating this diagnosis in a hemodynamically stable child who appears to be in good health is to
   a. Monitor urine and serum sodium and potassium levels every hour.
   b. Monitor the intake/output ratio closely.
   c. Monitor urine specific gravity every voiding.
   d. Restrict all fluids and monitor urine output and osmolality, body weight, and serum osmolality.

2. If the infant has DI, which of the following would be observed during a fluid restriction challenge?
   a. A reduction in urine output.
   b. No change in urine output but a drop in body weight.

   c. A marked increase in urine specific gravity.
   d. A decline in serum osmolality.

3. The dominant effect of antidiuretic hormone (ADH) on the kidney is to
   a. Increase the excretion of water and sodium and decrease urine specific gravity.
   b. Increase the reabsorption of water and increase urine specific gravity.
   c. Increase excretion of sodium and reabsorption of potassium.
   d. Increase serum osmolality by increasing reabsorption of sodium.

4. The nurse should recognize that a major complication of DI could include
   a. Dehydration and hypovolemic shock.
   b. Hyponatremia and seizures.
   c. Hyperkalemia and cardiac dysrhythmias.
   d. Bradycardia and hypertension.

5. Infants with DI are particularly at risk for dehydration and hypovolemic shock because
   a. Their gastrointestinal systems cannot accommodate the high volumes of fluids necessary to correct the condition.
   b. They depend on others to provide appropriate quantities of fluids to compensate for massive fluid losses.
   c. Cardiac overload with congestive heart failure is a frequent complication with administration of large volumes of fluids.
   d. They are more prone to renal failure because the renal system remains immature at this time.

CASE 13-4

An 8-month-old girl with an established diagnosis of bacterial meningitis is transferred to the PICU from the pediatric unit. The infant is demonstrating decreased urine output, with an elevated specific gravity and slight weight gain during the past 24 hours without peripheral edema. The laboratory results indicate that her K^+, Cl^-, CO_2, calcium (Ca^{2+}), and glucose (Glu) values are within normal limits. Other results, including creatine (Cr) and uric acid (UA), are

Na^+: 119 mEq/L	UA: 2 mg/dL
Osm: 250 mOsm/kg	BUN: 11 mg/dL
	Cr: 0.6 mg/dL

1. From this constellation of clinical findings, it is likely that this child is developing
   a. DI.
   b. Diabetes mellitus.
   c. SIADH.
   d. Renal failure.

2. In this case, the underlying cause of the SIADH is most likely
   a. An alteration in the renal threshold for ADH.
   b. An idiosyncratic response to anticonvulsants used to prevent seizures associated with meningitis.
   c. An effect of the infection on the central nervous system.
   d. Renal failure due to the infectious process.

3. The initial objective in the treatment of SIADH is to
   a. Treat the underlying cause.
   b. Correct the electrolyte imbalances.
   c. Provide a fluid challenge to increase renal output.
   d. Prevent seizures.

4. The primary treatment modality in the treatment of SIADH is
   a. Restricting fluids.
   b. Providing a fluid challenge.
   c. Administering anticonvulsants.
   d. Administering antibiotics.

5. A 3% solution of NaCl may be given intravenously to patients with SIADH because
   a. This solution rapidly replaces sodium to correct the hyponatremia.
   b. Normal saline is physiologically compatible with normal body sodium levels.
   c. This solution will provide a fluid challenge to increase renal output.
   d. The child cannot tolerate intravenous fluids containing dextrose.

6. Inappropriate ADH secretion results in
   a. Increased permeability of the distal and collecting tubules in the kidney.
   b. Decreased water reabsorption from the kidney.
   c. Decreased urine specific gravity.
   d. Increased serum electrolytes.

7. Prompt treatment is necessary to prevent which complication?
   a. Changes in mental status.
   b. Hypernatremia.
   c. Hyperglycemia.
   d. Hyperkalemia.

CASE 13-5

J., a 3-year-old boy, was the product of a term pregnancy without complications. His birth weight was 7 pounds 2 ounces, and the neonatal course was unremarkable. Previous hospitalizations included admission at 4 months of age for gastroenteritis and dehydration and repeated admissions since the age of 18 months for acute episodes of asthma. Treatment for his asthma included intravenous dexamethasone, followed by a continued course of oral steroids after discharge. On admission to the PICU from the emergency room, J. is limp, lethargic, pale, and small for his age. His skin is cool and clammy. His electrocardiogram indicates sinus tachycardia with peaked T waves. Vital signs include a temperature of 100°F, a pulse of 152, and a respiratory rate of 34 breaths per minute, although other physical examination findings are normal. The initial laboratory values are

$$Na^+: 122 \text{ mEq/L} \qquad Glu: 34 \text{ mg/dL}$$
$$K^+: 8.0 \text{ mEq/L} \qquad Ca2+: 4.8 \text{ mEq/L}$$
$$Cl^-: 96 \text{ mEq/L} \qquad CO_2: 18 \text{ mEq/L}$$

1. From this constellation of signs and symptoms, a presumptive diagnosis is
   a. DI.
   b. Cushing's disease.
   c. Pituitary dysfunction.
   d. Acute adrenal insufficiency.

2. In this case, the condition could have resulted from
   a. Poor renal function.
   b. Abrupt glucocorticoid withdrawal.
   c. Androgen imbalance.
   d. Malabsorption syndrome.

3. A primary objective in the emergency management of this child is
   a. Treatment for hypovolemic shock.
   b. Electrolyte replacement.
   c. Intravenous replacement of glucocorticoids.
   d. Prevention of hypoglycemia.

4. The electrocardiographic finding of elevated T waves indicates
   a. Hypovolemic shock.
   b. Congenital heart disease.
   c. Hyperkalemia.
   d. Hyponatremia.

CASE 13-6

Baby girl S., weighing 4230 g, was born at 6:30 A.M. to a mother with gestational diabetes controlled by insulin and diet. During the initial physical examination, the infant was observed to have respiratory distress and was transferred to the critical care unit for observation. Immediately after admission, the baby was alert and active. As the day progresses, the infant becomes increasingly irritable and jittery, cyanotic, and tachypneic. She feeds poorly and exhibits fine tremors. The nurse notices that the infant is becoming cool and clammy.

1. This infant is most likely manifesting
   a. Hyperglycemia.
   b. Hypoglycemia.
   c. Nonketotic hyperosmolar acidosis.
   d. An inherent seizure disorder.

Serum electrolytes are tested, and the laboratory findings reveal

Na^+:	133 mEq/L	Glu:	23 mg/dL
K^+:	3.7 mEq/L	HCO_3^-:	25 mg/dL
Cl^-:	100 mEq/L	Osm:	282 mOsm/kg

2. Based on this information, what treatment should be given to this infant?
   a. An insulin bolus, followed by a continuous infusion of regular insulin.
   b. An intravenous glucose bolus in the form of 10% dextrose in water, followed by a continuous infusion of fluids containing dextrose.
   c. A normal saline bolus that includes potassium.
   d. Intravenous glucocorticoids.

3. More highly concentrated dextrose infusions should be avoided primarily because of
   a. The danger of extravasation and potential tissue damage.
   b. The inability of a neonate to tolerate more highly concentrated solutions.
   c. The potential for rebound hypoglycemia secondary to stimulation of insulin secretion.
   d. The possibility of inducing hyperglycemia.

4. Preterm neonates are particularly susceptible to hypoglycemia because of
   a. An inability to ingest amounts of calories sufficent to maintain serum glucose within normal limits.
   b. Inadequate or inaccessible glycogen stores relative to body size.
   c. An excessive production of endogenous insulin during the early neonatal period.
   d. Difficulty metabolizing complex carbohydrates.

5. Which nursing action is most effective in preventing hypoglycemia in infants and children?
   a. Reducing the fasting time from birth to the onset of oral feedings of glucose-containing solutions.
   b. Identifying patients at risk and providing early interventions before symptoms occur.
   c. Closely observing infants for clinical manifestations of hypoglycemia.
   d. Providing oral and intravenous fluids at greater than maintenance rates.

6. The primary reason to maintain serum glucose within normal limits in the newborn is to
   a. Ensure weight gain in the first few days of life.
   b. Prevent central nervous system effects, because glucose is the major substrate used by the brain.
   c. Avoid depleting glycogen reservoirs, which are limited in the neonate.
   d. Maintain serum osmolality.

CASE 13-7

R., a 10-year-old girl, has been brought to the hospital by her parents, who state that "she isn't acting right." On admission, R. demonstrates a heart rate of 124 bpm, respiratory rate of 36 breaths per minute, blood pressure of 60/40 mmHg, temperature of 99°F, and an altered level of consciousness in response to verbal commands and questions. In addition, R. complains of blurred vision and headache. Blood is drawn for laboratory tests. There is no history of recent illness, trauma, or ingestion of unusual substances.

1. Until laboratory values are available, the safest intervention is to
   a. Provide intravenous fluids containing dextrose.
   b. Provide dextrose-free intravenous fluids.
   c. Administer Dextran.
   d. Administer vasopressors.

The laboratory values, including phosphorus (P), reveal the following information:

Na$^+$: 134 mEq/L   Glu: 650 mg/dL
K$^+$: 5.2 mEq/L   Osm: 312 mOsm/kg
Cl$^-$: 100 mEq/L   P: 3.0 mg/dL
CO$_2$: 15 mEq/L

2. In this case, the most immediate goal of therapy is to
   a. Reduce the serum osmolality.
   b. Reduce the serum glucose.
   c. Maintain electrolytes within normal limits.
   d. Treat the patient for shock.

3. Based on the laboratory data, the appropriate intervention at this point is to
   a. Continue the pre-existing treatment regimen.
   b. Add potassium to the intravenous fluids: one half as potassium chloride (KCl) and one half as potassium phosphate (K$_3$PO$_4$).
   c. Increase the intravenous rate to 30 mL/kg per hour.
   d. Change the intravenous fluids to normal saline and give at a rate of 20 mL/kg per hour.

4. During fluid resuscitation, care is taken to avoid reducing the blood glucose at a rate greater 100 mg/dL per hour to prevent
   a. Osmotic fluid shifts in the brain by a too rapid correction of hyperglycemia.
   b. Reducing the availability of circulating glucose to meet metabolic demands.
   c. Decreasing renal perfusion as a result of reduced hydrostatic pressure.
   d. Rebound hypoglycemia.

5. Polyuria occurs in instances of hyperglycemia because of
   a. An inability of the kidney to conserve fluid.
   b. An osmotic diuresis associated with glycosuria.
   c. Increased mobilization of fluids from the intracellular to the extracellular spaces.
   d. Fluid replacement in excess of body requirements.

ANSWERS ■ CASE 13-1

1. Answer (c). New-onset insulin-dependent diabetes mellitus (IDDM) leading to DKA occurs more often in the autumn and winter. Approximately 0.2% of patients are school-aged children (2 of every 1000 children). Almost one half the children with newly diagnosed IDDM present with ketoacidosis. On physical examination, the child with DKA exhibits lethargy, dehydration, Kussmaul breathing, abdominal pain, vomiting, and fever. Most children have a significant history of polydipsia, polyuria, and weight loss for weeks to months.

REFERENCES
Bonadio, W. (1992). Pediatric diabetic ketoacidosis: Pathophysiology and potential for outpatient management of selected children. *Pediatric Emergency Care,* 8 (5), 287–290.
Wood, E., Go-Wingkun, J., Luisiri, A., & Aceto, T. (1990). Symptomatic cerebral swelling complicating diabetic ketoacidosis documented by intraventricular pressure monitoring: Survival without neurologic sequela. *Pediatric Emergency Care,* 6 (4), 285–288.

2. Answer (d). The osmotic diuresis from DKA causes a vast fluid deficit. If the child has a low blood pressure and shows signs of hypovolemia, 10- to 20-mL/kg boluses of 0.9% normal saline should be given. Treating dehydration should be the initial treatment, as well as giving an insulin bolus and starting an insulin drip of regular insulin at 0.1U/kg per hour.

REFERENCE
Ellis, E. (1990). Concepts of fluid therapy in diabetic ketoacidosis and hyperosmolar hyperglycemia nonketotic coma. *Pediatric Clinics of North America,* 37 (2), 313–321.

3. Answer (b). A major consequence of insulin deficiency is uncontrolled ketogenesis. The accumulation of ketoacids and an overworked buffering system send the pH to low levels, leading to metabolic acidosis.

REFERENCE
Mullen-Monakil, M.L., & Feldman, S.R. (1993). Diabetic ketoacidosis. In J.E. Wright & B.K. Shelton (Eds.). *Desk reference for critical care nursing* (pp. 1051–1061). Boston: Jones & Bartlett Publishers.

4. Answer (c). Hyperglycemia and an accumulation of ketones induce osmotic diuresis. Ketoacids and the dehydration resulting from the osmotic diuresis cause metabolic acidosis. The decrease in circulating blood volume results in reduced tissue perfusion, causing a further accumulation of acids, leading to lactic acidosis.

REFERENCE

Bonadio, W. (1992). Pediatric diabetic ketoacidosis: Pathophysiology and potential for outpatient management of selected children. *Pediatric Emergency Care,* 8 (5), 287–290.

5. Answer (c). In DKA, metabolic acidosis is the result of cellular derangement of glucose, electrolytes, and an altered metabolic process to secure glucose. An insulin drip helps glucose to enter the cell and promotes electrolyte balance that allows cellular energy shifting and tissue metabolism. Metabolic acidosis from DKA should be treated with sodium bicarbonate if severe acidosis (serum pH <7.0) is associated with myocardial depression.

REFERENCE

Bonadio, W. (1992). Pediatric diabetic ketoacidosis: Pathophysiology and potential for outpatient management of selected children. *Pediatric Emergency Care,* 8 (5) 350–360.

6. Answer (d). A 5% glucose solution should be added to the crystalloid infusion when the serum glucose levels range from 250 to 300 mg/dL. By adding a 5% glucose solution at this point, hypoglycemia, further catabolism, and a rapidly occurring low serum osmolality are prevented. The goal is to avoid a rapid fluid administration that may lead to a rapid decline in the serum osmolality. There is a correlation between a rapid decline in serum osmolality and cerebral edema.

REFERENCES

Bonadio, W. (1992) Pediatric diabetic ketoacidosis: Pathophysiology and potential for outpatient management of selected children. *Pediatric Emergency Care,* 8 (5), 287–290.

Rosenbloom, A. (1990). Intracerebral crises during treatment of diabetic ketoacidosis. *Diabetes Care,* 13 (1), 22–33.

7. Answer (d). Restoration of fluid volume reverses dehydration and promotes the shifting of cations and glucose. Potassium levels fall as acidosis is corrected, and insulin moves glucose into the cells. Potassium levels must be watched closely for potential hypokalemia as the shift of potassium back into the intracellular space occurs. Phosphate deficit can also occur during the correction of ketoacidosis, and after renal function is determined, approximately 40 to 80 mEq/L of potassium is needed, and one half of that should be administered as phosphate and the remainder as chloride.

REFERENCES

Ellis, E. (1990). Concepts of fluid therapy in diabetic ketoacidosis and hyperosmolar hyperglycemic nonketotic coma. *Pediatric Clinics of North America,* 37 (2), 313–319.

Sauve, D., & Kessler, C. (1992). Hyperglycemic emergencies. *AACN Clinical Issues in Critical Care Nursing,* 3 (2), 350–360.

8. Answer (b). In a DKA patient, a massive amount of unusable glucose accumulates in the blood faster than the kidneys excrete it. As tissues "starve" from unusable sugar, the body tries to compensate and produces glucose in other forms. This precipitates the initial problem of hyperglycemia. Glycogenolysis, the hepatic breakdown of glycogen stores; gluconeogenesis, the restraint of protein synthesis; and lipolysis contribute to the hyperglycemic state. Hypovolemia and hyponatremia can activate the secretion of catecholamine, the renin-aldosterone system, and the release of vasopressin, which all lead to extracellular volume changes, not to the production of glucose.

REFERENCES

Bonadio, W. (1992). Pediatric diabetic ketoacidosis: Pathophysiology and potential for outpatient management of selected children. *Pediatric Emergency Care,* 8 (5), 287–290.

Tulassay, K., Miltenyi, M., Szucs, L., & Nagy, I. (1991). Urinary catecholamine in children with diabetic ketoacidosis. *Child Nephrology Urology,* 11, 79–83.

9. Answer (c). The onset of cerebral edema is usually between 4 and 16 hours after the onset of therapy. There are many hypotheses about the predisposing factors and pathophysiology of brain edema. Factors that have been related to cerebral edema during DKA are excessive fluid administration with a rapid decline in serum osmolality, rapid correction of hyperglycemia, and a rapid increase in sodium levels. Sodium and glucose are inversely related; as glucose levels decline, sodium levels rise. A rapid correction of hyperglycemia can cause this inverse ratio to become disproportional, leading to high sodium levels that could allow free water to enter brain cells.

REFERENCES

Bonadio, W. (1992). Pediatric diabetic ketoacidosis: Pathophysiology and potential for outpatient management of selected children. *Pediatric Emergency Care,* 8 (5), 287–290.

Greene, S., Jefferson, I., & Baum, J. (1990). Cerebral edema complicating diabetic ketoacidosis. *Development Medicine and Child Neurology, 32,* 633–638.

Shabbir, N., Oberfield, S., Corrales, R., Kairam, R., & Levine, L. (1992). Recovery from symptomatic brain swelling in diabetic ketoacidosis. *Clinical Pediatrics,* 31 (9), 570–573.

10. Answer (**c**). Cerebral swelling continues to be a potentially lethal complication of DKA. The mortality rate for this condition is still approximately 90%. The treatment should be prompt and directed at reducing intracranial pressure. When cerebral edema is suspected, treatment should include fluid restriction at one half to two thirds of maintenance levels, hyperventilation, administration of mannitol (approximately 0.5 g/kg), furosemide, or all three approaches. Draining ventricular fluid, monitoring intracranial pressure, obtaining serial computed tomography scans, and using steroids for reducing diffuse brain swelling are controversial methods.

REFERENCES

Shabbir, N., Oberfield, S., Corrales, R., Kairam, R., & Levine, L. (1992). Recovery from symptomatic brain swelling in diabetic ketoacidosis. *Clinical Pediatrics,* 3l (9), 570–573.

Wood, E., Go-Wingkun, J., Lusirir, A., & Aceto, T. (1990). Symptomatic cerebral swelling complicating diabetic ketoacidosis documented by intraventricular pressure monitoring: Survival without neurologic sequela. *Pediatric Emergency Care,* 6 (4), 285–288.

11. Answer (**a**). DKA is usually produced by a stressful physiologic or psychological event. Many children who have repeated episodes of ketoacidosis live in socially deprived situations and have poor coping abilities. Family therapy is recommended to help the child express negative feelings and defend her or his position in the family. In a controlled study in which psychological stress was reproduced, the study group demonstrated diabetic decompensation that was mainly precipitated by an increase in catecholamines.

REFERENCE

Kaye, R. (1992). Unforgettable patients. *The Journal of Pediatrics,* 120 (6), 995–997.

ANSWERS ■ CASE 13-2

1. Answer (**b**). DI is a condition that can be precipitated by trauma to or dysfunction of the pituitary gland, which may alter secretion of ADH or corticotropin. Diabetes mellitus is a pancreatic dysfunction; primary adrenal insufficiency arises from the adrenal glands themselves; and thyrotoxicosis is generally seen in children with an existing thyroid dysfunction with inadequate treatment.

REFERENCE

Whaley, L.F., & Wong, D.L. (1991). *Nursing care of infants and children* (4th ed., p. 1781). St. Louis: Mosby–Year Book.

2. Answer (**a**). After the physiologic effects of a hormone have been achieved, information is transmitted to the secreting gland to inhibit further secretion. This mechanism is called a negative effect on the further production of hormones.

REFERENCE

Whaley, L.F., & Wong, D.L. (1991). *Nursing care of infants and children* (4th ed., p. 1780). St. Louis: Mosby–Year Book.

3. Answer (**d**). DI is associated with inordinate fluid intake, coupled with the production of maximally dilute urine with low specific gravity, low urine sodium and osmolality, diuresis, hypernatremia, and serum hyperosmolality.

REFERENCE

Hill, J.L. (1990). SIADH, cerebral salt wasting, and central DI. In J.L. Blumer (Ed.). *A practical guide to pediatric intensive care* (3rd ed., pp. 535–543). St. Louis: Mosby–Year Book.

4. Answer (**b**). DDAVP is a synthetic analog of arginine vasopressin, an antidiuretic hormone produced by the pituitary. It is used for replacement therapy in DI and should result in the concentration of urine, characterized by a reduction in urine output and an elevation in urine specific gravity.

REFERENCE

Yucha, C., & Suddaby, P. (1991). David could have died of thirst, yet he never felt thirsty. *Nursing 91, 21,* (7), 42–45.

5. Answer (**a**). DDAVP has a rapid onset of action that produces a volume reduction and concentration of urine. Administration of exogenous DDAVP, or vasopressin, rapidly elevates urine osmolality. Retention of water through the action of the antidiuretic hormone reduces serum osmolality and serum sodium.

REFERENCE

Yucha, C., & Suddaby, P. (1991). David could have died of thirst, yet he never felt thirsty. *Nursing 91,* 21, (7), 42–45.

ANSWERS ■ CASE 13-3

1. Answer (**d**). The simplest test is fluid restriction and noticing changes in urine output and body weight. Comparison between urine and serum osmolality should also be monitored to identify an inverse correlation.

REFERENCE

Whaley, L.F., & Wong, D.L. (1991). *Nursing care of infants and children* (4th ed., p. 1791). St. Louis: Mosby–Year Book.

2. Answer (**b**). In DI, fluid restriction has no effect on polyuria, but it results in weight loss and dehydration. Weight loss of 3% to 5% is diagnostic. This test is followed with vasopressin to assess the alleviation of polyuria and polydipsia. In patients with a severe deficiency of ADH, a 3-hour period of dehydration induced by fluid restriction predisposes the patient to an elevation of plasma osmolality, although urine osmolality remains below plasma levels. In children without DI, the weight remains constant, urine specific gravity increases to at least 1.010, urine volume decreases, and the ratio of urine to plasma osmolality increases to 2:1. If diuresis continues in the absence of oral intake and if weight loss and serum hyperosmolality exist, DI should be suspected.

REFERENCES

Libber, S.M., & Plotnick, L.P. (1992). Polyuria. In R.A. Hoekelman (Ed.). *Primary pediatric care* (2nd ed., p. 1028). St. Louis: Mosby–Year Book.
Whaley, L.F., & Wong, D.L. (1991). *Nursing care of infants and children* (4th ed., p. 1791). St. Louis: Mosby–Year Book.

3. Answer (**b**). ADH acts on the kidney to increase reabsorption of filtered fluid into the cardiovascular system, which reduces urine output and increases urine specific gravity.

REFERENCE

Yucha, C., & Suddaby, P. (1991). David could have died of thirst, yet he never felt thirsty. *Nursing 91,* 21 (7), 42–45.

4. Answer (**a**). Dehydration and hypovolemic shock can result from massive fluid losses in the urine that are not replaced. In a patient who is polyuric and unable to maintain free access to fluids, a negative water balance results, often accompanied by weight loss, dehydration, electrolyte imbalances, and hypovolemic shock.

REFERENCE

Libber, S.M., & Plotnick. L.P. (1992). Polyuria. In R.A. Hoekelman (Ed.). *Primary pediatric care* (2nd ed., p. 1028). St. Louis: Mosby–Year Book.

5. Answer (**b**). Most children with an intact thirst mechanism can meet their water requirements by ingesting large volumes of fluids. Infants depend on others to provide their fluids.

REFERENCE

Marks, J.F., & Arant, B.S. (1990). Central DI. In D.L. Levine & F.C. Morriss (Eds.). *Essentials of pediatric intensive care* (pp. 432–433). St. Louis: Quality Medical Publishing.

ANSWERS ■ CASE 13-4

1. Answer (**c**). SIADH is associated with low urine output and elevated specific gravity despite serum hypo-osmolality and hyponatremia.

REFERENCE

Murphy, K., & Alter, C. (1996). Endocrine critical care problems. In M.A.Q. Curley, J.B. Smith, & P.A. Moloney-Harmon (Eds.). *Critical care nursing of infants and children* (pp. 777–792). Philadelphia: W.B. Saunders.

2. Answer (**c**). A possible etiologic agent of SIADH is infection, such as meningitis. An infection of the CNS may affect the pituitary gland and alter hormone response. In SIADH, ADH continues to be released despite progressive serum hypoosmolality.

REFERENCE

Weigle, C.G.M., & Tobin, J.R. (1992). Metabolic and endocrine disease in pediatric intensive care. In M. C. Rogers (Ed.). *Textbook of pediatric intensive care* (2nd ed., Vol. 2, pp. 1235–1289). Baltimore: Williams & Wilkins.

3. Answer (**b**). Electrolyte imbalances represent not a true depletion, but rather dilu-

tion by excess water in the extracellular fluid compartment. Continued decline can predispose the patient to seizures.

REFERENCE

Marks, J.F., & Arant, B.S. (1990). Syndrome of inappropriate antidiuretic hormone secretion. In D.L. Levine & F.C. Morriss (Eds.). *Essentials of pediatric intensive care* (pp. 430–431). St. Louis: Quality Medical Publishing.

4. Answer (**a**). Because the pathophysiologic consequence of SIADH is retention of excess body water, the primary treatment is to reduce total body water through fluid restriction. Fluid restriction is the cornerstone of treatment of SIADH to prevent progressive water intoxication.

REFERENCE

Marks, J.F., & Arant, B.S. (1990). Syndrome of inappropriate antidiuretic hormone secretion. In D.L. Levine & F.C. Morriss (Eds.). *Essentials of pediatric intensive care* (pp. 430–431). St. Louis: Quality Medical Publishing.

5. Answer (**a**). Hyponatremia can be a life-threatening situation, and it requires rapid correction with 3% sodium chloride, as appropriate.

REFERENCE

Kuhn, M. (1991). Colloids vs crystalloids. *Critical Care Nurse*, 11 (5), 37–51.

6. Answer (**a**). ADH plays a major role in the regulation of fluid balance by increasing the kidneys' permeability to water, which results in increased water reabsorption and reduced urine output.

REFERENCE

Poe, C.M., & Taylor, L.M. (1989). Syndrome of inappropriate antidiuretic hormone: Assessment and nursing implications. *Oncology Nursing Forum*, 16, 373–381.

7. Answer (**a**). Fluid overload in SIADH may produce cerebral edema, which results in alterations in the level of consciousness.

REFERENCE

Hill, J.L. (1990). SIADH, cerebral salt wasting, and central DI. In J.L. Blumer (Ed.). *A practical guide to pediatric intensive care* (3rd ed., pp. 535–545). St. Louis: Mosby–Year Book.

ANSWERS ■ CASE 13-5

1. Answer (**d**). Signs and symptoms of acute adrenal insufficiency include lethargy, poor muscle tone, shock-like state, hypo-natremia, hypoglycemia, and hyperkalemia.

REFERENCE

Marks, J. (1990). Acute adrenocortical insufficiency. In D.L. Levine & F.C. Morriss (Eds.). *Essentials of pediatric intensive care* (pp. 123–427). St. Louis: Quality Medical Publishing.

2. Answer (**b**). Acute adrenal insufficiency may be precipitated by an abrupt withdrawal of exogenous steroid therapy. Exogenous steroids inhibit adrenal function, producing glandular atrophy and an inability to meet endogenous demands, especially with stress.

REFERENCE

Marks, J. (1990). Acute adrenocortical insufficiency. In D.L. Levine & F.C. Morriss (Eds.). *Essentials of pediatric intensive care* (pp. 123–427). St. Louis: Quality Medical Publishing.

3. Answer (**a**). Although treatment objectives include replacement of absent adrenal corticosteroids, correction of electrolyte imbalances, and treatment of hypoglycemia, rapid intervention to treat hypovolemic shock is the first consideration, because shock is a life-threatening situation. Correction with intravenous fluids (5% dextrose in normal saline) is indicated to correct hypoglycemia and hypovolemia. Vasopressors may also be given to assist in the reversal of the shock-like state.

REFERENCE

Weigle, C.G.M., & Tobin, J.R. (1992). Metabolic and endocrine disease in pediatric intensive care. In M.C. Rogers (Ed.). *Textbook of pediatric intensive care* (2nd ed., Vol. 2, pp. 1235–1289). Baltimore: Williams & Wilkins.

4. Answer (**c**). The elevated levels of potassium are demonstrated on the electrocardiogram, reflected in peaked narrow T waves and a shortened QT interval.

REFERENCE

Perkin, R.M., & Levine, D.L. (1990). Mineral and glucose requirements and abnormalities. In D.L. Levine & F.C. Morriss (Eds.). *Essentials of pediatric intensive care* (pp. 121-136). St. Louis: Quality Medical Publishing.

ANSWERS ■ CASE 13-6

1. Answer (**b**). Hypoglycemia may be manifested by jitteriness, cyanosis, irritability, tachypnea, tachycardia, poor feeding, and cool, clammy skin. Infants of diabetic mothers are at particular risk.

REFERENCE

Murphy, K., & Alter, C. (1996). Endocrine critical care problems. In M.A.Q. Curley, J.B. Smith, & P.A. Moloney-Harmon (Eds.). *Critical care nursing of infants and children* (pp. 777–792). Philadelphia: W.B. Saunders.

2. Answer (**b**). A 10% glucose intravenous solution may prevent or correct hypoglycemia.

REFERENCE

Weigle, C.G.M., & Tobin, J.R. (1992). Metabolic and endocrine disease in pediatric intensive care. In M.C. Rogers (Ed.). *Textbook of pediatric intensive care* (2nd ed., Vol. 2, pp. 1235–1289). Baltimore: Williams & Wilkins.

3. Answer (**c**). Provision of exogenous glucose stimulates insulin production from the pancreas, which may produce a subsequent hypoglycemia in the absence of continued dextrose infusion. Continued intravenous glucose administration after an initial bolus is indicated to avoid the reactive hypoglycemia that can follow administration of large amounts of glucose.

REFERENCE

Perkin, R.M., & Levine, D.L. (1990). Mineral and glucose requirements and abnormalities. In D.L. Levine & F.C. Morriss (Eds.). *Essentials of pediatric intensive care* (pp. 121–136). St. Louis: Quality Medical Publishing.

4. Answer (**b**). Hypoglycemia is more likely to develop in infants because of low glycogen stores.

REFERENCE

Hazinski, M.F., & van Stralen, D. (1990). Physiologic and anatomic differences between children and adults. In D.L. Levine & F.C. Morriss (Eds.). *Essentials of pediatric intensive care* (pp. 5–17). St. Louis: Quality Medical Publishing.

5. Answer (**b**). The best treatment of hypoglycemia is early observation and identification of infants at risk, and prevention of the occurrence. After infants have been identified as being at risk, prevention of incipient hypoglycemia may be accomplished through early feeding, monitoring of blood glucose levels, and provision of intravenous glucose, as indicated.

REFERENCE

Merinstein, G.B., & Gardner, S.L. (1989). *Handbook of neonatal intensive care*. St. Louis: Mosby–Year Book.

6. Answer (**b**). All the body's countermeasures against hypoglycemia are an attempt to continue to supply the central nervous system. Glucose is the major substrate oxidized by the brain for energy production.

REFERENCE

Margraf, D. (1990). Metabolic encephalopathy. In J.L. Blumer (Ed.). *A practical guide to pediatric intensive care* (3rd ed., pp. 248–255). St. Louis: Mosby–Year Book.

ANSWERS ■ CASE 13-7

1. Answer (**a**). The symptoms may result from hypoglycemia or hyperglycemia. If the cause is in doubt, immediate administration of intravenous glucose (2–3 mL/kg of 50% dextrose) may prevent significant neurologic damage. Even if the blood glucose is elevated in this case, the effect of further raising an already elevated serum glucose is not significant relative to the total pool of available glucose. It is better to treat possible hypoglycemia by providing exogenous glucose and risk further elevating the serum glucose than to risk continuing hypoglycemia.

REFERENCE

Greenberg, R.E. (1992). Diabetic ketoacidosis. In R.A. Hoekelman (Ed.). *Primary pediatric care* (2nd ed., p. 1586). St. Louis: Mosby–Year Book.

2. Answer (**d**). The priority is immediate treatment of the shock-like state. Subsequent management is directed toward a gradual reduction of serum glucose, reversal of dehydration and hyperosmolality, and correction of electrolyte imbalances.

REFERENCE

Perkin, R.M., & Levine, D.L. (1990). Shock. In D.L. Levine & F.C. Morriss (Eds.). *Essentials of pediatric intensive care* (pp. 78–96). St. Louis: Quality Medical Publishing.

3. Answer (**d**). Saline boluses at a rate of 20 to 30 mL/kg per hour are recommended in the fluid resuscitation of hyperglycemia.

REFERENCE

Rice, V. (1991). Shock, a clinical syndrome: An update (Part 3). *Critical Care Nurse*, 11 (6), 34–39.

4. Answer (**a**). Cerebral edema may be related to excess fluid administration, an excessively rapid decline in serum glucose, or both conditions.

REFERENCE

Rosenbloom, A. (1990). Intracerebral crisis during treatment of diabetic ketoacidosis. *Diabetic Care,* 13 (1), 22–33.

5. Answer (**b**). Hyperglycemia that exceeds the reabsorption capacity of the renal tubule precipitates an osmotic diuresis and subsequent losses of free water and electrolytes.

REFERENCE

Castillo, L., & Chernow, B. (1993). Endocrine disorders. In P.R. Holbrook (Ed.). *Textbook of pediatric critical care* (pp. 703–724). Philadelphia: W.B. Saunders.

CHAPTER *14*

Hematologic Disorders

SHARON Y. IRVING-DANIELS, RN, MSN, CRNP, CCRN

CASE 14-1

T. is an 8-month-old black boy whose mother is known to have sickle cell disease (SCD). T.'s father was never tested, and although T. was screened at birth, his mother does not know the test results. T. presents to the emergency department with a 2-day history of abdominal pain and distention, a low-grade fever of 38°C (100.4°F), and extreme irritability. His mother states, "He acts like he hurts all the time." T.'s mother also notices that he has not been crawling and pulling himself up as he usually does. She points out that T.'s hands and feet are edematous.

1. T. may be exhibiting signs of
   a. Sequestration crisis.
   b. Vaso-occlusive crisis.
   c. Sepsis.
   d. Normal developmental changes.

2. T. is admitted to the general pediatric unit for crisis management and a diagnostic workup. Initial therapy includes
   a. Hydration and pain management.
   b. Red blood cell transfusion.
   c. A decrease in noxious stimuli to calm the patient.
   d. Separation of the patient from the parent or primary caregiver to initiate care.

3. T. is diagnosed with SCD, which is an autosomal recessive disorder. If T.'s mother has the disease and his father carries the trait,

a. 25% or 1 in 4 of their children will have SCD.
b. 100% or all of their children will only carry the trait.
c. 50% or 2 in 4 of their children will have SCD.
d. 25% or 1 in 4 of their children will carry the trait.

4. The most important aspect of ongoing treatment of T. is
   a. Prevention of infection.
   b. Anticipation of "crisis" episodes and administration of analgesia before his pain progresses.
   c. That no specific treatment is necessary.
   d. Prevention of injury to reduce the possibility of increasing the number of sickled cells.

CASE 14-2

D. is a 10-year-old black girl with SCD that was diagnosed in infancy. She presents to the emergency department with pain in her right thigh and across her chest. She also had joint pain at home during the previous 36 hours, and her usual pain management techniques have been unsuccessful. D. is febrile at 38.8°C (101.8°F) and has had one episode of emesis. She is complaining of increasing chest pain, and moderate intercostal retractions are observed with inspiration. Her respiratory rate is 46 breaths per minute, and she has an intermittent cough.

118

D.'s initial arterial blood gas determinations in room air include hydrogen ion concentration (pH), partial pressures of oxygen (Po_2) and carbon dioxide (Pco_2), and bicarbonate (HCO_3^-) level:

pH: 7.46	Po_2: 65 mmHg
HCO_3^-: 27 mEq/L	Pco_2: 38 mmHg

Her pulse oximeter reading is 86%. The chest radiograph is pictured in Figure 14–1. D. is placed on 50% oxygen delivered through a face mask, and she is transported to the pediatric intensive care unit (PICU).

1. D. appears to be experiencing
   a. Splenic sequestration crisis.
   b. Aplastic crisis.
   c. Acute chest syndrome.
   d. Vaso-occlusive crisis.

2. Imperative for D.'s immediate management is
   a. Pain relief.
   b. Red blood cell transfusion.
   c. Orotracheal intubation.
   d. That a child-life worker alleviate D.'s anxiety.

Even with aggressive management, D. continues to experience severe chest pain, and severe intracostal retractions occur with inspiration. Her oxygen is increased to 100% by means of a non-rebreathing face mask, and her chest x-ray film shows increasing infiltrates (see Fig. 14–1), indicating that her condition has worsened. Breath sounds are markedly decreased bilaterally in the bases,

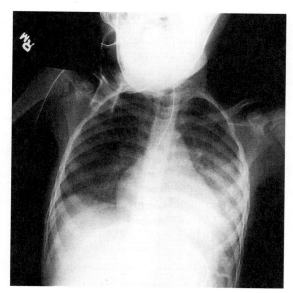

Figure 14-1 Chest radiograph of a child with acute chest syndrome.

and her Pco_2 has risen to 68 mmHg. The decision is made to perform an exchange transfusion with apheresis.

3. The type of apheresis procedure best suited for D. is
   a. Plasmapheresis.
   b. Leukopheresis.
   c. Erythropheresis.
   d. None, because an apheresis procedure is not appropriate.

4. Which of the following electrolyte disturbances are frequently associated with a large-volume blood transfusion?
   a. Hypernatremia and hyperchloremia.
   b. Hypocalcemia and hypophosphatemia.
   c. Hyperkalemia and hyponatremia.
   d. Hypocalcemia and hyperkalemia.

After her exchange transfusion is completed, D.'s oxygen requirement is reduced to 40%, her respiratory rate drops to 26 breaths per minute, and her oxygen saturation rises to 97%. The arterial blood gas determinations after the transfusion are

pH: 7.47	Po_2: 123 mmHg
HCO_3^-: 27 mEq/L	Pco_2: 46 mmHg

Intercostal retractions are no longer observed, and breath sounds, although still diminished in the lower lobes, are audible.

CASE 14-3

S., a 5-year-old girl, is brought to the emergency department by her parents. They tell the nurse that S. exhibited symptoms of a mild upper respiratory infection 10 days ago. Yesterday, she had a sudden onset of abdominal pain, vomiting, and diarrhea. One day before the onset of the vomiting and diarrhea, S.'s mother took her and some friends to a fast food restaurant for dinner. During the 2 days since then, S. had intermittent episodes of abdominal pain and vomiting with recurrent diarrhea. Early this morning, S.'s parents became even more concerned, because it has been 3 days since her abdominal symptoms started. The pain and vomiting have continued, and the diarrhea is now bloody. S.'s pediatrician instructed her parents to take her to the hospital.

On arrival in the emergency department, S. is alert, although somewhat irritable. She is very pale, and her mouth is dry. Her initial temperature is 38.2°C, heart rate is 125 beats per minute (bpm), blood pressure is 114/66 mmHg, respiratory rate is 22 breaths per minute, and oxygen saturation is 99%.

On physical examination, her abdomen is distended, is tender to the touch, and has hypoactive bowel sounds. On palpation, no hepatosplenomegaly or masses are found. While being prepared for a rectal examination, S. again has an episode of bloody diarrhea. A stool specimen is collected and sent for smear and culture. Additional tests include a complete blood count (CBC), including the percentage of granulocytes (Gran) and number of platelets (Plat); determination of the hemoglobin (Hgb) level, hematocrit (Hct), prothrombin time (PT), and partial thromboplastin time (PTT); determinations of electrolytes, including sodium (Na^+), potassium (K^+), chloride (Cl^-), carbon dioxide (CO_2), calcium (Ca), blood urea nitrogen (BUN), and creatinine (Cr); a blood culture; and a urinalysis with culture. Because of the persistence of her symptoms and a moderate degree of dehydration, S. is admitted to the general pediatric unit for monitoring, diagnosis, and treatment.

1. Using the history, presenting symptoms, and physical examination findings, which of the following is the most likely diagnosis for S.?
   a. Intussusception.
   b. "Classic" hemolytic-uremic syndrome (HUS).
   c. *Clostridium difficile* infection.
   d. Meckel's diverticulum.

2. HUS is commonly characterized by which of the following triads?
   a. Acute renal failure, severe respiratory distress, and neurologic insult.
   b. Microangiopathic hemolytic anemia, thrombocytopenia, and severe respiratory distress.
   c. Neurologic insult, respiratory distress, and thrombocytopenia.
   d. Microangiopathic hemolytic anemia, thrombocytopenia, and acute renal failure.

3. The initial management of S.'s condition is directed toward
   a. Meticulous management of fluid and electrolyte status.
   b. Initiation of peripheral hyperalimentation to enhance S.'s nutritional status.

   c. Immediate intubation to manage the airway, anticipating respiratory insult.
   d. Administration of anticonvulsants as prophylaxis for possible seizures.

Urinalysis revealed proteinuria and casts. Results from S.'s initial laboratory studies are as follows:

WBC: 28,000/μL	Na^+: 154 mEq/L
Gran: 76%	K^+: 4.8 mEq/L
Plat: 66,000/μL	Cl^-: 115 mmol/L
Hct: 30%	CO_2: 20 mmol/L
Hgb: 9.4 g/dL	Ca: 7.8 mg/dL
PT: 13 sec	Cr: 2.0 mg/dL
PTT: 32 sec	BUN: 20 mg/dL

Despite hydration and management of S.'s vomiting and diarrhea, the morning laboratory results reveal the following:

Hct: 24%	CO_2: 18 mmol/L
Hgb: 6.8 g/dL	Ca: 6.9 mg/dL
Na^+: 128 mEq/L	Cr: 2.8 mg/dL
K^+: 5.6 mEq/L	BUN: 34 mg/dL
Cl^-: 89 mmol/L	

Overnight, S. becomes oliguric, with a urine output of less than 0.3 mL/kg per hour, and her respiratory rate increases to 44 breaths per minute. The stool sample sent on admission is positive for *Escherichia coli* 0157:H7. She is transferred to the PICU.

4. The nurse caring for S. should understand
   a. *E. coli* 0157:H7 is the most common pathogen associated with HUS, and a positive finding is diagnostically definitive.
   b. Only 5% to 10% of children with questionable HUS have a stool culture positive for *E. coli* 0157:H7.
   c. There is no relevance to the finding of *E. coli* 0157:H7.
   d. *Salmonella typhi* is the definitive pathogen associated with the HUS syndrome.

5. The most common route of transmission of the *E. coli* 0157:H7 pathogen is
   a. Ingestion of unpasteurized dairy products.
   b. Ingestion of improperly prepared or undercooked beef.
   c. Direct fecal-oral contamination.
   d. Raw or undercooked seafood.

6. Based on the morning laboratory data, the overnight decrease in urine output, and the increase in the respiratory rate, S. is exhibiting signs of

a. Hemorrhagic colitis.
b. Neurologic insult, causing renal damage.
c. Acute renal failure.
d. Hepatic dysfunction.

During the next 3 weeks, S. requires aggressive medical and nursing management, including hemodialysis, mechanical ventilation, and inotropics for cardiac function support. She does, however, make a full recovery.

7. Full recovery from typical or classic HUS is considered
    a. Extremely fortunate, for which S. and her family should be very grateful.
    b. A random occurrence that may depend on the overall health of the child before the HUS illness.
    c. A common occurrence, because more than 90% of children who present with classic HUS experience full recovery.
    d. Extremely unlikely, because more than 90% of children with HUS go on to have chronic renal disease.

CASE 14-4

M. is a 12-year-old white boy who was diagnosed 3 weeks ago with acute lymphocytic leukemia. He had a double-lumen Hickman catheter placed 2 days ago in preparation for aggressive, rapid-induction chemotherapy to be administered on an alternate-day basis for 7 days.

On day 4 of his chemotherapy course, M. becomes febrile to 39.8°C and tachypneic, with a respiratory rate of 38 breaths per minute. His oxygen saturation rate is 88% on room air, and he is moderately hypotensive. On examination, he is lethargic, has generalized pallor, and is tachycardiac, with a heart rate of 120 bpm. Because of his overall appearance and the oxygen requirement, M. is transferred to the PICU. The CBC shows blastocytes on the peripheral smear, and the results of his laboratory studies are

WBC: 2.2/mm³	PO_4: 1.7 mmol/L
Hct: 19%	Cl^-: 98 mmol/L
Hgb: 7.3 g/dL	CO_2: 18 mmol/L
Plat: 33,000/μL	Ca: 7.1 mg/dL
PT: 16 sec	Mg^+: 1.5 mEq/L
PTT: 43 sec	Cr: 0.4 mg/dL
Na^+: 132 mEq/L	BUN: 13 mg/dL
K^+: 3.8 mEq/L	

Additional coagulation studies determine a fibrinogen level of 63 mg/dL, D-dimer level greater than 1000 mg/mL, and fibrin split product level greater than 100 μg/mL. The blood culture indicates gram-negative cocci, although the specific organism is not yet identified. The urine culture is negative for pathogens.

M. is placed on 2 L/minute of oxygen by means of a nasal cannula. His initial arterial blood gas results are

pH: 7.34 PO_2: 97 mmHg
HCO_3^-: 17 mEq/L PCO_2: 29 mmHg

Because of the identification of gram-negative cocci, M. is placed on vancomycin and ceftazidime.

1. Based on the history, laboratory information, and M.'s appearance, the nurse should suspect
    a. Disseminated intravascular coagulation (DIC) secondary to sepsis.
    b. Vitamin K deficiency, causing the coagulopathy.
    c. The intravenous fluid infusing through the Hickman catheter diluted the blood specimen drawn, and another should be drawn.
    d. The chemotherapy is stimulating tumor lysis, causing the abnormalities in the laboratory results.

2. One of the primary nursing goals to consider in planning care for the patient with DIC is
    a. Interaction with family and friends to maintain a positive attitude toward hospitalization.
    b. Incorporation of appropriate developmental tasks and activities in the patient's daily routine.
    c. Adequate tissue perfusion and oxygen delivery.
    d. Maintenance of adequate nutritional intake.

3. Which of the following laboratory tests are considered most specific for diagnosing DIC?
    a. PT and PTT.
    b. Levels of fibrin split products or D-dimer.
    c. Levels of factors V and VIII.
    d. Fibrinogen level.

4. DIC can be described as
    a. Inactivation of the reticuloendothelial system.

b. Deficiency of platelet function, inhibition of thrombin and clotting factors, and activation of complement and fibrinolysis.

c. Neutropenia, thrombocytopenia, and hemolytic anemia.

d. Leukopenia, deficiency of platelet function, and factor II deficiency.

5. Which of the following laboratory tests reflects rapid cell lysis?
   a. Decreased factor XI level.
   b. Increased lactate level.
   c. Less than 2% reticulocytes.
   d. Increased BUN and uric acid levels.

M. has begun to have heme-positive stools and nasogastric drainage that is grossly bloody. He is intubated and mechanically ventilated to manage ventilation and oxygenation, control pulmonary edema, and re-establish the integrity of his airway. He is ordered to receive blood and blood products to correct his DIC and control the bleeding.

6. Which of the following blood products should be administered if the goal is to correct the fibrinogen level?
   a. White blood cells.
   b. Fresh-frozen plasma.
   c. Cryoprecipitate.
   d. Platelets.

7. A standard guideline used for the administration of platelets in DIC is
   a. To treat any patient who is actively bleeding, regardless of the platelet count.
   b. To treat if the platelet count is less than 50,000/μL without active bleeding.
   c. To treat if the platelet count is less than 20,000/μL with active bleeding.
   d. To treat if the platelet count is greater than 50,000/μL with active bleeding.

8. Because M. is receiving multiple transfusions of blood and blood products, he is at risk for
   a. Hemolytic transfusion reaction.
   b. Anaphylactic reaction.
   c. Non-hemolytic transfusion reaction.
   d. Alloimmunization.

ANSWERS ■ CASE 14-1

1. Answer (**b**). Vaso-occlusive crisis is the earliest and most frequent presentation of SCD. The disease typically does not

manifest until the second half of the first year of life because of the large amounts of fetal hemoglobin (Hgb F) in younger infants. In patients with SCD, a hemolytic process is usually evident by 2 months, but clinical symptoms before 6 months of age are unusual. Symmetric, painful swelling of the hands and feet, also known as sickle cell dactylitis, may be the initial clinical presentation of the disease in infants. It is caused by infarction of the small bones of the hands and feet, producing bony destruction that can be depicted by radiographic films.

REFERENCES
Behrman, R.E., & Vaughan, V.C. (1992). Diseases of the blood. In W.E. Nelson (Sr. Ed.). *Nelson's textbook of pediatrics* (13th ed., pp. 1049–1051). Philadelphia: W.B. Saunders.
Martin, P.L., & Pearson, H.A. (1994). Diseases of the blood. In F.A. Oski, C.D. DeAngelis, R.D. Feigin, J.A. McMillan, & J.B. Warshaw (Eds.). *Principles and practice of pediatrics* (2nd ed., pp. 1660–1661). Philadelphia: J.B. Lippincott.

2. Answer (**a**). The diagnosis of a crisis usually is based on the history and presenting symptoms. Therapy is directed to removal of the cause, treatment of the crisis, and prevention of complications and further vaso-occlusive events. Red blood cell transfusion is not the first mode of therapy in uncomplicated pain crisis. However, this therapy is indicated for prolonged or extreme pain or when involvement of the lungs or central nervous system is evident. Fluid therapy to prevent dehydration, pain management, and treatment and prevention of infection are the mainstays of therapy.

REFERENCES
Cohen, A. (1989). Hematology. In R.A. Polin & M.F. Ditmar (Eds.). *Pediatric secrets* (pp. 151–152). Philadelphia: Hanley & Belfus.
Martin, P.L., & Pearson, H.A. (1994). Diseases of the blood. In F.A. Oski, C.D. DeAngelis, R.D. Feigin, J.A. McMillan, & J.B. Warshaw (Eds.). *Principles and practice of pediatrics* (2nd ed., pp. 1660–1661). Philadelphia: J.B. Lippincott.

3. Answer (**c**). To exhibit SCD, the child must inherit a hemoglobin S gene from each parent. If one parent has the disease, the other parent, whether carrying the trait or expressing the disease, must also carry the gene. If one parent has the disease and the other has the trait, 2 of 4 or 50% of their children will inherit one hemoglobin S gene from each parent and have the disease. The other 2 will inherit one hemoglobin S and one hemoglobin A gene and therefore only carry the trait.

REFERENCE

Cahill, C.A., & McDermott, B. (1996). Hematologic critical care problems. In M.A.Q. Curley, J.B. Smith, & P.A. Moloney-Harmon (Eds.). *Critical care nursing of infants and children*. (pp. 793–817). Philadelphia: W.B. Saunders.

4. Answer (**a**). Prevention of infection is the most important aspect of care for patients with SCD. Administration of the pneumococcal and *Haemophilus* vaccines, regular childhood immunizations, and prophylactic penicillin have prevented possibly life-threatening infections in patients younger than 5 to 6 years of age.

REFERENCE

Nugent, D.J., & Tarantino, M.D. (1992). Hematology-oncology problems in the intensive care unit. In B.P. Fuhrman & J.J. Zimmerman (Eds.). *Pediatric critical care* (pp. 815–827). St. Louis: Mosby–Year Book.

ANSWERS ■ CASE 14-2

1. Answer (**c**). Acute chest syndrome is typified by tachypnea, chest pain, cough, hypoxemia, and an infiltrate seen on the chest radiograph. It results from sickling of cells in the pulmonary vasculature.

REFERENCE

Gordon, J.B., Bernstein, M.L., & Rogers, M.C. (1992). Hematologic disorders in the pediatric intensive care unit. In M.C. Rogers (Ed.). *Textbook of pediatric intensive care* (2nd ed., Vol. 2, pp. 1357–1401). Baltimore: Williams & Wilkins.

2. Answer (**a**). Pain relief is critical for the child with acute chest syndrome to allow effective pulmonary toilet. Continuous narcotic infusion is the treatment of choice.

REFERENCE

Gordon, J.B., Bernstein, M.L., & Rogers, M.C. (1992). Hematologic disorders in the pediatric intensive care unit. In M.C. Rogers (Ed.). *Textbook of pediatric intensive care* (2nd ed., Vol. 2, pp. 1357–1401). Baltimore: Williams & Wilkins.

3. Answer (**c**). Erythropheresis is used for the removal or exchange of red blood cells. It has been especially successful in the treatment of acute chest syndrome. Transfusion of packed red blood cells is indicated in patients with symptomatic anemia to increase oxygen delivery.

REFERENCES

Cahill, C.A., & McDermott, B. (1996). Hematologic critical care problems. In M.A.Q. Curley, J.B. Smith, & P.A. Moloney-Harmon (Eds.). *Critical care nursing of infants and children*. (pp. 793–817). Philadelphia: W.B. Saunders.
Luban, N.L. (1992). Basics of transfusion medicine. In B.P. Fuhrman & J.J. Zimmerman (Eds.). *Pediatric critical care* (pp. 829–840). St. Louis: Mosby–Year Book.

4. Answer (**d**). With a large-volume blood transfusion, metabolically adverse effects such as hypocalcemia and hyperkalemia can occur. Because of the association with depressed myocardial contractility, hypocalcemia may be the more critical abnormality. The preservatives used to bank and store blood may add to the electrolyte imbalance, especially if the blood is transfused cold; 0.5 kcal/1°C is required to raise the blood temperature as blood enters the body, causing the release of potassium.

REFERENCES

Gordon, J.B., Bernstein, M.L., & Rogers, M.C. (1992). Hematologic disorders in the pediatric intensive care unit. In M.C. Rogers (Ed.). *Textbook of pediatric intensive care* (2nd ed., Vol. 2, pp. 1357–1401). Baltimore: Williams & Wilkins.
Luban, N.L. (1992). Basics of transfusion medicine. In B.P. Fuhrman & J.J. Zimmerman (Eds.). *Pediatric critical care* (pp. 829–840). St. Louis: Mosby–Year Book.

ANSWERS ■ CASE 14-3

1. Answer (**b**). Classic HUS commonly has a prodromal illness consisting of nausea, vomiting, abdominal pain, and bloody diarrhea. It occurs in children between the ages of 6 months and 10 years, most commonly affecting those between 18 months and 5 years of age. An upper respiratory infection may be part of the initial history, but it is not part of the presenting symptoms. Intussusception presents with nausea, vomiting, and the passage of "currant jelly" stools, and it is more common within the first 2 years of life. *Clostridium difficile* infection, most often associated with antibiotic administration, results from suppression of the normal flora by antibiotics, and the damaging effects result from the production of toxin by the bacteria. Meckel's diverticulum manifests with painless rectal bleeding.

REFERENCES

Brown, M.R. (1994). Gastrointestinal bleeding. In F.A. Oski, C.D. DeAngelis, R.D. Feigin, J.A. McMillan, &

J.B. Warshaw (Eds.). *Principles and practice of pediatrics* (2nd ed., pp. 1097–1098). Philadelphia: J.B. Lippincott.

Friedman, A.L. (1992). Acute renal failure. In B.P. Fuhrman & J.J. Zimmerman (Eds.). *Pediatric critical care* (pp. 723–739). St. Louis: Mosby–Year Book.

Neumann, M., & Urizar, R. (1994). Hemolytic uremic syndrome: Current pathophysiology and management. *American Nephrology Nurses Association Journal, 21* (2), 137–143.

2. Answer (**d**). HUS is characterized by the triad of microangiopathic hemolytic anemia, thrombocytopenia, and acute renal failure after a prodromal illness involving gastroenteritis and possibly including an upper respiratory infection. The microangiopathy activates platelet aggregation and fibrin deposits in small vessels, primarily in the kidneys and intestine, causing impairment of renal function, bloody diarrhea, and a decrease in the platelet count. Shearing or hemolysis of red blood cells as they pass through the involved vessels results in hemolytic anemia.

REFERENCES

Friedman, A.L. (1992). Acute renal failure. In B.P. Fuhrman & J.J. Zimmerman (Eds.). *Pediatric critical care* (pp. 723–739). St. Louis: Mosby–Year Book.

Klee, K.M., McAfee, N., & Greenleaf, K. (1993). Hemolytic uremic syndrome. *American Nephrology Nurses Association Journal, 20* (4), 505–506.

3. Answer (**a**). Initial management of HUS is mainly supportive, with the emphasis on close control of fluid and electrolyte balance. For dehydration, reestablishment of euvolemia is essential, regardless of the renal function status. Achieving a euvolemic balance with an electrolyte steady-state level may result in overhydration and may then require fluid restriction, diuretic therapy, or dialysis. Initiation of dialysis as necessary to manage electrolyte or fluid imbalances, metabolic acidosis, and renal failure may be lifesaving, but it is not usually first-line treatment.

REFERENCES

Neumann, M., & Urizar, R. (1994). Hemolytic uremic syndrome: Current pathophysiology and management. *American Association of Nurse Anesthetists Journal, 21* (2), 137–143.

Terhune-Louis, P. (1994). Hemolytic-uremic syndrome. In F.A. Oski, C.D. DeAngelis, R.D. Feigin, J.A. McMillan, & J.B. Warshaw (Eds.). *Principles and practice of pediatrics* (2nd ed., pp. 1097–1098). Philadelphia: J.B. Lippincott.

4. Answer (**a**). Between 40% and 50% of stools cultured from patients suspected of having HUS carry *E. coli* 0157:H7. It is the most common pathogen linked to the HUS triad. Less frequently identified are *Shigella dysenteriae* type I, *Salmonella typhi, Campylobacter jejuni, Yersinia pseudotuberculosis, Streptococcus pneumoniae,* and various viruses. Critical to the isolation and identification of the *E. coli* 0157:H7 pathogen is obtaining a stool culture within 1 week of the onset of symptoms. Identification of *E. coli* 0157:H7 in the stool of patients with symptoms related to the HUS triad is diagnostically definitive.

REFERENCES

Cahill, C.A., & McDermott, B. (1996). Hematologic critical care problems. In M.A.Q. Curley, J.B. Smith, & P.A. Moloney-Harmon (Eds.). *Critical care nursing of infants and children* (pp. 793–817). Philadelphia: W.B. Saunders.

Tarr, P.I., Neill, M.A., Clausen, C.R., Watkins, S.L., Christie, D.L., & Hickman, R.O. (1990). *Escherichia coli* 0157:H7 and the hemolytic uremic syndrome: Importance of early cultures in establishing etiology. *The Journal of Infectious Diseases, 162,* 553–556.

5. Answer (**b**). Undercooked beef is the most likely route of transmission of the *E. coli* 0157:H7 pathogen to humans. This bacterium lives in the intestine of some cattle and can be transferred in the normal slaughtering process. The bacterium also is present in some dairy cows and is transmitted by the ingestion of unpasteurized milk and milk products. If inadequate hygiene occurs between an infected person and one who is not infected, there is a chance for spread of the bacterium.

REFERENCE

Griffin, P.M., & Tauxe, R.V. (1993). Escherichia coli 0157:H7: Human illness in North America, food vehicles and animal reservoirs. *International Food Safety News, 2* (2), 15–17.

6. Answer (**c**). HUS is the leading cause of acquired acute renal failure in children. The kidneys are the principal sites of insult. The predominant causes are glomerular capillary obstruction resulting from endothelial cell edema and fibrin and platelet deposition, which reduce glomerular filtration.

REFERENCES

Cahill, C.A., & McDermott, B. (1996). Hematologic critical care problems. In M.A.Q. Curley, J.B. Smith, & P.A. Moloney-Harmon (Eds.). *Critical care nursing of infants and children* (pp. 793–817). Philadelphia: W.B. Saunders.

Friedman, A.L. (1992). Acute renal failure. In B.P. Fuhrman & J.J. Zimmerman (Eds.). *Pediatric critical care* (pp. 723–739). St. Louis: Mosby–Year Book.

7. Answer (**c**). More than 90% of children with classic HUS experience complete recovery without long-term sequelae.

REFERENCES

Cahill-Alsip, C., & McDermott, B. (1996). Hematologic critical care problems. In M.A.Q. Curley, J.B. Smith, & P.A. Moloney-Harmon (Eds.). *Critical care nursing of infants and children* (pp. 793–817). Philadelphia: W.B. Saunders.

Friedman, A.L. (1992). Acute renal failure. In B.P. Fuhrman & J.J. Zimmerman (Eds.). *Pediatric critical care* (pp. 723–739). St. Louis: Mosby–Year Book.

ANSWERS ■ CASE 14-4

1. Answer (**a**). DIC is a constellation of laboratory and clinical abnormalities that occurs as a complication secondary to a disease process. The most common cause of DIC is gram-negative infections. Endotoxin released by the organism can directly injure the vessel wall, causing exposure of the subendothelial surface. This exposure is enough to initiate contact activation of coagulation. Endotoxin release can also mobilize factor XII and initiate the coagulation cascade.

REFERENCES

Casella, J.F. (1994). Disorders of coagulation. In F.A. Oski, C.D. DeAngelis, R.D. Feigin, J.A. McMillan, & J.B. Warshaw (Eds.). *Principles and practice of pediatrics* (2nd ed., pp. 1685–1699). Philadelphia: J.B. Lippincott.

Shelton, B.K. (1994). Disorders of hemostasis in sepsis. *Critical Care Nursing Clinics of North America,* 6 (2), 373–387.

2. Answer (**c**). Interventions are supportive and aimed at the underlying cause. The major goal of nursing care is to enhance tissue perfusion. This may include correction of shock and acidosis, antibiotic administration to combat the underlying bacterial infection, and replacement of coagulation factors and blood products as necessary.

REFERENCES

Brown, K.K. (1994). Part 1: Critical intervention in septic shock. *American Journal of Nursing,* 94 (10), 20–25.

Shelton, B.K. (1994). Disorders of hemostasis in sepsis. *Critical Care Nursing Clinics of North America,* 6 (2), 373–387.

3. Answer (**b**). The fibrin split product, also called the fibrin degradation product, is considered most specific for DIC. This level indicates the clot breakdown products and is elevated if excessive clots are lysing. The D-dimer is specific for fibrin proteolysis and confirms the diagnosis of DIC when the fibrin split product value is elevated. Factor VIII assay results and other factor levels, especially factor IX, are used to monitor clotting abnormalities. PT and PTT are useful in monitoring the response to treatment, but they are not specific for changes in coagulation factor levels. A decrease in the fibrinogen level may be the earliest indicator of subclinical changes in the patient's clotting ability. However, it may also reflect other conditions, such as chemotherapy administration, which can cause hepatic disease.

REFERENCES

Kedar, A., & Gross, S. (1990). Disseminated intravascular coagulation. In J.L. Blumer (Ed.). *A practical guide to pediatric intensive care* (3rd ed., pp. 517–519). St. Louis: Mosby–Year Book.

Shelton, B.K. (1994). Disorders of hemostasis in sepsis. *Critical Care Nursing Clinics of North America,* 6 (2), 373–387.

4. Answer (**b**). A patient with DIC has excessive production of thrombin, which leads to consumption of clotting factors, microcirculatory fibrin deposits, and excessive fibrinolysis. This causes an inadequacy of platelets and clotting factors, microcirculatory thrombi, and fibrinolysis. The patient can show signs of clotting and bleeding simultaneously.

REFERENCES

Cahill-Alsip, C., & McDermott, B. (1996). Hematologic critical care problems. In M.A.Q. Curley, J.B. Smith, & P.A. Moloney-Harmon (Eds.). *Critical care nursing of infants and children* (pp. 793–819). Philadelphia: W.B. Saunders.

Shelton, B.K. (1994). Disorders of hemostasis in sepsis. *Critical Care Nursing Clinics of North America,* 6 (2), 373–387.

5. Answer (**d**). Elevated BUN and uric acid levels indicate cell lysis secondary to the breakdown products produced. An increase in the lactate level reflects cell conversion to anaerobic metabolism due to the presence of microthrombi. A reticulocyte level of less than 2% may indicate an anemia, but it has little diagnostic relevance to the rate of cell lysis. Factor XI deficiency is characteristic for hemophilia C; the deficiency has an autosomal recessive pattern of inheritance.

REFERENCES

Casella, J.F. (1994). Disorders of coagulation. In F.A. Oski, C.D. DeAngelis, R.D. Feigin, J.A. McMillan, &

J.B. Warshaw (Eds.). *Principles and practice of pediatrics* (2nd ed., pp. 1685–1699). Philadelphia: J.B. Lippincott.

Shelton, B.K. (1994). Disorders of hemostasis in sepsis. *Critical Care Nursing Clinics of North America,* 6 (2), 373–387.

6. Answer (**c**). Cryoprecipitate contains fibrinogen, factor VIII, and factor XIII. It is the treatment of choice for the correction of low fibrinogen levels to control bleeding. Patients who are thrombocytopenic, have decreased clotting proteins, have prolonged PT and PTT, and are bleeding are often treated with platelet transfusions because platelets are suspended in fresh-frozen plasma. The addition of cryoprecipitate slows the consumption of clotting proteins and platelets and controls fibrinolysis. WBC transfusion is reserved for patients with retracted neutropenia (or anticipation of neutropenia) with a good chance of bone marrow recovery and long-term survival. There are numerous risks associated with WBC transfusion; the most critical is acute respiratory distress syndrome, causing deoxygenation and respiratory failure.

REFERENCES

Kedar, A., & Gross, S. (1990). Disseminated intravascular coagulation. In J.L. Blumer (Ed.). *A practical guide to pediatric intensive care* (3rd ed., pp. 517–519). St. Louis: Mosby–Year Book.

Nugent, D.J., & Tarantino, M.D. (1992). Hematology-oncology problems in the intensive care unit. In B.P. Fuhrman & J.J. Zimmerman (Eds.). *Pediatric critical care* (pp. 815–827). St. Louis: Mosby–Year Book.

7. Answer (**c**). When the platelet count is less than $20,000/\mu L$ and active bleeding persists, platelets are administered to raise the count to $60,000/\mu L$. If the platelet count is greater than $50,000/\mu L$ and active bleeding persists, fresh-frozen plasma is indicated.

REFERENCES

Kedar, A., & Gross, S. (1990). Disseminated intravascular coagulation. In J.L. Blumer (Ed.). *A practical guide to pediatric intensive care* (3rd ed., pp. 517–519). St. Louis: Mosby–Year Book.

Nugent, D.J., & Tarantino, M.D. (1992). Hematology-oncology problems in the intensive care unit. In B.P. Fuhrman & J.J. Zimmerman (Eds.). *Pediatric critical care* (pp. 815–827). St. Louis: Mosby–Year Book.

8. Answer (**d**). Alloimmunization is a risk for patients who receive multiple blood transfusions. These patients develop antibodies against antigens that they intrinsically lack but that are present in the transfused product. This reaction is evidenced by the development of antibodies against the transfused product, rendering future transfusions ineffective, and may be demonstrated by hemolysis of donor cells. The patient becomes refractory to a particular product. The newly formed antibodies destroy transfused cells with the targeted antigen. In these cases, platelet transfusions have no therapeutic effect, and red cell hemolysis may occur.

REFERENCE

Cahill, C.A., & McDermott, B. (1996). Hematologic critical care problems. In M.A.Q. Curley, J.B. Smith, & P.A. Moloney-Harmon (Eds.). *Critical care nursing of infants and children* (pp. 793–819). Philadelphia: W.B. Saunders.

CHAPTER *15*

Shock

SANDRA J. CZERWINSKI, RN, MS, CCRN
BONNIE LYSY-NESTLER, RN, BSN, CCRN

CASE 15-1

J., a 3-week-old girl, was admitted directly to the pediatric intensive care unit (PICU) this evening with a history of vomiting for the past 24 hours. The infant is lethargic and cool to touch, and she has had no wet diapers since early morning. Assessment reveals a temperature of 38°C; heart rate of 160 beats per minute (bpm), with weak and thready peripheral and central pulses; a respiratory rate of 35 breaths per minute, with shallow and irregular breathing; blood pressure of 60 mmHg/palpation only; and a capillary refill time of more than 3 seconds. The fontanelle is soft and slightly depressed, and the skin is mottled, pale, and cool. J. is difficult to arouse, and her mucous membranes are dry. Examination reveals a soft abdomen with hyperactive bowel sounds, and there is no urine output.

1. Based on J.'s history and assessment, which category of shock applies to her?
   a. Septic shock.
   b. Cardiogenic shock.
   c. Hypovolemic shock.
   d. Distributive shock.

2. The primary metabolic abnormality in all types of shock is
   a. Metabolic acidosis.
   b. Metabolic alkalosis.
   c. Aerobic metabolism.
   d. Severely decreased lactic acid.

3. Which of the following parameters from J.'s initial assessment would be most useful in identifying her shock category?

   a. Level of consciousness.
   b. Blood pressure.
   c. Weak cry and poor suck.
   d. Sunken fontanelle.

4. The pathophysiology of hypovolemic shock is most accurately described by which of the following series of events?
   a. Decreased intravascular volume → decreased venous return → increased stroke volume → inadequate tissue perfusion.
   b. Decreased intravascular volume → increased left atrial pressure → increased pulmonary venous return → inadequate tissue perfusion.
   c. Decreased intravascular volume → venous dilatation → increased left atrial pressure → inadequate tissue perfusion.
   d. Decreased intravascular volume → decreased ventricular filling → decreased stroke volume → inadequate tissue perfusion.

5. What would the nurse expect J.'s hemodynamic profile to look like?
   a. Decreased systemic vascular resistance index (SVRI).
   b. Increased cardiac index.
   c. Decreased pulmonary artery occlusion pressure (PAOP).
   d. Increased systemic venous oxygen concentration (Svo_2).

6. The most appropriate intervention after initial assessment is to
   a. Administer normal saline (0.9% NaCl).

b. Administer 5% dextrose in 0.45% NaCl with 20 mEq of potassium chloride (KCl).

c. Administer 5% dextrose in water intravenously.

d. Administer 0.45% NaCl in water.

7. The fluid resuscitation regimen frequently includes the use of colloids as well as crystalloids. One of the advantages of including colloids in the treatment regimen is that
a. They help maintain normal serum ionized calcium levels.
b. They are less likely to cause sensitivity reactions.
c. They provide greater improvement in the cardiac index and stroke work index.
d. They increase the likelihood of hyponatremia.

Since admission, J. has been rehydrated with isotonic crystalloids (20 mL/kg) four times and one administration of 5% albumin (20 mL/kg). After J. has been in the PICU for 2 hours, assessment findings include a temperature of 37.8°C; heart rate of 150 bpm; respiratory rate of 48 breaths per minute, with labored breathing and rales; blood pressure of 85 mmHg/palpation only; pale and diaphoretic skin; and a capillary refill of less than 2 seconds. The infant is restless and responsive. Her mucous membranes are moist. Examination reveals a soft abdomen with hyperactive bowel sounds, and hepatomegaly is detected.

8. J. may be exhibiting signs of
a. Left ventricular constriction.
b. Pulmonary edema.
c. Renal failure.
d. Liver failure.

9. After J. is rehydrated and her metabolic acidosis corrected, she is most at risk for
a. Hyponatremia.
b. Hyperkalemia.
c. Hypocalcemia.
d. Hypernatremia.

CASE 15-2

C., a 10-year-old boy, was stung by a wasp 30 minutes before arriving at the emergency center. He has significant swelling at the site, and he is hypotensive and mildly agitated.

1. Shock is a progressive syndrome that results from the loss of integrity of one or more of the four essential components of circulation. Which of the following best describes anaphylactic shock?
a. Sufficient circulating blood volume in relation to the vascular space.
b. Insufficient cardiac output despite adequate ventricular preload.
c. Inappropriate systemic or pulmonary vascular tone, or both.
d. Ineffective tissue use of oxygen and nutrients.

2. The pathophysiology of anaphylactic shock is best characterized by which of the following events?
a. Vasodilation and increased capillary permeability.
b. Vasoconstriction and decreased capillary permeability.
c. Venous and arteriolar dilation.
d. Decreased stroke volume and inadequate systolic emptying.

3. C.'s hemodynamic findings may include
a. Increased cardiac index.
b. Increased right atrial pressure.
c. Decreased PAOP.
d. Elevated pulmonary artery pressures.

4. Which of the following drugs may play a role in C.'s treatment?
a. Fortaz.
b. Methylprednisolone.
c. Albumin.
d. Dobutamine.

CASE 15-3

M., a 3-month-old girl, was just admitted to the PICU. She has a large, uncorrected ventricular septal defect and is in severe congestive heart failure and cardiogenic shock. M. has been treated with digoxin and diuretics for the past 2 months and has been stable. She developed a respiratory illness several days ago and has become progressively worse.

1. Which of the following changes would be seen in M.'s oxygen profile?
a. Increased oxygen delivery (DO_2).
b. Decreased oxygen consumption (VO_2) initially and then increased.
c. Low, continuous mixed-venous oxygen saturation ($S\bar{v}O_2$).
d. Decreased arteriovenous difference in the oxygen gradient ($avDO_2$).

2. What findings may be seen on assessment?
   a. Poor skin turgor.
   b. Jugular venous distention.
   c. Normal capillary refill.
   d. Warm and dry skin.

3. Which of the following hemodynamic profiles may M. have?
   a. Increased heart rate, decreased cardiac index, increased SVRI, and increased PAOP.
   b. Decreased heart rate, increased cardiac index, decreased SVRI, and decreased PAOP.
   c. Increased heart rate, increased cardiac index, increased right atrial pressure, and increased SVRI.
   d. Decreased heart rate, decreased cardiac index, increased right atrial pressure, and decreased SVRI.

4. If M. is started on a dobutamine drip, her hemodynamic profile may include
   a. Increased cardiac output.
   b. Decreased PAOP.
   c. Decreased systemic vascular resistance.
   d. Significantly increased heart rate.

5. Which of the following therapies would have an adverse effect on M.'s oxygenation status?
   a. Administration of fentanyl.
   b. Administration of oxygen through a nasal cannula.
   c. Administration of epinephrine.
   d. Administration of furosemide.

CASE 15-4

A., a 5-year-old girl, presents in the emergency department with a history of flu-like symptoms for 4 days. She has a heart rate of 160 bpm, blood pressure of 95/53 mmHg, respiratory rate of 40 breaths per minute, and temperature of 38.2°C. Her diagnosis is "fever of unknown origin, possible sepsis." Her initial treatment in the emergency department includes blood and urine cultures, a chest x-ray, a lumbar puncture, and administration of acetaminophen.

A. is transferred to the PICU for further evaluation and treatment. Initial assessment in the PICU reveals a temperature of 38.3°C and warm, dry skin; respiratory rate of 44 breaths per minute; a heart rate of 170 bpm, with bounding, full pulses; blood pressure of 98/48 mmHg; and a widened pulse pressure. A. is restless with dilated pupils, peripheral edema and has a brisk capillary refill time.

1. A. is experiencing the initial stage of what type of shock?
   a. Maldistributive.
   b. Obstructive.
   c. Cardiogenic.
   d. Low-flow.

2. In A.'s assessment, the nurse understands that the symptoms are the result of
   a. Massive vasodilation.
   b. Decreased venous capacity.
   c. Local vasodilation.
   d. Decreased capillary permeability.

3. What would be a red flag in this phase of shock?
   a. Normal to high blood pressure.
   b. Cool, pale, moist skin.
   c. Low urine output.
   d. Weak, thready pulses.

4. What compensatory mechanism is activated to maintain A.'s cardiac output and tissue perfusion?
   a. Baroreceptor reflex stimulation.
   b. Constriction of coronary arteries.
   c. Parasympathetic stimulation.
   d. Release of fibrinogen.

5. A significant assessment parameter for this type of shock is
   a. White blood cell (WBC) count greater than 12,000/mm^3 or less than 4000/mm^3.
   b. Temperature greater than 38°C.
   c. Serum sodium level less than 135 mEq/L.
   d. Serum glucose level less than 100 mg/dL.

6. The most important intervention at this point is to
   a. Reculture blood.
   b. Administer one-half maintenance intravenous fluids.
   c. Administer oxygen.
   d. Administer fluid boluses at 10 mL/kg.

After she has been in the PICU for 2 hours, A.'s sensorium, respiratory, and hemodynamic status begins to rapidly deteriorate. The assessment findings at this time include a decreased response to procedures, an SaO$_2$ of 70%, poor capillary refill, weak pulses, mottling of the lower extremities, tachycardia, palpable-only blood pressure, tachypnea, and a temperature of 38°C.

7. Based on these findings, A. is in what stage of shock?
   a. Compensated.
   b. Uncompensated.
   c. Irreversible.
   d. Low-flow.

8. An essential goal of treatment for this stage would be
   a. Inotropic support.
   b. Maintenance of intravenous fluids.
   c. Narcan administration.
   d. Nasal cannula.

9. A.'s therapeutic regimen includes trending what parameter?
   a. PAOP.
   b. Blood pressure.
   c. Pulse pressure.
   d. Oxygen saturation.

10. What factor can increase A.'s V_{O_2}?
   a. Blood pressure.
   b. Temperature.
   c. Hemoglobin.
   d. Hypoxia.

A. is showing signs of increased respiratory effort. Her arterial blood gas results indicate metabolic acidosis and respiratory alkalosis. She is intubated and mechanically ventilated.

11. A.'s deteriorating respiratory status probably results from
   a. Increased alveolar surface tension.
   b. Pulmonary beds that are less permeable.
   c. Redistribution of blood to priority organs.
   d. Increased capillary blood flow.

A.'s blood culture results indicate a gram-negative bacterial infection.

12. Immediately after starting antibiotics, A.'s heart rate increases to 250 bpm, and her blood pressure drops to 50 mmHg/palpation only. This is happening because the
   a. WBC count rises.
   b. Endotoxin levels rise.
   c. Cytokine levels decrease.
   d. WBC count drops.

To assist with the management of A.'s septic shock, central lines are inserted. Her initial central venous pressure reading is

1 mmHg. Fluid therapy is re-evaluated at this time.

13. What is the intravenous solution of choice?
   a. One-half normal saline.
   b. 0.9 sodium chloride.
   c. 50% dextrose.
   d. 0.45 NaCl in water.

A.'s immune system plays an important role in the septic shock cascade and in the inflammatory response. Significant detrimental hemodynamic changes occur when these systems become overactive.

14. What major hemodynamic change occurs when mediators are activated?
   a. Widespread vasoconstriction.
   b. Decreased capillary permeability.
   c. Insufficient distribution of blood.
   d. Bradycardia.

15. Children in septic shock frequently exhibit derangements in their
   a. Antigen cascade.
   b. Lipid profile.
   c. Hormone response.
   d. Coagulation cascade.

16. The main intervention for the prevention of septic shock is
   a. Handwashing.
   b. Meticulous manipulation of lines.
   c. Observing for signs of septic shock.
   d. Aseptic technique used with dressing changes.

17. The potent vasodilator effects of the kallikrein/kinin system (e.g., bradykinin) are evidenced by what clinical parameter?
   a. Fever.
   b. Increased microvascular permeability.
   c. Platelet aggregation.
   d. Excessive intravascular coagulation.

18. Understanding that tumor necrosis factor is the major endogenous mediator of the septic cascade, what pathophysiologic event results from its release?
   a. Decreased capillary permeability.
   b. Widespread vasoconstriction.
   c. Increased responsiveness to catecholamines.
   d. Modulation of the inflammatory response.

19. Overactivation of the systemic inflammatory response syndrome and the in-

flammatory/immune response systems activates what major mediator?
a. Complement.
b. Anticoagulation.
c. Renin-angiotensin.
d. Insulin pump.

A. has been in septic shock for more than 20 hours, and most of that time, she has been in an uncompensated state. Her management includes careful monitoring for the onset of complications. At this time, the results of her laboratory tests for platelet (Plat) concentration, prothrombin time (PT), partial thromboplastin time (PTT), thrombin time (TT), fibrin split products (FSP), and fibrinogen (Fib) are

Plat: 85,000/mm^3	TT: 27 sec
PT: 19 sec	FSP: 40 μg/mL
PTT: 80 sec	Fib: 188 mg/mL

20. Which of the following would indicate that A. was experiencing uncompensated septic shock?
a. Hypertension.
b. Pulmonary edema.
c. Metabolic alkalosis.
d. Poor respiratory effort.

21. What is the most likely complication that A. is exhibiting?
a. Thrombocytopenia.
b. Disseminated intravascular coagulation (DIC).
c. Stress ulcer.
d. Factor X deficiency.

The septic syndrome puts A. at risk for numerous complications, including adult respiratory distress syndrome (ARDS).

22. Why is ARDS frequently a complication of septic shock?
a. Decreased clotting.
b. Decreased capillary permeability.
c. Decreased carbon dioxide (CO_2) level.
d. Decreased surfactant.

The mortality rate continues to be high for patients who develop septic shock in the presence of certain conditions.

23. One of the conditions that contribute to this high mortality is
a. Low cardiac output.
b. High cardiac output.
c. Increased systemic vascular resistance.
d. Increased oxygen extraction ratio (O_2ER).

24. When hypotension exists with shock, it is related to
a. Increased ventricular ejection fraction.
b. Decreased venous return.
c. Increased venous return.
d. Increased afterload.

A.'s nutritional needs have been met with intravenous hyperalimentation for the last 72 hours. This form of nutrition should be reassessed, and enteral feeding should be considered.

25. What role do enteral feedings play in the management of septic shock?
a. They facilitate volume expansion.
b. They impede bacteria from leaving the gut.
c. They increase gastrointestinal motility.
d. They keep the systemic inflammatory response syndrome and the inflammatory/immune response from becoming overactive.

A.'s rate of healing is influenced by her psychological reaction to the PICU environment. She was moved to a private room in the PICU 72 hours after admission.

26. How does the PICU environment influence A.'s shock state?
a. It alters cardiac function.
b. It decreases capillary blood flow.
c. It decreases activation of the inflammatory/immune response.
d. It decreases levels of adrenal hormones.

27. One of the factors in the PICU environment that the nurse should consider as she or he plans A.'s care is
a. Neighboring patients.
b. Sleep intervals.
c. Parameter of bed space.
d. Meal times.

ANSWERS ■ CASE 15-1

1. Answer (c). Shock can be divided into two main categories: low-flow shock and maldistributive shock. Low-flow shock may result from hypovolemia, cardiac failure, or critical obstruction of blood flow. Maldistributive forms of shock include neurogenic, anaphylactic, and septic shock. Hypovolemic low-flow shock is the most common shock syndrome seen in infants

and children. It can result from any illness or injury that causes an acute reduction in circulating blood volume (i.e., blood, plasma, or body fluid). The warning signs of low-flow shock are symptoms of increased systemic vascular resistance and decreased cardiac output. The warning signs of maldistributive shock are symptoms of decreased systemic vascular resistance and increased cardiac output.

REFERENCE

Curley, M.A.Q. (1996). Shock. In M.A.Q. Curley, J.B. Smith, & P.A. Moloney-Harmon (Eds.). *Critical care nursing of infants and children* (pp. 874–892). Philadelphia: W.B. Saunders.

2. Answer (**a**). Shock can be described as inadequate tissue perfusion that leads to anaerobic metabolism, accumulation of lactic acid, and metabolic acidosis. Oxygen delivery (Do_2) is inadequate and altered from the accelerated metabolic processes and alterations in microcirculation. Cellular processes occur anaerobically, and lactic acid accumulates.

REFERENCE

Curley, M.A.Q. (1995). Shock. In M.A.Q. Curley, J.B. Smith, & P.A. Moloney-Harmon (Eds.). *Critical care nursing of infants and children* (pp. 874–892). Philadelphia: W.B. Saunders.

3. Answer (**d**). Assessment findings for children with low-flow forms of shock include cool skin, mottled or gray extremities, sluggish capillary refill, and peripheral pulses that are difficult to palpate. Urine output is an important assessment parameter, and it may decrease before other signs of impaired tissue perfusion are evident. A thorough, ongoing neurologic assessment is important because signs and symptoms of inadequate cerebral perfusion are often elusive in the early stages. Response to stimuli may be diminished, and children may be anxious, irritable, or lethargic. Infants often have a weak cry, poor suck, or both manifestations. Certain assessment findings are characteristic of *hypovolemic* low-flow shock, such as poor skin turgor, dry mucous membranes, a sunken fontanelle, crying without tears, and weight loss. The patient with *cardiogenic* low-flow shock may have a gallop rhythm and often appears "wet." Children with low-flow shock as the result of an outflow obstruction may present with a low-voltage electrocardiogram and electromechanical dissociation. As the low-flow state progresses, neurologic deterioration, hypotension, and bradycardia result.

REFERENCES

Curley, M.A.Q. (1995). Shock. In M.A.Q. Curley, J.B. Smith, & P.A. Moloney-Harmon (Eds.). *Critical care nursing of infants and children* (pp. 874–892). Philadelphia: W.B. Saunders.
Russell, S. (1994). Hypovolemic shock. *Nursing 94, 13* (4), 34–39.

4. Answer (**d**). Hypovolemic shock produces intravascular volume deficits. The resulting volume is not enough to maintain adequate circulation. Venous blood return to the heart falls, and the ventricular chambers do not fill completely, resulting in decreased diastolic filling and decreased systolic ejection volume. As stroke volume decreases, so does cardiac output and blood flow; oxygen delivery to the cells is inadequate.

REFERENCE

Rice, V. (1991). Shock, a clinical syndrome: An update. Part 1. *Critical Care Nurse,* 11 (4), 20–24.

5. Answer (**c**). Heart rate increases in all shock states. Mean arterial pressure remains normal during effective compensation, but it falls when compensatory mechanisms fail. PAOP, which reflects the left ventricular preload, is decreased in hypovolemic shock because of inadequate circulating blood volume. SVRI reflects the left ventricular afterload and is increased in an attempt to maintain blood pressure in low-flow shock. The cardiac index is decreased, and the Svo_2 is low, reflecting decreased cardiac output and increased O_2ER.

REFERENCES

Curley, M.A.Q. (1995). Shock. In M.A.Q. Curley, J.B. Smith, & P.A. Moloney-Harmon (Eds.). *Critical care nursing of infants and children* (pp. 874–892). Philadelphia: W.B. Saunders.
Rice, V. (1991). Shock, a clinical syndrome: An update. Part 2. *Critical Care Nurse,* 11 (5), 74–85.

6. Answer (**a**). Fluid administration must begin quickly after perfusion is compromised. Isotonic crystalloid solutions, such as normal saline or lactated Ringer's solution, should be used initially. A bolus of 20 mL/kg is given and repeated as necessary until systemic perfusion improves. Hypotonic fluids such as 5% dextrose in water and 5% dextrose in 0.45% NaCl should not be used for volume expansion,

because free water remains in the vascular space as glucose is metabolized. The use of 5% dextrose in 0.45% NaCl with 20 mEq KCl is not appropriate, because J. has had no urine output since admission.

REFERENCES

Hazinski, M.F. (1990). Shock in the pediatric patient. *Critical Care Nursing Clinics of North America, 2* (2), 309–324.
Perkin, R.M., & Levine, D.L. (1990). Shock. In D.L. Levine & F.C. Morriss (Eds.). *Essentials of pediatric intensive care* (pp. 78–97). St. Louis: Quality Medical Publishing.

7. Answer (**c**). Colloid solutions have large molecules that are generally confined to the intravascular compartment. The oncotic effect of these substances maintains a balance between intravascular and interstitial water. This balance is disrupted when oncotic pressure in the vascular bed is increased. Fluid is pulled from the interstitial compartment, and total plasma volume is increased. Colloids increase the hemodynamic parameters (e.g., cardiac index, left ventricular stroke work index, oxygen transport, oxygen consumption) more than crystalloids. Administration of certain colloids (e.g., albumin) may lower serum ionized calcium levels and inhibit sodium ion diuresis. Sensitivity reactions such as urticaria and hypotension have occurred.

REFERENCES

Kuhn, M. (1991). Colloids vs crystalloids. *Critical Care Nurse,* 11 (5), 37–51.
Perkin, R.M., & Levine, D.L. (1990). Shock. In D.L. Levine & F.C. Morriss (Eds.). *Essentials of pediatric intensive care* (pp. 78–97). St. Louis: Quality Medical Publishing.

8. Answer (**b**). Excessive fluid administration is a potential complication of fluid replacement therapy. It is a particularly worrisome complication that can result in ventricular dilatation and in systemic and pulmonary edema. Because pulmonary edema is a frequent complication of shock resuscitation, appropriate respiratory monitoring and support must be provided.

REFERENCE

Hazinski, M.F. (1990). Shock in the pediatric patient. *Critical Care Nursing Clinics of North America, 2* (2), 309–324.

9. Answer (**c**). As the metabolic acidosis is corrected, electrolytes shift. As the pH increases, ionized calcium levels fall, and potassium shifts into the intracellular space. This results in a decreased serum potassium level.

REFERENCE

Curley, M.A.Q. (1995). Shock. In M.A.Q. Curley, J.B. Smith, & P.A. Moloney-Harmon (Eds.). *Critical care nursing of infants and children* (pp. 874–892). Philadelphia: W.B. Saunders.

ANSWERS ■ CASE 15-2

1. Answer (**c**). Anaphylactic shock is a form of maldistributive shock that occurs after a severe allergic reaction. The antigen-antibody reaction is characterized by massive vasodilation and increased capillary permeability. This change in vascular tone and capillary permeability results in insufficient tissue perfusion.

REFERENCES

Curley, M.A.Q. (1995). Shock. In M.A.Q. Curley, J.B. Smith, & P.A. Moloney-Harmon (Eds.). *Critical Care Nursing of Infants and children* (pp. 874–892). Philadelphia: W.B. Saunders.
Rice, V. (1991). Shock, a clinical syndrome: An update. Part 1. *Critical Care Nurse,* 11 (4), 20–24.

2. Answer (**a**). When an antigen enters the body, it is attacked by antibodies. This antigen-antibody reaction stimulates the release of chemical mediators from the inflammatory immune cells. The immune mediators produce massive vasodilation and increased capillary permeability, which permits fluid to leak from capillaries into the interstitial compartment. A relative hypovolemia develops as fluids move from the intravascular space to the interstitial space.

REFERENCE

Rice, V. (1991). Shock, a clinical syndrome: An update. Part 1. *Critical Care Nurse,* 11 (4), 20–24.

3. Answer (**c**). The massive vasodilation and increased capillary permeability seen in anaphylactic shock leads to decreased filling pressures, which result in reduced right atrial pressure and PAOP. Cardiac output and arterial blood pressure are low, and pulmonary artery pressures are normal or low because of decreased blood volume.

REFERENCES

Curley, M.A.Q. (1995). Shock. In M.A.Q. Curley, J.B. Smith, & P.A. Moloney-Harmon (Eds.). *Critical care nursing of infants and children* (pp. 874–892). Philadelphia: W.B. Saunders.

Rice, V. (1991). Shock, a clinical syndrome: An update. Part 4. *Critical Care Nurse,* 11 (7), 28–42.

4. Answer (**b**). Methylprednisolone is given in severe cases to reverse the adverse effects of immune mediators and decrease capillary permeability Epinephrine is used to restore vascular tone and raise arterial blood pressure. Antihistamines can reverse the adverse effects of histamine, and aminophylline may be needed to decrease respiratory distress.

REFERENCE
Rice, V. (1991). Shock, a clinical syndrome: An update. Part 3. *Critical Care Nurse,* 11 (6), 34–39.

ANSWERS ■ CASE 15-3

1. Answer (**c**). $S\bar{v}o_2$ is decreased in low-flow shock as the result of the decreased cardiac output and O_2ER. Similarly, $avDo_2$ increases because tissues extract more oxygen during low cardiac output. Do_2 is decreased in low-flow states, and Vo_2 is initially increased but eventually becomes dependent on Do_2 and decreases.

REFERENCES
Carcillo, J.A., Pollack, M.M., Ruttimann, E.E., & Fields, A.I. (1989). Sequential physiologic interactions in pediatric cardiogenic and septic shock. *Critical Care Medicine,* 17 (1), 12–16.
Curley, M.A.Q. (1995). Shock. In M.A.Q. Curley, J.B. Smith, & P.A. Moloney-Harmon (Eds.). *Critical care nursing of infants and children* (pp. 874–892). Philadelphia: W.B. Saunders.

2. Answer (**b**). Children in cardiogenic shock secondary to congestive heart failure may have a gallop rhythm and appear wet. They may be diaphoretic and may have periorbital and sacral or dependent edema, hepatomegaly, jugular venous distention, and rales with increased work of breathing. These children also show signs of poor systemic perfusion, such as cool extremities, diminished peripheral pulses, and decreased urine volume.

REFERENCES
Curley, M.A.Q. (1995). Shock. In M.A.Q. Curley, J.B. Smith, & P.A. Moloney-Harmon (Eds.). *Critical care nursing of infants and children* (pp. 874–892). Philadelphia: W.B. Saunders.
Rimar, J.M. (1988). Recognizing shock syndromes in infants and children. *MCN: American Journal of Maternal Child Nursing,* 13, 32–37.

3. Answer (**a**). When the ventricular chambers do not adequately propel blood forward, two problems occur. First, stroke volume is decreased, which results in decreased cardiac output, blood pressure, and tissue perfusion. The second problem is related to the blood that remains in the left ventricle after systolic ejection. This blood increases ventricular filling pressures, elevating the pulmonary venous pressure, and the PAOP rises. The increased pulmonary capillary pressures cause fluid to move from the vascular space into the interstitial and intraalveolar spaces. The high pulmonary pressure is transmitted passively to the right heart and systemic venous circulation, which can lead to congestive heart failure.

REFERENCES
Curley, M.A.Q. (1995). Shock. In M.A.Q. Curley, J.B. Smith, & P.A. Moloney-Harmon (Eds.). *Critical care nursing of infants and children* (pp. 874–892). Philadelphia: W.B. Saunders.
Rice, V. (1991). Shock, a clinical syndrome: An update. Part 1. *Critical Care Nurse,* 11 (4), 20–24.

4. Answer (**a**). Dobutamine is a beta stimulant that increases cardiac contractility but causes only a slight increase in heart rate. In cardiogenic shock, dobutamine increases cardiac output and decreases PAOP and systemic vascular resistance.

REFERENCE
Curley, M.A.Q. (1995). Shock. In M.A.Q. Curley, J.B. Smith, & P.A. Moloney-Harmon (Eds.). *Critical care nursing of infants and children* (pp. 874–892). Philadelphia: W.B. Saunders.

5. Answer (**c**). Epinephrine is an endogenous catecholamine that provides a balance between alpha and beta stimulation. Catecholamines increase myocardial oxygen consumption, and signs of myocardial hypoxia or ischemia may occur during drug administration. All the other options are aimed at decreasing oxygen consumption.

REFERENCE
Curley, M.A.Q. (1995). Shock. In M.A.Q. Curley, J.B. Smith, & P.A. Moloney-Harmon (Eds.). *Critical care nursing of infants and children* (pp. 874–892). Philadelphia: W.B. Saunders.

ANSWERS ■ CASE 15-4

1. Answer (**a**). Shock can be divided into two major categories: low-flow shock and maldistributive shock. The findings in

A.'s assessment indicate the beginning of septic shock, a subcategory of maldistributive shock. Two other forms that fall into this category are neurogenic shock and anaphylactic shock. The hallmarks of early septic shock are displayed in A.'s assessment; they reflect activation of the *compensatory mechanisms* to maintain the cardiac output and tissue perfusion, accompanied by a maldistribution of blood. The hemodynamic characteristics of septic shock, which are evident in A.'s assessment findings, are a low preload and afterload, accompanied by a high cardiac output. Anaphylactic shock and neurogenic shock are characterized by low preload, afterload, and cardiac output. The outstanding hemodynamic factor in septic shock is the high to normal cardiac output. This is a direct result of stimulation of the sympathetic nervous system (SNS), which improves cardiac output by increasing heart rate and contractility (i.e., stroke volume). This is particularly significant in children, because the child's cardiac output is related to the heart rate; therefore, a high heart rate initially maintains the cardiac output. The exception is a heart rate greater than 200 bpm, which may be ineffective in maintaining the cardiac output. Cardiac output is considered a poor indicator for measuring the severity of hemodynamic changes occurring in septic shock, because the primary problem lies in the delivery, use, and extraction of oxygen, not in the cardiac output.

REFERENCES

Curley, M.A.Q. (1995). Shock. In M.A.Q. Curley, J. B. Smith, & P.A. Moloney-Harmon (Eds.). *Critical care nursing of infants and children* (pp. 874–892). Philadelphia: W.B. Saunders.
Hazinski, M. (1990). Shock in the pediatric patient. *Critical Care Nursing Clinics of North America,* 2 (2), 309–324.
Klein, D. (1991). Shock. *Nursing 91,* 21 (11), 74–76.
Vincent, J., Van Der Linden, P. (1990). Septic shock: Particular type of acute circulatory failure. *Critical Care Medicine,* 18, S70–S74.

2. Answer (**a**). In early septic shock, *three major changes* occur that create a confusing and falsely reassuring picture. The changes are related to the release of mediators that are produced in infection and inflammation. The changes are vasodilation, increased capillary permeability, and the abnormal distribution of blood flow. Overactivation of the sys-

temic inflammatory response syndrome and the inflammatory/immune response also plays a vital role in this reaction. When these systems are activated, multiple mediators (i.e., cytokines, plasma enzyme cascade, lipid mediators, and toxic oxygen metabolites) are released to fight infection and maintain homeostasis. The activation of the inflammatory response is beneficial at the local site of infection; it is when regulation of this response *does not occur* that the result can be devastating.

REFERENCE

Secor, V. (1994). The inflammatory/immune response in critical illness. *Critical Care Nursing Clinics of North America,* 6 (2), 251–273.

3. Answer (**a**). The primary red flags of shock in the compensated-hyperdynamic phase include normal or high blood pressure, bounding pulses, high urine output, and warm, flushed skin. Blood pressure changes are a late sign in pediatric shock; a low blood pressure may not occur until cardiogenic shock develops. During the compensated-hyperdynamic phase, compensatory mechanisms are intricately interrelated and include neural, hormonal, and chemical changes. When activated, these compensatory mechanisms successfully maintain cardiac output and tissue perfusion to vital organs. The mean arterial pressure continues to be normal as long as compensatory mechanisms continue to be effective. As the shock state progresses, systolic blood pressure falls as cardiac output decreases, and the diastolic blood pressure remains within normal range because of vasoconstriction. This results in a narrowed pulse pressure.

REFERENCES

Hazinski, M. (1990). Shock in the pediatric patient. *Critical Care Nursing of North America,* 2 (2), 309–324.
Rice, V. (1991). Shock, a clinical syndrome: An update. Part 2. *Critical Care Nurse,* 11 (4), 74–85.
Rice, V. (1991). Shock, a clinical syndrome: An update. Part 4. *Critical Care Nurse,* 11 (7), 28–42.
Strodtbeck, F., & Joyce, B. (1988). Shock in the newborn and children. *Critical Care Nursing Quarterly,* 11 (1), 75–83.

4. Answer (**a**). Neural compensation includes the activation of SNS by means of baroreceptor stimulation. When the cardiac output falls, the pressor receptors are immediately stimulated in the carotid and aorta; this sends a message to the medulla, leading to activation of the SNS. Activation of the SNS improves cardiac output by increasing heart rate, improving contractility, and releasing catecholamines.

REFERENCES

Klein, D. (1991). Shock. *Nursing 91, 21* (11), 74–76.
Rice, V. (1991). Shock, a clinical syndrome: An update. Part 2. *Critical Care Nurse,* 11 (5), 74–85.

5. Answer (**a**). The fluctuation in the WBC count is based on the individual's immune response to the infection. When infection is present, an *intact* immune system is evidenced by an elevated WBC count. The blood glucose concentration is typically elevated in septic shock as a result of the anterior pituitary gland secreting adrenocorticotropic hormone (ACTH), which increases the production of glucocorticoid. Sodium and potassium retention occurs and is the result of aldosterone being released and acting on the renal tubules. Temperature can range from fever to hypothermia, which is reflected by the metabolic rate and the direct action of mediators on the hypothalamus. Hypothermia may exist in late stages secondary to thermoregulatory failure of hypothalamus and decreased metabolic activity, which causes decreased heat production. Sepsis has been thought to be the result of a systemic response from an infecting organism; however, the same septic picture can be exhibited without an infection.

REFERENCES

Rice, V. (1991). Shock, a clinical syndrome: An update. Part 2. *Critical Care Nurse,* 11 (5), 74–85.
Secor, V. (1994). The inflammatory/immune response in critical illness. *Critical Care Nursing Clinics of North America,* 6 (2), 251–273.

6. Answer (**c**). The patient in shock needs to receive high concentrations of oxygen to prevent tissue hypoxia. In any type of shock, there is a problem with inadequate blood perfusion, which results in an alteration in oxygen uptake and consumption (Vo_2) and oxygen transport and delivery (Do_2). During septic shock, the relation between Vo_2 and Do_2 becomes dependent. This occurs as a result of the systemic circulation's inability to adequately deliver the oxygenated blood to the tissues and the cells' inability to adequately use the oxygen that does be-

come available. This is observed when compensatory mechanisms fail; oxygen delivery to the cells becomes inadequate, causing cell metabolism to switch from aerobic to anaerobic, forming lactic acid. In septic shock, oxygen requirements are increased, oxygen extraction is altered, and myocardial function is depressed even when the cardiac output is unchanged. Although difficult, the most beneficial intervention at this stage would be to correct the ratio of oxygen uptake over supply (O_2ER). The easiest and most effective means of assisting this intervention is to increase the oxygen supply. This is why the administration of oxygen is one of the most vital components in treating septic shock.

REFERENCES

Klein, D. (1991). Shock. *Nursing 91, 21* (11), 74–76.
Rice, V. (1991). Shock, a clinical syndrome: An update. Part 3. *Critical Care Nurse,* 11 (6), 34–39.
Vincent, J., & Van Der Linden, P. (1990). Septic shock: Particular type of acute circulatory failure. *Critical Care Medicine,* 18, S70–S74.

7. Answer (**b**). The uncompensated stage is thought to correlate with decompensation; this stage occurs when the symptoms of shock last longer than 1 hour despite significant treatment, and vasopressors are added to the regimen. When the compensatory mechanisms become ineffective, despite fluid administration, temperature control, and the use of supplemental oxygen, concerns surface about whether the vital organs are being adequately perfused. The development of multiple organ dysfunction syndrome is a great fear at this point. Manifestations of the uncompensated phase are hypotension (i.e., systolic pressure dropping below the 5th percentile for age) despite adequate fluid resuscitation, poor capillary refill, inadequate perfusion that may include oliguria, lactic acidosis, and an acute change in sensorium.

REFERENCES

Ackerman, M. (1994). The systemic inflammatory response, sepsis, and multiple organ dysfunction. *Critical Care Nursing Clinics of North America,* 6 (2), 243–250.
Curley, M.A.Q. (1995). Shock. In M.A.Q. Curley, J.B. Smith, & P.A. Moloney-Harmon (Eds.). *Critical care nursing of infants and children* (pp. 874–892). Philadelphia: W.B. Saunders.
Llorens, X., & McCracken, G. (1994). Sepsis syndrome and septic shock in pediatrics: Current concepts of

terminology, pathophysiology, and management. *Journal of Pediatrics*, 4, 497–508.

Rice, V. (1991). Shock, a clinical syndrome: An update. Part 2. *Critical Care Nurse*, 11 (5), 74–85.

8. Answer (**a**). The goal is to maintain hemodynamic stability and oxygenation of vital tissues. After the compensatory mechanisms fail and volume resuscitation is ineffective, exogenous support is needed. The use of inotropic support at this time is imperative to control contractility, preload, and afterload. Dopamine, epinephrine, norepinephrine, and dobutamine are the drugs most often used to treat shock. Epinephrine is often one of the first drugs to be used to improve ventricular function and afterload. Epinephrine improves the pumping of the heart indirectly by reducing preload and afterload. When epinephrine is used in treating shock, there is an increase in oxygen delivery. This reflects an increase in the cardiac index without altering the systemic vascular resistance. Concern is warranted when dopamine at high doses (>10 μg/kg/minute) is used in treating septic shock. It can cause tachycardia, renal vasoconstriction, and an increased systemic vascular resistance. The increased afterload that is produced by dopamine may decrease cardiac output, which would further compromise the patient. The use of Narcan in treating septic shock is unclear at this time. Several research studies involving animals, adults, and neonates have shown a positive response to Narcan when treating patients with refractory hypotension in septic shock. These studies showed an association between Narcan administration and improved blood pressure, cardiac output, and stroke volume measurements. However, the results of other studies do not agree with these findings.

REFERENCES

Hazinski, M. (1990). Shock in the pediatric patient. *Critical Care Nursing of North America*, 2 (2), 309–324.

Llorens, X., & McCracken, G. (1994). Sepsis syndrome and septic shock in pediatrics: Current concepts of terminology, pathophysiology, and management. *Journal of Pediatrics*, 4, 497–508.

Nash, P. (1990). Naloxone and its use in neonatal septic shock. *Neonatal Network*, 8, 29–35

Rice, V. (1991). Shock, a clinical syndrome: An update. Part 3. *Critical Care Nurse*, 11 (6), 34–39.

Russell, S. (1994). Septic shock: Can you recognize the clues? *Nursing*, 24 (4), 40–47.

9. Answer (**d**). Oxygen consumption, delivery, and extraction have been proven to be significant parameters to trend in septic shock. Continuous mixed-venous oxygen saturation monitoring (($S\bar{v}O_2$) and the arteriovenous difference in oxygen ($avDO_2$) can be used to measure tissue perfusion. The $S\bar{v}O_2$ in septic shock reflects the adequacy of the cardiac output to manage the hemodynamics. The $avDO_2$ is inversely related to cardiac output. During septic shock, a *dependent* relationship develops between VO_2 and DO_2, leading to a low oxygen extraction rate (O_2ER). To assist in the management of the O_2ER, it is necessary to consider the patient's hemoglobin level. By maintaining an adequate hematocrit, oxygen delivery is optimized. This effect may increase the oxygen uptake, which then improves the O_2ER. The patient's metabolic demands also should be considered and controlled to manage the O_2ER. Interventions that can assist with this are managing the patient's work of breathing, temperature, sleep intervals, and pain control. Blood pressure and pulse pressures by themselves are *unreliable* indicators of tissue perfusion during shock.

REFERENCES

Ackerman, M. (1994). The systemic inflammatory response, sepsis, and multiple organ dysfunction. *Critical Care Nursing Clinics of North America*, 6 (2), 243–250.

Curley, M.A.Q. (1995). Shock. In M.A.Q. Curley, J.B. Smith, & P.A. Moloney-Harmon (Eds.). *Critical care nursing of infants and children* (pp. 874–892). Philadelphia: W.B. Saunders.

Vincent, J., & Van Der Linden, P. (1990). Septic shock: Particular type of acute circulatory failure. *Critical Care Medicine*, 18, S70–S74.

10. Answer (**b**). Managing A.'s temperature helps to minimize the oxygen delivery and consumption mismatch. An elevated temperature in septic shock is detrimental to the already present hyperdynamic state. As the temperature increases, so do the inflammatory response, cytokine-mediated host defense mechanisms, carbon dioxide production, cardiac output, and oxygen consumption. The increased cardiac output is of great concern for the child who is already having difficulty maintaining an adequate cardiac output. It is during septic shock that VO_2 becomes dependent on DO_2, leading to tissue hypoxia; this dependent relationship reflects an O_2ER problem and indicates the cells' inability to adequately use the oxygen that does reach them. This pattern also indicates the maldistribution and interference of the circulating blood. Additional aspects that should be considered when addressing A.'s VO_2 are catecholamine release, pain control, environmental stimulation, and work of breathing.

REFERENCES
Cain, S. (1983). Peripheral oxygen uptake and delivery in health and disease. *Clinics in Chest Medicine, 4,* 139–148.
Russell, S. (1994). Septic shock: Can you recognize the clues? *Nursing,* 24 (4), 40–47.
Saltiel, A., Sanfilippo, D., Hendler, R., & Lister, G. (1992). Oxygen transport during anemic hypoxia in pigs: Effects of digoxin on metabolism. *American Journal of Physiology, 263,* H208–H217.

11. Answer (**c**). In shock, pulmonary capillary blood flow is decreased in relation to the shunting of blood to vital organs. This reduction causes an increase in the physiologic dead space and alters gas exchange. Alveolar cells lack sufficient oxygen, and the production of surfactant is reduced. Pulmonary edema arises from the increase in capillary permeability. The combination of a massive atelectasis, widespread interstitial edema, and reduced pulmonary compliance profoundly decreases ventilation and gas exchange and leads to respiratory failure.

REFERENCES
Rice, V. (1991). Shock, a clinical syndrome: An update. Part 2. *Critical Care Nurse,* 11 (4), 74–85.
Secor, V. (1994). The inflammatory/immune response in critical illness. *Critical Care Clinics of North America,* 6 (2), 251–273.

12. Answer (**b**). Antibiotic therapy is essential in the treatment of septic shock and should be started as soon as possible. The release of endotoxins from the rapid destruction of the bacteria may cause an accelerated systemic inflammatory response syndrome and inflammatory/immune response to occur. This is of great concern when an outlying hospital administers the first dose of antibiotics before transferring the patient. During the transfer, the patient's condition can rapidly deteriorate from the accelerated release of endotoxins. Studies are being conducted to determine how to slow the release of endotoxins in gram-negative bacteria and to define the rates of cytokine activation.

REFERENCE
Llorens, X., & McCracken, G. (1994). Sepsis syndrome and septic shock in pediatrics: Current concepts of terminology, pathophysiology, and management. *Journal of Pediatrics,* 4, 497–508.

13. Answer (**b**). Volume resuscitation is essential to improve cardiac output and oxygen delivery and to prevent the progression of shock. Children in shock have an enormous fluid requirement from peripheral vasodilation and capillary leaking. Controversy continues over what fluid is the best to use in the treatment of hypovolemia in septic shock. The main crystalloid intravenous solutions used are isotonic saline or Ringer's lactate. They are instrumental in increasing volume and cardiac output. If a single agent fails to do this, a combination of crystalloids and colloids is recommended.

REFERENCES
Hazinski, M. (1990). Shock in the pediatric patient. *Critical Care Nursing Clinics of North America,* 2 (2), 309–324.
Rice, V. (1991). Shock, a clinical syndrome: An update. Part 3. *Critical Care Nurse,* 11 (6), 34–39.

14. Answer (**c**). Humoral mediators, cytokines, and lipopolysaccharides activate the systemic inflammatory response syndrome. These mediators contribute to the massive vasodilation, increased capillary permeability, and insufficient distribution of blood. When an infection occurs, various cells become activated and participate in phagocytosis and inflammatory activities. The detrimental effects occur only when the cytokine and mediator functions carry over into other areas and cause extension of the injury and systemic effects. Mediators are responsible for the damage that occurs in systemic inflammation, sepsis, and multiple organ dysfunction syndrome. The increased stimulation of the sympathetic nervous system leads to an osmotic shift of interstitial fluid to the intravascular space. This is a particular concern in a child, because the extracellular fluid volume is already high and an addition to it may lead to dilution of the hematocrit and plasma.

REFERENCES
Curley, M.A.Q. (1995). Shock. In M.A.Q. Curley, J.B. Smith, & P.A. Moloney-Harmon (Eds.). *Critical care*

nursing of infants and children (pp. 874–892). Philadelphia: W.B. Saunders.

Hazinski, M. (1994). Mediator-specific therapies for the systemic inflammatory response syndrome, sepsis, severe sepsis, and septic shock. *Critical Care Nursing Clinics of North America,* 6 (2), 309–317.

Secor, V. (1994). The inflammatory/immune response in critical illness. *Critical Care Clinics of North America,* 6 (2), 251–273.

15. Answer (**d**). The most serious derangement associated with septic shock is an alteration in the coagulation cascade. It is one of the major systems activated when the inflammatory response is initiated. The events that occur when the coagulation cascade is activated are vasodilation, increased microvascular permeability, cellular activation, and adhesion. These events, which are beneficial at the local level, present problems when they are generalized. The goal of coagulation is to stabilize blood loss and restrict the area of injury. Accelerating this process causes rapid clotting and a depletion of the body's supply of platelets, fibrinogen, and other clotting factors. This may result in DIC. There are many mediators and cells that are involved in the coagulation process; some of the major components are platelets, complement, Hageman factor, the kallikrein/kinin system, tumor necrosis factor, and arachidonic acid metabolites.

REFERENCES

Corisco, M. (1994) DIC. *RN,* 57 (8), 35–41.

Klein, D. (1991). Shock. *Nursing 91,* 21 (11), 74–76.

Secor, V. (1994). The inflammatory/immune response in critical illness. *Critical Care Clinics of North America,* 6 (2), 251–273.

16. Answer (**a**). Septic shock continues to be an increasing problem in ICUs, despite advancements in medicine. More than one half the children who are hospitalized in an ICU for more than 3 weeks have developed nosocomial infections. The nosocomial infections that children acquire are usually related to bacteremias, cutaneous infections, and pulmonary infections. Inadequate handwashing is a main contributor to the spread of infection. The goal is to perform effective handwashing before and after contact with each patient.

REFERENCES

Hazinski, M. (1990). Shock in the pediatric patient. *Critical Care Nursing Clinics of North America,* 2 (2), 309–324.

Rice, V. (1991). Shock, a clinical syndrome: An update. Part 4. *Critical Care Nurse,* 11 (7), 28–42.

17. Answer (**b**). The activities that bradykinin brings to the inflammatory response include accelerated inflammation, accelerated fibrinolysis, and regulation of renal blood flow and blood pressure. The injuries that occur from these activities include massive vasodilation, increased microvasculature permeability, and excessive inflammation. The child shows signs of third spacing and appears hypervolemic, although relative hypovolemia exists. The significant clinical parameter that correlates with the massive vasodilation is a low systemic vascular resistance.

REFERENCES

Llorens, X., & McCracken, G. (1994). Sepsis syndrome and septic shock in pediatrics: Current concepts of terminology, pathophysiology, and management. *Journal of Pediatrics,* 4, 497–508.

Secor, V. (1994). The inflammatory/immune response in critical illness. *Critical Care Nursing Clinics of North America,* 6 (2), 251–273.

18. Answer (**d**). Tumor necrosis factor enhances immune cell activity. The outcome of this can be fever, endothelial changes, anorexia, decreased responsiveness to catecholamine, and increased WBC adhesion to endothelium. Tumor necrosis factor is responsible for almost all the same actions that occur with endotoxin, and it plays a major role in the septic cascade, stimulation of arachidonic acid metabolism, and clotting cascade. The level of tumor necrosis factor has been correlated with the severity of symptoms experienced in septic shock.

REFERENCES

Curley, M.A.Q. (1995). Shock. In M.A.Q. Curley, J.B. Smith, & P.A. Moloney-Harmon (Eds.). *Critical care nursing of infants and children* (pp. 874–892). Philadelphia: W.B. Saunders.

Hazinski, M. (1994). Mediator-specific therapies for the systemic inflammatory response syndrome, sepsis, severe sepsis, and septic shock. *Critical Care Nursing Clinics of North America,* 6 (2), 309–317.

Secor, V. (1994). The inflammatory/immune response in critical illness. *Critical Care Nursing Clinics of North America,* 6 (2), 251–273.

19. Answer (**a**). Complement is a mediator that is responsible for excessive cellular activation and inflammation. It is a component of the plasma enzyme cascade. Under normal conditions, the complement system, along with phagocytic leukocytes and antibodies, protects the host from bacterial and fungal infections. It is an important system, although it can cause tissue injury and provoke inflammation. Increased activation of the complement system can produce pulmonary leukostasis, which is a necessary factor in the development of ARDS.

REFERENCES

Llorens, X., & McCracken, G. (1994). Sepsis syndrome and septic shock in pediatrics: Current concepts of terminology, pathophysiology, and management. *Journal of Pediatrics,* 4, 497–508.
Secor, V. (1994). The inflammatory/immune response in critical illness. *Critical Care Nursing Clinics of North America,* 6 (2), 251–273.

20. Answer (**b**). Pulmonary edema occurs during the hyperdynamic-uncompensated stage of septic shock as a result of increased capillary permeability, pulmonary venous constriction, and pulmonary capillary pressure. The severity of the pulmonary edema increases if left ventricular dysfunction becomes evident.

REFERENCE

Hazinski. M. (1992). Cardiovascular disorders. In M.F Hazinski (Ed.). *Nursing care of the critically ill child* (pp. 117–394). St. Louis: Mosby–Year Book.

21. Answer (**b**). DIC commonly occurs in septic shock from overstimulation of the systemic inflammatory response syndrome and inflammatory/immune response, leading to activation of the coagulation cascade. This is evidenced by simultaneous widespread bleeding and clotting. The laboratory values in DIC reflect a platelet count that is decreased as a result of massive intravascular clotting. The PT and PTT values are elevated because of the consumption of fibrinogen, factor V, and factor VII and from the fibrin degradation products. The prolonged thrombin time indicates the defect in the rate of fibrin formation. Fibrinogen is also low because of the consumption of fibrin. FSPs are abundant; this indicates that microvascular clots have formed. The result of this abnormal coagulation process is the accumulation of microemboli within small blood vessels throughout the body. These blood clots interfere with blood flow and lead to peripheral and central ischemia. The rapid clotting depletes the supply of platelet, fibrinogen, and other clotting factors, which causes uncontrolled bleeding.

REFERENCES

Corisco, M. (1994) DIC. *RN,* 57 (8), 35–41.
Emery, M. (1992). Disseminated intravascular coagulation in the neonate. *Neonatal Network,* 11, 5–14.
Llorens, X., & McCracken, G. (1994). Sepsis syndrome and septic shock in pediatrics: Current concepts of terminology, pathophysiology, and management. *Journal of Pediatrics,* 4, 497–508.

22. Answer (**d**). Surfactant is depleted in ARDS. This change in surfactant contributes to an increased surface tension in the alveoli and leads to atelectasis. As alveolar cells become ischemic, the production of surfactant is reduced. ARDS results from a combination of atelectasis, interstitial edema, and decreased gas exchange, which leads to respiratory failure. Indications of ARDS are tachypnea, dyspnea, cyanosis, resistant hypoxia, and a general decrease in pulmonary compliance.

REFERENCES

Carroll, P. (1988). A.R.D.S. *Nursing 88,* 18 (10), 74–75.
Rice, V. (1991). Shock, a clinical syndrome: An update. Part 2. *Critical Care Nurse,* 11 (5), 74–85.

23. Answer (**a**). Children who experience a low cardiac output, minimal left ventricular dysfunction, and a low Vo_2 throughout shock have been shown to have a higher mortality rate. Blood flow to the heart, brain, and other vital organs is compromised when all three conditions are present. The cardiac output must be adequate during shock to maintain tissue oxygenation and delivery; the O_2ER must be adequate to promote tissue oxygenation. Children who do not survive septic shock demonstrate left ventricular dysfunction, progressive acidosis, low cardiac output, inadequate oxygen uptake, and severe pulmonary edema.

REFERENCES

Curley, M.A.Q. (1995). Shock. In M.A.Q. Curley, J.B. Smith, & P.A. Moloney-Harmon (Eds.). *Critical care nursing of infants and children* (pp. 874–892). Philadelphia: W.B. Saunders.
Hazinski, M. (1990). Shock in the pediatric patient. *Critical Care Nursing Clinics of North America,* 2 (2), 309–324.
Klein, D. (1991). Shock. *Nursing 91,* 21 (11), 74–76.

24. Answer (**b**). After compensatory mechanisms fail, the blood pressure begins to drop. This occurs when autoregulation of the microcirculation becomes less effective and capillary permeability is increased. Blood flow to the right side of the heart (i.e., venous return) is reduced, and the child's heart rate is no longer able to contribute to maintenance of the cardiac output. A low blood pressure indicates that the coronary arteries are less oxygenated and the heart rate can no longer contribute to maintenance of the cardiac output. This results in an imbalance between myocardial oxygen demand and supply. Bradykinin also plays a role in producing hypotension by means of the vasodilator effect.

REFERENCES

Rice, V. (1991). Shock, a clinical syndrome: An update. Part 4. *Critical Care Nurse,* 11 (7), 28–42.
Rice, V. (1991). Shock, a clinical syndrome: An update. Part 2. *Critical Care Nurse,* 11 (5), 74–85.
Secor, V. (1994). The inflammatory/immune response in critical illness. *Critical Care Nursing Clinics of North America,* 6 (2), 251–273.

25. Answer (**b**). Nutritional support of a child in sepsis through enteral feedings, even at 1 mL/kg per hour, has been proven to slow the translocation of gram-negative bacteria or endotoxins in the intestinal lumen. The gut has been identified as a key organ in the progression and initiation of sepsis. Under normal conditions, the gram-negative bacteria in the intestinal lumen are isolated from the rest of the body. In sepsis, the gastrointestinal immune function is compromised, allowing the gram-negative bacteria to leave the gastrointestinal system and enter the blood stream. Nutritional support has a significant effect on the permeability of the gastrointestinal mucosa. Gram-positive bacteria and viruses also may increase gastrointestinal permeability, and enteral feeding is appropriate therapy for patients with these organisms, too.

REFERENCES

Ackerman, M. (1994). The systemic inflammatory response, sepsis, and multiple organ dysfunction. *Critical Care Nursing Clinics of North America,* 6 (2), 243–250.
Hazinski, M. (1994). Mediator-specific therapies for the systemic inflammatory response syndrome, sepsis, se-

vere sepsis, and septic shock. *Critical Care Nursing Clinics of North America,* 6 (2), 309–317.

26. Answer (**a**). The PICU environment can be highly stressful for the patient. The ambient noise in the PICU environment has been correlated with a busy restaurant at prime time. A strong correlation exists between the environment and healing, and a significant alteration in cardiac function has been identified. Being exposed to a *continuous* complex environment activates the SNS to deal with the stressors encountered. Continuous activation of the SNS can be detrimental to the condition already compromised by septic shock or any other disease. The common physiologic responses that occur with activation of the SNS are increased salt retention, increased myocardial contractility, and increased platelet aggregation.

REFERENCE

Clark, S. (1994). Psychiatric and mental health concerns in the patient with sepsis. *Critical Care Nursing Clinics of North America,* 6 (2), 389–401.

27. Answer (**b**). Noise made by personnel can be more devastating than that made by equipment. An ICU environment has an abundance of both. It is believed that the patient's healing may significantly correlate with environmental stimuli. The startle response is activated frequently in the ICU patient, causing altered sleep intervals. This alteration leads to a decreased production of growth hormone, which can be the catalyst for the delayed healing. The assumption is that a patient would heal sooner if the ICU environment was conducive to long periods of sleep. There are enough data to support the idea that a relationship exists between stress in the ICU environment and the immune system response.

REFERENCE

Clark, S. (1994). Psychiatric and metal health concerns in the patient with sepsis. *Critical Care Nursing Clinics of North America,* 6 (2), 389–401.

CHAPTER 16

Trauma

PATRICIA A. MOLONEY-HARMON, RN, MS, CCRN

CASE 16-1

J., a 6.5-year-old girl, was hit by a car while crossing the street with her father. She pulled away from her father and ran into the path of a car that was traveling at 30 to 40 mph. She was thrown 20 feet into the path of an oncoming car and run over.

At the scene, she was alert and crying, tachycardiac, tachypneic, and hypotensive. She experienced loss of consciousness immediately, but she regained consciousness after a few moments. She opened her eyes spontaneously, cried for her mother, and moved her arms on command. She was given oxygen by face mask, and her cervical spine was immobilized. An intravenous line was placed, and lactated Ringer's solution was started. She was transported by air to the children's hospital. In the emergency department, she exhibited signs of acute respiratory distress and was hypotensive. She had a heart rate of 90 beats per minute (bpm) and a respiratory rate of 15 breaths per minute.

1. Based on this information, what is the first priority for J.'s resuscitation?
   a. Insert an intravenous line and start fluid resuscitation at 20 mL/kg.
   b. Insert an intravenous line, but because of the possibility of a head injury, fluid resuscitation should be only 10 mL/kg.
   c. Intubate the child and provide artificial ventilation.
   d. Send the child for a computed tomography (CT) scan to determine the extent of her injuries.

After intubation and ventilation with 100% oxygen, J. is still hypotensive and cyanotic. Her left-sided chest excursion is poor, and her breath sounds are markedly diminished on that side.

2. What is the treatment of choice at this time?
   a. A chest x-ray film is obtained to confirm the position of the tube.
   b. A needle decompression is performed, and a chest tube is inserted.
   c. A second intravenous line is inserted, and additional fluids administered.
   d. The child is immediately taken to the operating room for a thoracentesis.

J. responds well after her initial resuscitation and is stabilized. From the emergency department, she is sent for a CT scan, which reveals the following: diffuse cerebral swelling, a left rib fracture, splenic laceration with hemoperitoneum, and left renal subcapsular hematoma. An extremity x-ray film taken in the emergency room had also revealed a left distal femur fracture.

J. is sent to the pediatric intensive care unit (PICU), where she has a Camino catheter inserted for intracranial pressure (ICP) monitoring. Her initial ICP is 25 mmHg.

3. What is the goal of ICP monitoring?
   a. To prevent the development of a secondary head injury due to intracranial hypertension.
   b. To reverse the effects of brain damage that have already occurred.

c. To determine the best treatment for intracranial hypertension.

d. To determine the need for fluid resuscitation to maintain cerebral perfusion pressure.

4. Secondary injury is
   a. Injury that develops when the child has experienced more than one blow to the head.
   b. Bleeding that occurs with the initial injury and enters the epidural space.
   c. Skull fractures that occur concomitantly with a scalp laceration.
   d. A process that is produced by the brain's response to trauma.

5. What is the immediate intervention to treat J.'s ICP of 25 mmHg?
   a. Hyperventilate her to bring the ICP down to less than 20 mmHg.
   b. Administer mannitol at 1.0 g/kg intravenously.
   c. Administer pentobarbital at 5.0 mg/kg intravenously.
   d. Restrict fluids to one-half maintenance levels.

6. What would be an important nursing concern when hyperventilating J.?
   a. Monitor the Pao_2 to ensure that it does not go above 100 mmHg.
   b. Monitor the $Paco_2$ to ensure that it does not go below 20 mmHg.
   c. Monitor the $Paco_2$ to ensure that it stays above 45 mmHg.
   d. Monitor the Pao_2 to ensure that it stays above 150 mmHg.

7. An independent nursing intervention for J. when her ICP increases is to
   a. Provide hyperventilation.
   b. Administer mannitol.
   c. Provide nonprocedural touch.
   d. Administer pentobarbital.

8. Indicators of splenic injury include
   a. Pain in the right shoulder and right upper quadrant, decreased hematocrit, and leukocytosis.
   b. Pain in the left shoulder and left upper quadrant, decreased hematocrit, and leukocytosis.
   c. Pain in the left flank, elevated levels of serum glutamic oxaloacetic transaminase (SGOT) and serum glutamic pyruvic transaminase (SGPT), and signs of peritoneal irritation.

   d. Diffuse abdominal tenderness, decreased white blood cell count, and decreased SGOT and SGPT.

9. The diagnostic method of choice to rule out a splenic or liver injury is
   a. Diagnostic peritoneal lavage (DPL).
   b. Exploratory laparotomy.
   c. CT scan.
   d. Abdominal x-ray film.

10. J.'s splenic and renal injuries are managed nonoperatively. What would indicate the development of complications related to nonoperative management?
   a. Unstable vital signs, decreasing hematocrit and hemoglobin levels, and a worsening abdominal examination.
   b. Bile accumulation leading to hepatic necrosis or abscess formation.
   c. Development of a pancreatic fistula or pseudocyst formation.
   d. Decrease in abdominal pain and diminished sensitivity to touch.

Approximately 12 hours after J.'s admission to the PICU, she is in acute respiratory distress. J. is being ventilated with the Servo 300C on an intermittent mandatory ventilation (IMV) of 15, fraction of inspired oxygen (Fio_2) of 0.5, and positive end-expiratory pressure (PEEP) of 7 cmH_2O. Blood is drawn, and the arterial blood gas determinations include hydrogen ion concentration (pH), partial pressures of oxygen (Po_2) and carbon dioxide (Pco_2), and the bicarbonate (HCO_3^-) level:

$$pH: 7.32 \qquad Po_2: 60 \text{ mmHg}$$
$$HCO_3^-: 22 \text{ mEq/L} \quad Pco_2: 49 \text{ mmHg}$$

11. Based on this information, what does the nurse suspect is occurring?
   a. Abdominal bleeding.
   b. Intracranial hypertension.
   c. Agitation and pain.
   d. Pulmonary contusion.

12. What diagnostic test can confirm the diagnosis of pulmonary contusion?
   a. Additional arterial blood gas determinations.
   b. Chest radiograph.
   c. Pulmonary function tests.
   d. Pulse oximetry.

13. The chest radiograph confirms a severe bilateral pulmonary contusion. Appropriate interventions include
   a. Massive fluid resuscitation.
   b. Administration of antifungal agents.

c. Lung biopsy.
d. Use of high-flow oxygen and PEEP.

14. What is a complication of fluid administration in a child with a pulmonary contusion?
    a. Peripheral edema may develop.
    b. Congestive heart failure may develop.
    c. Overhydration may extend the area of contusion.
    d. The spread of infection may be augmented.

15. The nurse is considering the appropriate positioning for J. to optimize oxygenation and ventilation. She should position her
    a. With the injured lung up.
    b. With the injured lung down.
    c. In the right lateral decubitus position.
    d. In the prone position.

J.'s ventilatory settings are adjusted, and she begins to improve after several days. Her ICP remains within normal limits, and her Camino catheter is removed on day 4. She is extubated on day 7 and sent to the floor on day 8. She is discharged to home 23 days after her injury.

CASE 16-2

F., a 3-year-old boy, was a passenger in a car that was hit from behind and rolled several times. He was thrown about 30 feet. His mother was also critically injured in the accident. At the scene, F.'s heart rate was 120 bpm, respiratory rate was 40 breaths per minute, and blood pressure was 100/60 mmHg. His capillary refill time was less than 2 seconds, and his extremities were warm. No alteration in his level of consciousness was reported. He was transported by air, with a cervical collar and long backboard in place. In the admitting area, his vital signs remain stable. He is in no acute distress, has a Glasgow Coma scale (GSC) score of 15/15, and complains of neck pain.

1. F.'s symptoms indicate a strong possibility of
   a. Spinal cord injury (SCI).
   b. Compensated hypovolemic shock.
   c. Mild head injury.
   d. Abdominal injury.

2. SCI in children differs from that in adults in that

a. Children experience SCI more commonly than adults.
b. Children experience a higher incidence of cervical injuries and spinal cord injury without radiographic abnormality (SCIWORA).
c. The development of the pediatric spine is complete by 1 year of age.
d. The vertebral facets in children have a more vertical orientation and are ossified between 7 and 10 years of age.

3. Which of the features listed is the most critical determinant of SCI in F.?
   a. Degree of ossification.
   b. Shape of the vertebrae.
   c. Hypermobility of the spine.
   d. Closure of epiphyseal plates.

F.'s cervical spine x-ray film reveals a C1-C2 fracture and anterior dislocation of the vertebrae. Immediate reduction of the cervical spine fracture is required, because there appear to be some slight neurologic changes. He is intubated and anesthetized, and halo traction is placed. He is admitted to the PICU.

4. Priority nursing concerns for F. at this time include
   a. Prevention of decubiti.
   b. Placement of the halo.
   c. Fluid administration.
   d. Maintenance of the airway.

F. stabilizes and is extubated the next day. He remains in the PICU for 1 month and is then discharged to home. His halo is removed 16 days later. His mother also completely recovers from her injuries.

5. Assessment of a 4-year-old child with a fresh SCI shows that the child is cool to touch, with a heart rate of 90 bpm and a blood pressure of 70/50 mmHg. There is a strong suspicion of
   a. Spinal neurogenic shock.
   b. Increased ICP.
   c. Third spacing into the abdomen.
   d. Dissecting aortic aneurysm.

6. Appropriate treatment for spinal neurogenic shock is
   a. Isuprel and fluids.
   b. Fluids and Neo-Synephrine.
   c. Dobutamine.
   d. Amrinone and epinephrine.

7. A child involved in a high-speed crash in which the child was thrown a distance of 30 feet is admitted to the PICU. Radio-

graphic studies are normal. Can SCI be completely ruled out?

a. Yes, after the appropriate radiographs are completed and show normal patterns, SCI is ruled out.
b. No, the child should remain in a cervical collar for 1 week.
c. Yes, but the child should have another cervical radiograph in 1 week.
d. No, a CT scan should be obtained, and a thorough neurologic examination should be done.

ANSWERS ■ CASE 16-1

1. Answer (c). The first priority for treating the pediatric trauma victim is establishment of a patent airway. The child is observed for signs of respiratory distress, such as tachypnea, nasal flaring, retractions, stridor, the use of accessory muscles, and decreased level of consciousness. These symptoms require immediate intervention. Even though fluid resuscitation occurs simultaneously with airway management, the primary focus is the airway.

REFERENCES

Moloney-Harmon, P.A., Srnec, P., & Muir, R. (1996). Trauma. In M.A.Q. Curley, J.B. Smith, & P.A. Moloney-Harmon (Eds.). *Critical care nursing of infants and children* (pp. 893–923). Philadelphia: W.B. Saunders.
Yaster, M. (1991). Airway management. In D.G. Nichols, et al. (Eds.). *Golden hour: The handbook of advanced pediatric life support* (pp. 9–46). St. Louis: Mosby–Year Book.

2. Answer (b). Based on the mechanism of injury and symptoms, J. probably has a tension pneumothorax. Signs of a tension pneumothorax include severe respiratory distress, absence of breath sounds and hyper-resonance over the affected lung, lack of chest excursion on the affected side, cardiovascular instability, and tracheal shift to the unaffected side. The immediate treatment of choice is a needle decompression to relieve the tension. After the air is evacuated, a chest tube is inserted.

REFERENCES

Dickenson, C.M. (1991). Thoracic trauma in children. *Critical Care Nursing Clinics of North America, 3* (3), 423–432.
Hurn, P.D., & Hartsock, R.L. (1993). Blunt thoracic injuries. *Critical Care Nursing Clinics of North America,* 5 (4), 673–686.

3. Answer (a). The only absolute means of ascertaining the presence and evaluating treatment of intracranial hypertension is direct monitoring. The most important alteration to control in the head-injured child following resuscitation is increased ICP. Children are more susceptible to a secondary head injury caused by intracranial hypertension than to a primary injury.

REFERENCES

Ghajar, J., & Hariri, R.J. (1992). Management of pediatric head injury. *Pediatric Clinics of North America,* 39 (5), 1093–1125.
Vernon-Levett, P. (1991). Head injuries in children. *Critical Care Nursing Clinics of North America,* 3 (3), 411–421.

4. Answer (d). Secondary injury is produced by the brain's response to trauma and involves the loss of cerebral autoregulation, development of extracellular and intracellular edema, and breakdown of the blood-brain barrier.

REFERENCE

Walker, M.L., Storrs, B.B., & Mayer, T.A. (1985). Head injuries. In T.A. Mayer (Ed.). *Emergency management of pediatric trauma* (pp. 272–286). Philadelphia: W.B. Saunders.

5. Answer (a). In this situation, hyperventilation is the treatment of choice. Hyperventilation provides a rapid means of reducing ICP by causing vasoconstriction of the cerebral blood vessels. Mannitol may also diminish the ICP in the short term, but it must be used with caution in the head-injured child, because it may exacerbate cerebral edema. If it is used, a dose of 0.25 g/kg is recommended.

REFERENCES

Bruce, D.A., Alavi, A., Bilaniuk, L., et al. (1981). Diffuse cerebral swelling following head injuries in children: The syndrome of "malignant brain edema." *Journal of Neurosurgery,* 54, 170.
Fackler, J.C., & Yaster, M. (1992). Multiple trauma in the pediatric patient. In M.C. Rogers (Ed.). *Textbook of pediatric intensive care* (2nd ed., Vol. 2, pp. 1443–1475). Baltimore: Williams & Wilkins.

6. Answer (b). An important nursing action is to monitor the $Paco_2$ when using hyperventilation as an intervention, because $Paco_2$ levels of less than 20 mmHg can have a negative effect on cerebral blood flow.

REFERENCES

Davis, R.J., Tait, V.F., Dean, J.M., et al. (1992). Head and spinal cord injury. In M.C. Rogers (Ed.). *Textbook of pediatric intensive care* (2nd ed., Vol. 2, pp. 805–857). Baltimore: Williams & Wilkins.

Curley, M.A.Q., & Vernon-Levett, P. (1996). Intracranial dynamics. In M.A.Q. Curley, J.B. Smith, & P.A. Moloney-Harmon (Eds.). *Critical care nursing of infants and children* (pp. 336–384). Philadelphia: W.B. Saunders.

7. Answer (**c**). Touch, although it may not decrease ICP, does not increase ICP to a life-threatening level and provides comfort to the child. Mitchell and colleagues (1985) examined the effects of touch on children with intracranial hypertension. They found that, because touch never increased the ICP to a life-threatening level, the fear of doing harm by gentle touch is not well founded. They suggested that nurses increase the amount of nonprocedural touch and encourage parents to touch their children.

REFERENCE

Mitchell, P.H., Haberman-Little, B., Johnson, F., et al. (1985). Critically ill children: The importance of touch in a high-technology environment. *Nursing Administration Quarterly, 9* (3), 38–46.

8. Answer (**b**). Children with splenic injury most often experience pain in the left shoulder, in the left upper quadrant, or in the left chest with breathing. Laboratory study results may often be normal, but if abnormalities are seen, they are usually a decreased hematocrit and leukocytosis of 20,000 to 30,000/mm^3. Right-sided pain and elevated SGOT and SGPT are associated with liver injuries.

REFERENCES

Lebet, R.M. (1991). Abdominal and genitourinary trauma in children. *Critical Care Nursing Clinics of North America, 3* (3), 433–443.

Scorpio, R.J., & Wesson, D.E. (1993). Splenic trauma. In M.R. Eichelberger (Ed.). *Pediatric trauma: Prevention, acute care, rehabilitation* (pp. 456–463). St. Louis: Mosby–Year Book.

9. Answer (**c**). The CT scan is the method of choice for the diagnosis of splenic and liver trauma in the hemodynamically stable child. DPL is not usually indicated for the child who is managed nonoperatively, because a positive DPL does not mandate surgery. DPL is most useful for the child who is hypotensive and who is not responding to fluid resuscitation.

REFERENCES

Pearl, R.H., Wesson, D.E., Spence, L.J., et al. (1989). Splenic injury: A 5-year update with improved results

and changing criteria for conservative management. *Journal of Pediatric Surgery, 24* (5), 428–431.

Scorpio, R.J., & Wesson, D.E. (1993). Splenic trauma. In M.R. Eichelberger (Ed.). *Pediatric trauma: Prevention, acute care, rehabilitation* (pp. 456–463). St. Louis: Mosby–Year Book.

Taylor, G.A., Fallat, M.E., Potter, B.M., et al. (1988). The role of computed tomography in blunt abdominal trauma in children. *The Journal of Trauma, 289* (12), 1660–1664.

10. Answer (**a**). The major complication of nonoperative management of a splenic injury is rupture of a subcapsular splenic hematoma, causing massive bleeding. Complications resulting from nonoperative management of a renal injury may include persistent or recurrent bleeding, parenchymal infarction, or segmental hydronephrosis.

REFERENCES

Hensle, T.W., & Dillon, P. (1990). Renal injuries. In R.J. Touloukian (Ed.). *Pediatric trauma* (2nd ed., pp. 358–370). St. Louis: Mosby–Year Book.

Lebet, R.M. (1991). Abdominal and genitourinary trauma in children. *Critical Care Nursing Clinics of North America, 3* (3), 433–443.

Touloukian, R.J. (1990). Splenic injuries. In R.J. Touloukian (Ed.). *Pediatric trauma* (2nd ed., pp. 332–348). St. Louis: Mosby–Year Book.

11. Answer (**d**). Pulmonary contusion is common in children and is suspected whenever the child has a thoracic injury, especially if there is bruising on the chest. Signs of pulmonary contusion such as development of respiratory distress may not appear until several hours after the injury.

REFERENCES

Allhouse, M.J., & Eichelberger, M.R. (1993). Patterns of thoracic injury. In M.R. Eichelberger (Ed.). *Pediatric trauma: Prevention, acute care, rehabilitation* (pp. 437–450). St. Louis: Mosby–Year Book.

Dickenson, C.M. (1991). Thoracic trauma in children. *Critical Care Nursing Clinics of North America, 3* (3), 423–431.

Moloney-Harmon, P.A., Srnec, P., & Muir, R. (1996). Trauma. In M.A.Q. Curley, J.B. Smith, & P.A. Moloney-Harmon (Eds.). *Critical care nursing of infants and children* (pp. 893–923). Philadelphia: W.B. Saunders.

12. Answer (**b**). The chest radiograph demonstrates patchy densities indicative of a pulmonary contusion, but this may not occur for 24 to 48 hours after the initial injury.

REFERENCES

Allhouse, M.J., & Eichelberger, M.R. (1993). Patterns of thoracic injury. In M.R. Eichelberger (Ed.). *Pediatric trauma: Prevention, acute care, rehabilitation* (pp. 437–450). St. Louis: Mosby–Year Book.

Dickenson, C.M. (1991). Thoracic trauma in children. *Critical Care Nursing Clinics of North America, 3* (3), 423–431.

13. Answer (**d**). Severe pulmonary contusions, which significantly alter respiratory function, require intubation and mechanical ventilation. These ventilatory interventions include the use of high-flow oxygen and PEEP.

REFERENCES

Cooper, A. (1993). Critical management of chest, abdomen, and extremity trauma. In P.R. Holbrook (Ed.). *Textbook of pediatric critical care* (pp. 1060–1081). Philadelphia: W.B. Saunders.

Hurn, P.D., & Hartsock, R.L. (1993). Blunt thoracic injuries. *Critical Care Nursing Clinics of North America,* 5 (4), 673–696.

14. Answer (**c**). Overhydration during fluid administration may spread the area of contusion. A Swan-Ganz catheter is useful to closely monitor the fluid status of the child.

REFERENCES

Dickenson, C.M. (1991). Thoracic trauma in children. *Critical Care Nursing Clinics of North America, 3* (3), 423–431.

Luchtefield, W.B. (1990). Pulmonary contusion. *Focus on Critical Care,* 17, 482–485.

15. Answer (**c**). The child with bilateral contusions, such as J., is placed in the right lateral decubitus position. The child receiving positive pressure ventilation with a unilateral contusion benefits from having the injured lung up. The child with a unilateral contusion who is spontaneously breathing is placed with the injured lung down.

REFERENCE

Luchtefield, W.B. (1990). Pulmonary contusion. *Focus on Critical Care,* 17, 482–485.

ANSWERS ■ CASE 16-2

1. Answer (**a**). Any child who experiences head or facial trauma or who complains of neck pain is suspected of having SCI. The mechanism of injury should also alert the caregivers.

REFERENCES

Dickman, C.A., & Rekate, H.L. (1993). Spinal trauma. In M.R. Eichelberger (Ed.). *Pediatric trauma: Prevention, acute care, rehabilitation* (pp. 362–377). St. Louis: Mosby–Year Book.

Dickman, C.A., Rekate, H.L, Sonntag, V.K.H., et al. (1989). Pediatric spinal trauma: Vertebral column and spinal cord injuries in children. *Pediatric Neuroscience,* 15, 237–256.

Moloney-Harmon, P.A., Srnec, P., & Muir, R. (1996). Trauma. In M.A.Q. Curley, J.B. Smith, & P.A. Moloney-Harmon (Eds.). *Critical care nursing of infants and children* (pp. 893–923). Philadelphia: W.B. Saunders.

2. Answer (**b**). Children experience a higher incidence of cervical injuries and SCIWORA because of several factors. Development of the pediatric spine is a continuous, dynamic process. The vertebral bodies are wedge shaped, and the vertebrae are mostly cartilaginous. The vertebral facets are more horizontally oriented; they become more vertical and ossify between 7 and 10 years of age. Before this time, they provide minimal stability to the vertebral column. The head of the infant or young child is large in relation to the neck, paraspinous muscles are not well developed, and vertebral ligaments and soft tissue are more elastic. These features contribute to a tendency toward SCIWORA and upper cervical spine injuries.

REFERENCE

Dickman, C.A., Rekate, H.L., Sonntag, V.K.H., et al. (1989). Pediatric spinal trauma: Vertebral and spinal cord injuries in children. *Pediatric Neuroscience,* 15, 237–256.

3. Answer (**c**). Hypermobility is the most critical determinant of SCI in F. Hypermobility protects the spinal cord in the child from injury, because force is dispersed over several vertebrae. Hypermobility also accounts for a low incidence of spinal injury among children and in patterns of injury seen.

REFERENCES

Dickman, C.A., & Rekate, H.L. (1993). Spinal trauma. In M.R. Eichelberger (Ed.). *Pediatric trauma: Prevention, acute care, rehabilitation* (pp. 362–377). St. Louis: Mosby–Year Book.

Dickman, C.A., Rekate, H.L., Sonntag, V.K.H., et al. (1989). Pediatric spinal trauma: Vertebral column and spinal cord injuries in children. *Pediatric Neuroscience,* 15, 237–256.

4. Answer (**d**). Airway maintenance is the primary concern when F. is admitted. Other concerns are addressed as F. stabilizes.

REFERENCES

Johnson, D.L. (1993). Spinal cord injury in children. In P.R. Holbrook (Ed.). *Textbook of pediatric critical care* (pp. 209–217). Philadelphia: W.B. Saunders.

Richmond, T.S. (1989). Spinal cord injury. In C. Joy (Ed.). *Pediatric trauma nursing* (pp. 79–90). Rockville, MD: Aspen Publishers.

5. Answer (a). Spinal neurogenic shock, often resulting from complete upper spinal cord injury, may occur at the time of injury. The triad of symptoms is hypotension, bradycardia, and hypothermia, and they occur within 30 to 60 minutes of injury. These symptoms are the result of the sudden loss of sympathetic outflow from the cervicothoracic region.

REFERENCES

Dickman, C.A., & Rekate, H.L. (1993). Spinal trauma. In M.R. Eichelberger (Ed.). *Pediatric trauma: Prevention, acute care, rehabilitation* (pp. 362–377). St. Louis: Mosby–Year Book.
Richmond, T.S. (1989). Spinal cord injury. In C. Joy (Ed.). *Pediatric trauma nursing* (pp. 79–90). Rockville, MD: Aspen Publishers.

6. Answer (b). The loss of vasomotor tone that results from the sudden loss of sympathetic outflow can be treated with Neo-Synephrine (50 mg in 250 mL of 5% dextrose in water titrated to 50 to 100 μg/hour). Volume expansion with fluid is also appropriate.

REFERENCE

Dickman, C.A., & Rekate, H.L. (1993). Spinal trauma. In M.R. Eichelberger (Ed.). *Pediatric trauma: Prevention, acute care, rehabilitation* (pp. 362–377). St. Louis: Mosby–Year Book.

7. Answer (d). In approximately 35% of pediatric injuries, SCIWORA is encountered. It occurs most commonly in children younger than 8 years of age who have severe spinal injuries, although it can occur with mild spinal injuries. SCI exists even though the x-ray films are normal. CT scans may also be normal. SCIWORA occurs because the immature pediatric spine has experienced momentary intersegmental damage, causing disruption of the cord without disrupting the bones or ligaments. Children with SCIWORA often present with delayed onset of neurologic deficit, which may occur hours to days after the injury. Children with head and neck injuries should have a thorough history and physical and neurologic examinations to determine the presence of transient neurologic symptoms.

REFERENCES

Johnson, D.L. (1993). Spinal cord injury in children. In P.R. Holbrook (Ed.). *Textbook of pediatric critical care* (pp. 209–217). Philadelphia: W.B. Saunders.
Osenbach, R.K., & Menezes, A.H. (1989). Spinal cord injury with radiographic abnormality in children. *Pediatric Neurosurgery, 15,* 168–175.
Pang, D., & Pollack, I.F. (1989). Spinal cord injury without radiographic abnormality in children—the SCIWORA syndrome. *Journal of Trauma, 29* (5), 654–664.

CHAPTER 17

Transplantation

AIMEE C. LYONS, RN, BSN, CCRN
KATHLEEN A. MARINE, RN, BSN
KAREN MAGGIO, RN
RITA BROSNAHAN, RN, BSN
SUSAN LINEHAN, RN, BSN

CASE 17-1

M. is a 10-year-old boy with chronic renal failure secondary to membranous nephropathy. His dry weight is 24 kg. He has been treated with steroids and synthetic erythropoietin for several years without a positive response. He was dialyzed only three times selectively before transplantation to keep his serum electrolytes and other blood values normal. He is admitted to the pediatric intensive care unit (PICU) after receiving a living-related donor renal transplant from his mother. He is admitted with a central venous catheter, 6.0-mm oral endotracheal tube (OETT), two Jackson-Pratt tubes, a Penrose drain, a Foley catheter, an epidural catheter, two peripheral intravenous lines, and a nasogastric tube.

1. Because M. has received a living-related donor graft, he has a greater than _____ chance of 1-year graft survival.
   a. 33%
   b. 50%
   c. 80%
   d. 95%

2. As part of testing before transplantation, M. and his mother, as donor, underwent
   a. CT scans.
   b. Histocompatibility testing.
   c. Pyelograms.
   d. Upper gastrointestinal series.

M.'s native kidneys were not removed during surgery because they were shown to have a small amount of function before transplantation.

3. The risk of leaving in M.'s native kidney's is that
   a. Cardiac output may be insufficient to perfuse the old kidneys and new graft.
   b. There may not be enough abdominal space to accommodate the native and transplanted kidneys, resulting in pulmonary insufficiency.
   c. There is an increased risk of peritonitis because of the native kidneys.
   d. There is an increased risk of infection of the transplanted kidney.

On arrival at the PICU, M. has a renal ultrasound done to use as a baseline for future comparison, and he has a radionuclide scan.

4. The nurse explains to M.'s father that a radionuclide scan is done at this time to
   a. Look for ileus secondary to abdominal surgery.
   b. Confirm and evaluate placement of the new graft.
   c. Evaluate perfusion and vascular supply to the new graft.
   d. Ensure proper placement and patency of drains.

5. M.'s postoperative orders include "maintain CVP at 5 to 10 mmHg." The nurse knows that the rationale for this order is to
   a. Determine if rejection is occurring.

b. Ensure the presence of adequate circulating blood flow.

c. Ensure the absence of intra-abdominal bleeding.

d. Compare with pulmonary artery pressures.

On postoperative day 2, the nurse at the bedside notices a significant decrease in M.'s urine output.

6. The nurse, knowing that acute rejection or renal failure is always a possibility, uses which independent nursing action initially to determine the reason for the oliguria?
   a. Recalculate the intake and output values to verify the decrease.
   b. Weigh the patient to assess third spacing.
   c. Gently irrigate the Foley to assess patency.
   d. Give a fluid challenge of 10 mL/kg to ensure hydration.

The catheter irrigates easily, but urine output does not increase. M. is afebrile, with a heart rate of 160 beats per minute (bpm), blood pressure of 110/60 mmHg, central venous pressure (CVP) of 3 to 4 mmHg, and capillary refill time of 4 seconds in all extremities. The urine specific gravity is 1.030. The complete blood count reveals a hematocrit of 34%, which is increased from 32%.

7. With this assessment, the nurse realizes the patient is showing symptoms of
   a. Acute tubular necrosis.
   b. Hypovolemia.
   c. Hypervolemia.
   d. Renal vascular complication.

8. Based on these findings, the next intervention is to
   a. Administer a fluid challenge of 240 mL of normal saline.
   b. Prepare the patient for renal scan.
   c. Restrict fluids to insensible losses.
   d. Transfuse the patient with packed red blood cells.

9. Because M. has had a living-related donor, he is at decreased risk for acute tubular necrosis. The nurse explains to M.'s father that this is because of
   a. The large size of the donor organ.
   b. The minimal ischemic time of the graft.
   c. The preoperative immunosuppression.
   d. The lack of long-term dialysis.

Before transplantation, M. was found to be cytomegalovirus (CMV) positive, and his mother CMV negative.

10. Based on this information, the nurse would
    a. Give CMV immune globulin per protocol before transplantation.
    b. Start the patient on antiviral therapy before transplantation.
    c. Place the patient on universal precautions.
    d. Convert the room air flow to positive air flow for isolation.

As the nurse reviews M.'s orders, she notices "cyclosporine, 40 mg IV over 4 hours every 8 hours."

11. The nurse understands that the rationale for slow administration of cyclosporine is
    a. To avoid acute nephrotoxic reaction.
    b. To avoid anaphylaxis.
    c. To aid in consistent cyclosporine clearance.
    d. To maintain a consistent serum level.

12. M. progresses well during the next day. The nurse explains to M.'s father that, with good allograft function, M. will have normal blood urea nitrogen (BUN) and creatinine levels
    a. By 2 weeks after transplantation.
    b. By the third to fourth day after transplantation.
    c. At the 2-month point after transplantation.
    d. At day 10 after transplantation.

M. is discharged to the general pediatric unit 4 days after his transplantation and to home 4 days later. His mother is discharged to home 4 days after her surgery. M. has been able to resume all of his normal activities.

CASE 17-2

T. is a 10-year-old boy who was diagnosed at birth with cystic fibrosis. His medical history includes one hospital admission for a "clean out" (i.e., chest physiotherapy and nebulized medications) and a 9-week course of antibiotics. He has experienced progressive respiratory deterioration over the last year and now requires continuous oxygen therapy of 2 L/min by nasal cannula. T. is admitted for bilateral lung transplantation. After a 13-hour surgery, T. comes to the PICU for recovery and postoperative care.

T. was intubated with a double-lumen OETT throughout the operation. Just before coming to the PICU, the OETT is changed to a 6.0-mm single-lumen tube with the cuff deflated. T. also has a pulmonary artery catheter in place, two Jackson-Pratt drains, two chest tubes that show no air leaks, and a nasogastric tube.

1. The nurse who admits T. to the PICU knows that a double-lumen endotracheal tube was used during the transplantation procedure to
    a. Allow for unilateral lung ventilation.
    b. Allow for an easier transition to extracorporeal membrane oxygenation during surgery.
    c. Allow for unilateral tracheal lavage of the lungs.
    d. Monitor and compare the pulmonary function tests of each lung.

Diminished breath sounds are heard in the left lobes. The arterial blood gas determinations include hydrogen ion concentration (pH), partial pressures of oxygen (Po_2) and carbon dioxide (Pco_2), oxygen saturation (Sao_2), and carbon dioxide (CO_2) level. T.'s admission arterial blood gas determinations are

pH: 7.31 Po_2: 142 mmHg
CO_2: 28 mEq/L Pco_2: 56 mmHg
Sao_2: 99%

2. The nurse's initial intervention is to
    a. Manipulate T.'s ventilator settings.
    b. Repeat the arterial blood gas determination.
    c. Repeat the chest radiograph for OETT placement.
    d. Suction T. and proceed with pulmonary toilet.

As the nurse is reviewing the physician's orders, she notices that cyclosporine and Imuran are the drugs of choice for T.'s immunosuppressive therapy.

3. The nurse knows that steroids are not included in the postoperative orders because steroids
    a. Increase the chance of clotting.
    b. Increase pulmonary edema in the new lungs.
    c. Increase postoperative hypertension.
    d. Impede the vascular supply to the new bronchus.

Chest physiotherapy (CPT) is ordered for T. every 2 hours. After initial stabilization,

T. receives CPT and is suctioned. Before suctioning, the nurse confirms the distance that the suction catheter can pass. After suctioning, auscultation of the lungs reveals that the lower lobes have rales. The chest tubes are draining large amounts of serosanguineous fluid.

4. CPT is performed every 2 hours to
    a. Prevent mucus plugging, which can lead to lung volume loss and consolidation.
    b. Stimulate the hyperreflexive cough, which helps move secretions.
    c. Mobilize chest tube drainage, which prevents the possibility of clotting.
    d. Minimize mediastinal shifting related to increased fluid collection.

5. The nurse considers T.'s chest tube drainage normal; however, what would she consider if the drainage were bright red?
    a. Normal status after operative drainage.
    b. Signs and symptoms of hemorrhage.
    c. Hyperacute rejection.
    d. Reimplantation response.

6. The nurse confirms the distance that the suction catheter can pass to
    a. Minimize oxygen consumption.
    b. Prevent the chance of trauma to the carina.
    c. Prevent injury to the anastomosis site.
    d. Provide optimal airway clearance with suctioning.

Three hours postoperatively, the nurse notices that T. is experiencing changes in systemic perfusion.

7. The nurse confirms these changes through a rapid physical examination by
    a. Assessing T.'s skin turgor.
    b. Assessing T.'s peripheral pulses and capillary refill time.
    c. Obtaining a pulmonary capillary wedge pressure.
    d. Obtaining serum electrolyte levels and the hematocrit.

T. is extubated on postoperative day 2. Six hours after extubation, he complains of shortness of breath and becomes increasingly agitated. Auscultation reveals that the rales heard earlier in T.'s lung fields have increased.

8. The nurse's first response to these findings is to
   a. Obtain a chest x-ray film.
   b. Position T. with his right side down.
   c. Provide pulmonary toilet and administer furosemide.
   d. Reintubate T. with an OETT.

9. The differential diagnosis for T.'s symptoms is
   a. Acute hemorrhage.
   b. Disruption of the bronchial anastomosis.
   c. Lymphatic interruption.
   d. Reimplantation response.

T. progresses rapidly and is discharged to home 3 weeks after transplantation. Six months after transplantation, T. experiences a low-grade fever, increased coughing episodes, and increased sputum production.

10. T. is experiencing
    a. Bronchiolitis obliterans.
    b. OKT3 toxicity.
    c. Hyperacute rejection.
    d. Pulmonary edema.

T. is readmitted to the hospital for treatment and is discharged 3 days later. He is doing well at home.

CASE 17-3

S., a 3.5-year-old boy, was diagnosed with biliary atresia at 5 weeks of age. He underwent a Kasai procedure soon after the diagnosis. He was listed for liver transplantation 6 months ago because of rising bilirubin levels, increasingly abnormal liver function test results, and bleeding from esophageal varices.

S. is admitted to the PICU after undergoing a 12-hour cadaver liver transplantation. His dry weight is 14 kg. His estimated blood loss throughout the procedure is 800 mL. He arrives in the PICU orally intubated. He has two large-bore peripheral intravenous lines, a central venous line, a nasogastric tube, a Foley catheter, two Jackson-Pratt drains, and a T-tube in place. His intravenous fluid, 5% dextrose in 0.45% normal saline, is running at 48 mL/hour. His oxygen saturation on admission is 88%.

1. The nurse's first priority is to
   a. Adjust the ventilator setting to maximize ventilatory support.
   b. Administer 140 mL of Ringer's lactate as a fluid bolus.

c. Auscultate breath sounds and obtain a chest x-ray film to check for the OETT position.
d. Repeat all serum and blood work and readjust fluid rates.

Within the first few minutes of stabilization postoperatively, a blood sample is sent for analysis. S.'s arterial blood gas results are

pH: 7.19 PO_2: 260 mmHg
CO_2: 16 mEq/L PCO_2: 45 mm

His ventilator settings include a peak inspiratory pressure of 24 cmH$_2$O, positive end-expiratory pressure of 5 cmH$_2$O, FIO_2 of 1.0, and a respiratory rate of 20 breaths per minute. He has a rectal temperature of 37.0°C, heart rate of 130 bpm, blood pressure of 80/40 mmHg, and a CVP of 6 mmHg. S. has a hematocrit of 34%, prothrombin time of 15.1 seconds, aspartate aminotransferase (AST) level of 469 U/L, alanine aminotransferase (ALT) level of 674 U/L, alkaline phosphatase level of 195 U/L, and direct and total bilirubin levels of 2.0 and 3.0 mg/dL, respectively.

2. S.'s liver function test results indicate
   a. Acute graft rejection.
   b. Expected laboratory values postoperatively.
   c. Normal liver function.
   d. Overwhelming infection.

Two hours postoperatively, the blood work is repeated, revealing a hematocrit of 30%, prothrombin time of 16.0 seconds, partial thromboplastin time of more than 50 seconds, and a platelet count of 45,000 cells/mm^3. S. has a rectal temperature of 37.0°C, heart rate of 140 bpm, and blood pressure of 110/60 mmHg. The two Jackson-Pratt drains have collected a total of 140 mL of serosanguineous fluid. The T-tube has drained 5 mL, and his urine output is 5 mL over the last 2 hours. His CVP range is 3 to 4 mmHg.

3. What is S. experiencing?
   a. Acute rejection.
   b. Hypervolemia.
   c. Hypovolemia.
   d. Infection.

4. What is the most appropriate intervention for the nurse to initiate?
   a. Administer 140 mL of colloid.
   b. Administer 14 mg of furosemide and restrict fluids.
   c. Increase fluids to run at 72 mL/hour.

d. Place S. in the Trendelenburg position.

5. When S.'s nurse initiates her nursing care plan, what is her goal for monitoring CVP for S.?
   a. To monitor for arteriovenous shunting.
   b. To monitor S.'s cardiac output.
   c. To monitor S.'s diuresis.
   d. To monitor S.'s hydration status.

6. In assessing S.'s T-tube drainage, the nurse is expecting
   a. Clear, thick drainage.
   b. Dark brown, viscous drainage.
   c. Green, thin drainage.
   d. Serosanguineous, clotted drainage.

On postoperative day 2, S. is successfully extubated. Eight hours later, he is tachypneic and tachycardiac. His abdominal girth is increased by 6 cm. The drainage from the Jackson-Pratt drains has increased. S.'s blood pressure is 110/60 mmHg, and his heart rate is 150 bpm.

7. The appropriate intervention is to
   a. Administer a 140-mL bolus of packed red blood cells.
   b. Elevate the head of the bed to 30 degrees and irrigate the nasogastric tube.
   c. Obtain arterial blood gas values and prepare for intubation.
   d. Obtain the Jackson-Pratt drainage hematocrit, serum hematocrit, and coagulation values.

After intervention to decrease S.'s discomfort, S. has a few quiet days. On postoperative day 4, S. has increasing AST and ALT values, confusion, and tenderness in his right upper quadrant, and he is febrile to 40°C. S.'s cyclosporine dose is increased because of a low trough level. Imuran and steroid pulses (i.e., high doses of steroids for a set amount of doses) are begun.

8. At this time, the nurse suspects
   a. Acute rejection.
   b. Hypervolemia
   c. Hypovolemia.
   d. Cyclosporine toxicity.

9. The nurse should monitor closely for
   a. Hemorrhage.
   b. Hypoglycemia.
   c. Polyuria.
   d. Seizures.

Acute rejection is diagnosed by liver biopsy, and S. is started on OKT3.

10. The most appropriate intervention before dosing S. is to
   a. Administer a fluid bolus and then give the full dose of OKT3.
   b. Administer a test dose, watch for a reaction, and then give the full dose of OKT3.
   c. Administer Tylenol and Benadryl and then give a test dose of OKT3.
   d. Administer Tylenol and Benadryl and then give the full dose of OKT3.

11. The major purpose to give OKT3 to S. is to
   a. Block his T cell function.
   b. Enhance his macrophage function.
   c. Increase his platelet proliferation.
   d. Increase his bone marrow activity.

12. What is the likely complication of OKT3 in a child with a significant positive fluid balance?
   a. It creates significant hypotension.
   b. It decreases the seizure threshold.
   c. It increases generalized edema.
   d. It increases the risk of pulmonary edema.

S. finishes his course of OKT3 and is transferred to the floor. He recovers from the transplantation slowly and remains in the hospital for 6 weeks. He is discharged to home with a well-functioning liver.

ANSWERS ■ CASE 17-1

1. Answer (**c**). The 1-year graft survival rate is 88% for grafts from living-related donors and 71% for cadaver grafts. The 1-year patient survival rate is 96%.

REFERENCE
Perryman, J.P., & Silverman, P.U. (1990). Kidney transplantation. In S.L. Smith (Ed.). *Tissue and organ transplantation: Implications for professional nursing practice* (pp. 176–209). St. Louis: Mosby–Year Book.

2. Answer (**b**). Histocompatibility testing is always done and is used to minimize graft foreignness and to reduce donor responses to the transplanted organ. The type (or types) of histocompatibility testing performed varies according to the organ transplanted.

REFERENCE
Smith, S.L. (1990). Immunologic aspects of transplantation. In S.L. Smith (Ed.). *Tissue and organ transplantation* (pp. 15–47). St. Louis: Mosby–Year Book.

3. Answer (**a**). Patients who do not require long-term dialysis before transplantation probably have better native renal function and higher urine output. It is possible that urine output from mature native kidneys and the transplanted kidney may cause the small recipient to become intravascularly depleted more readily in the postoperative state. The cardiac output also may not be sufficient to perfuse the relatively well-functioning native kidneys and the larger graft.

REFERENCE
Harmen, W.E., Stablein, D., Alexander, S.R., & Jejani, A. (1991). Graft thrombosis in pediatric renal transplant recipients. *Transplantation, 51,* 406–412.

4. Answer (**c**). Renal ultrasound is a simple diagnostic test that is commonly done in concurrence with a renal nuclide scan as a baseline within the first 24 hours after surgery. The renal nuclide scan is performed to evaluate vascular supply and perfusion to the transplanted kidney.

REFERENCE
Paltella, P.S., & Weiskittle, P.D. (1993). Kidney transplantation. In M.K. Gaedeke Norris & M.A. House (Eds.). *Organ and tissue transplantation: Nursing care from procurement through rehabilitation* (p. 59). Philadelphia: F.A. Davis Co.

5. Answer (**b**). The CVP is usually maintained at 5 to 10 mmHg to ensure adequate circulatory blood volume. Care should be taken to maintain CVP within normal parameters, because hypovolemia further compromises renal function.

REFERENCE
Kennedy, J. (1992). Renal disorders. In M.F. Hazinski (Ed.). *Nursing care of the critically ill child* (2nd ed., pp. 629–714). St. Louis: Mosby–Year Book.

6. Answer (**c**). If the Foley catheter ceases to drain, the patency of the catheter is assessed first by aseptic irrigation with normal saline or sterile water. The irrigation is done with extreme caution because of the potentially fragile anastomosis of the ureter into the bladder. Failure of the catheter to irrigate requires replacement of the catheter.

REFERENCE
Cunningham, N., & Smith, S.L. (1993). Postoperative care of the renal transplant patient. *Critical Care Nurse, 10* (9), 74–81.

7. Answer (**b**). The signs and symptoms consistent with significant hypovolemia are poor systemic perfusion, oliguria with increased specific gravity, dry mucous membranes, CVP of less than 5 mmHg, tachycardia, and a rise in the serum sodium level and the hematocrit.

REFERENCE
Samson, L., & Ouzts, K. (1995). Fluid and electrolytes. In M.A.Q. Curley, J.B. Smith, & P.A. Moloney-Harmon (Eds.). *Critical care nursing of infants and children* (pp. 385–409). Philadelphia: W.B. Saunders.

8. Answer (**a**). When urine output falls and the patient has signs and symptoms of decreased intravascular volume status, a fluid challenge of 10 mL/kg of normal saline may be initially provided. Mannitol and furosemide also may be administered to encourage diuresis.

REFERENCE
Samson, L., & Ouzts, K. (1995). Fluids and electrolytes. In M.A.Q. Curley, J.B. Smith, & P.A. Moloney-Harmon (Eds.). *Critical care nursing of infants and children* (pp. 385–409). Philadelphia: W.B. Saunders.

9. Answer (**b**). Ischemic times are decreased with transplants from living-related donors. Long, cold storage times that may occur with cadaver transplants generally correlate with delayed graft function and acute tubular necrosis.

REFERENCE
Harmen, W.E., Stablein, D., Alexander, S.R., & Jejani, A. (1991). Graft thrombosis in pediatric renal transplant recipients. *Transplantation, 51,* 406–412.

10. Answer (**c**). CMV is the major viral pathogen in renal transplant recipients. Most often, CMV-seronegative patients receive a kidney from a seropositive donor. However, M. needs no treatment, because he is seropositive. Even with no treatment, universal precautions are indicated.

REFERENCE
Snydman, D.R., Werner, B.G., & Tilney, N.L. (1991). Final analysis of primary CMV disease prevention in renal transplant recipients with a CMV-immune globulin: Comparison of randomized and open-label trials. *Transplantation Proceedings, 23* (1), 1357–1360.

11. Answer (**a**). The use of cyclosporine has been associated with an array of complications. The most common and clinically important is nephrotoxicity. Acute nephrotic reactions may occur after rapid administration of an intravenous dose.

REFERENCE
Hooks, M.A. (1990). Immunosuppressive agents used in transplantation. In S.L. Smith (Ed.). *Tissue and organ transplantation: Implications for professional nursing practice* (pp. 48–80). St. Louis: Mosby–Year Book.

12. Answer (**b**). Most patients with good allograft function have normal BUN and serum creatinine levels by the third or fourth day postoperatively.

REFERENCE
Gill, B., O'Brien, P., Zamberlan, K., et al. (1996). Organ transplantation. In M.A.Q. Curley, J.B. Smith, & P.A. Moloney-Harmon (Eds.). *Critical care nursing of infants and children* (pp. 821–860). Philadelphia: W.B. Saunders.

ANSWERS ■ CASE 17-2

1. Answer (**a**). A double-lumen endotracheal tube permits isolation of each lung and permits independent lung therapy. Continuous positive airway pressure (CPAP) and mechanical ventilation can be directed to provide the support necessary to each lung.

REFERENCE
Banner, M.J., & Desautels, D.A. (1990). Special ventilatory techniques and considerations. *Clinical Applications of Ventilatory Support,* 8, 239–241.

2. Answer (**c**). Considering the symptoms, the position of the OETT is checked by an x-ray film. If the tip of the OETT is too near the carina, it could easily slip into the child's right mainstem bronchus.

REFERENCE
Hazinski, M.F. (1992). Chest x-ray interpretation. In M. Hazinski (Ed.). *Nursing care of the critically ill child* (2nd ed., pp. 499–520). St. Louis: Mosby–Year Book.

3. Answer (**d**). Bronchial healing is markedly impaired by the administration of corticosteroids. Cyclosporine and Imuran do not have this effect.

REFERENCE
Patterson, A., & Cooper, J. (1988). Status of lung transplantation. *Surgical Clinics of North America,* 168 (3), 545–558.

4. Answer (**a**). The importance of aggressive CPT every 2 to 4 hours while the patient is awake cannot be overemphasized. Missing just one or two treatments can lead to mucus plugging, lung volume loss, and consolidation of the transplanted lung.

REFERENCE
Malen, J., & Bocchuck, J. (1989). Nursing perspectives on lung transplantation. *Critical Care Nursing Clinics of North America,* 1 (4), 707–722.

5. Answer (**b**). A large amount of bright red drainage through chest tubes, falling hemoglobin and hematocrit levels, hypotension, tachycardia, and tachypnea are indicative of hemorrhage.

REFERENCE
Lekander, B.J. (1988). Preventing complications for the heart and lung transplant recipient. *Dimensions of Critical Care Nursing,* 7 (1), 18–26.

6. Answer (**c**). To ensure safe suctioning techniques and prevent damage to the tracheal anastomosis site, a sample suction catheter is marked at the level designated by the surgeon after the first bronchoscopy. This level indicates the point to which the catheter can be inserted during suctioning.

REFERENCE
Ahern, T.S., & Powers, C. (1990). Heart-lung transplantation. In S.L. Smith (Ed.). *Tissue and organ transplantation: Implications for professional nursing practice* (pp. 245–272). St. Louis: Mosby–Year Book.

7. Answer (**b**). When cardiac output is inadequate to maintain oxygen and substrate delivery to the tissues, signs of poor systemic perfusion are usually observed. These include tachycardia, mottled or pale skin color, peripheral vasoconstriction, cool temperature of the extremities, delayed capillary refill, decreased urine output, and development of metabolic acidosis. Even though the pulmonary capillary wedge pressure also gives information about the cardiac output, measurement of this value is not part of a rapid physical examination.

REFERENCE
Hazinski, M. (1992). Cardiovascular disorders. In M.F. Hazinski (Ed.). *Nursing care of the critically ill child* (p. 149). St. Louis: Mosby–Year Book.

8. Answer (**a**). Radiologic surveillance is of value in assessing the lungs' postoperative performance. It is a noninvasive procedure that can determine the presence of pulmonary edema.

REFERENCE
McGoldrick, J.P., & Scott, J.P. (1990). Early graft function after heart-lung transplantation. *Journal of Heart Transplantation,* 693–698.

9. Answer (**d**). Reimplantation response is defined as the morphologic, radiologic, and functional changes that occur in a transplanted lung in the early postoperative period. The patient becomes anxious and complains of shortness of breath, and the examiner may see diffuse infiltrates on the x-ray film.

REFERENCE

Gill, B., O'Brien, P., Zamberlan, K., et al. (1996). Organ transplantation. In M.A.Q. Curley, J.B. Smith, & P.A. Moloney-Harmon (Eds.). *Critical care nursing of infants and children* (pp. 821–860). Philadelphia: W.B. Saunders.

10. Answer (**a**). Bronchiolitis obliterans is a late complication of lung transplantation. The pathogenesis is not well understood. Unfortunately, the condition is irreversible and generally progressive. Potential causes may include mucociliary transport abnormalities with the inability to clear foreign antigens, chronic infection, pulmonary rejection, and the loss of bronchial blood supply.

REFERENCE

Aherns, T., & Powers, C. (1990). Heart-lung transplantation. In S.L. Smith (Ed.). *Tissue and organ transplantation: Implications for professional nursing practice* (pp. 245–272). St. Louis: Mosby–Year Book.

ANSWERS ■ CASE 17-3

1. Answer (**c**). A right pleural effusion is a common postoperative complication. Liver transplant patients are also susceptible to pulmonary problems because of the long operative procedure, anesthesia time, and large abdominal incision. A chest x-ray film and auscultation of breath sounds are initial nursing considerations in the postoperative period.

REFERENCE

Williams, L. (1991). Liver transplantation. In M.K. Gaedeke Norris & M.A. House (Eds.). *Organ and tissue transplantation: Nursing care from procurement through rehabilitation.* Philadelphia: F.A. Davis Co.

2. Answer (**b**). Hypersplenism secondary to portal hypertension resolves slowly over time but may cause neutropenia and thrombocytopenia. Liver function test results, including the prothrombin time, are elevated initially because of the ischemic period before transplantation of the donor liver.

REFERENCE

Williams, L. (1991). Liver transplantation. In M.K. Gaedeke Norris & M.A. House (Eds.). *Organ and tissue transplantation: Nursing care from procurement through rehabilitation.* Philadelphia: F.A. Davis Co.

3. Answer (**c**). Losing excessive amounts of fluid and electrolytes is the most frequent cause of hypovolemia. The fluid loss through the Jackson-Pratt drains and the third spacing of fluid after surgery increased this patient's chance of having hypovolemia.

REFERENCE

Baer, C. (1993). Fluid and electrolyte balance. In M. Kinney, D. Packa, & S. Dunbar (Eds.). *Clinical reference for critical care nursing* (3rd ed., pp. 173–208). St. Louis: Mosby–Year Book.

4. Answer (**a**). Frequently after liver transplantation, patients have an excess of total body water despite low or normal intravascular volume. Patients requiring volume replacement receive colloid solution rather than crystalloid to restore the intravascular volume.

REFERENCE

Williams, L. (1991). Liver transplantation. In M.K. Gaedeke Norris & M.A. House (Eds.). *Organ and tissue transplantation: Nursing care from procurement through rehabilitation.* Philadelphia: F.A. Davis Co.

5. Answer (**d**). CVP is important for accurate and continuous monitoring of fluid status, because fluid accuracy is vital in the acute phase of recovery to prevent other complications. A normal CVP range is between 5 and 10 mmHg. A high CVP indicates circulatory overload, and a low CVP indicates reduced blood volume.

REFERENCE

Thomas, C.L. (Ed.) (1993). *Tabers cyclopedic medical dictionary* (17th ed., p. 348). Philadelphia: F.A. Davis Co.

6. Answer (**b**). When assessing the T-tube drainage postoperatively, the bile of a functional liver graft should be dark brown and viscous.

REFERENCE

Smith, S., & Ciferni, M. (1992). Liver transplantation. *Critical Care Nursing Clinics of North America,* 4 (1), pp. 131–148.

7. Answer (**d**). Hemorrhage is a complication after liver transplantation that is related to vascularity of the organ and

the number of anastomoses. The signs and symptoms of hemorrhage are hypotension, narrowed pulse pressures, oliguria, and peripheral vasoconstriction. Abdominal drains should be assessed for excessive bloody drainage, and the hematocrit and hemoglobin levels are obtained daily.

REFERENCE

Smith, S.L. (1985). Liver transplantation: Indications for critical care nursing. *Heart & Lung,* 14 (6), 617–628.

8. Answer (**a**). Symptoms of rejection include decreased bile flow, a change in the color of bile to colorless, jaundice, increase in prothrombin time, vacuoles, fever, tachycardia, right upper quadrant or flank pain, and increase in serum bilirubin, transaminases, and alkaline phosphatase levels. Rejection signs occur 4 to 10 days postoperatively.

REFERENCE

Scheve, P., Bendon, P., & Perler, R. (1991). Liver transplantation in the recovery phase. *Critical care Nursing Quarterly,* 13 (4), 51–58.

9. Answer (**d**). Seizures occur in 30% of transplantation patients as a side effect of cyclosporine. It is reversible by decreasing the dose of cyclosporine.

REFERENCE

Sorenson, S. (1990). Care of the critically ill child after liver transplantation. *Focus on Critical Care,* 17 (4), 301–308.

10. Answer (**c**). Medications that are given to lessen untoward effects of OKT3 include hydrocortisone, acetaminophen, and diphenhydramine. The patient must have a chest radiograph and have no evidence of fluid overload. A significant side effect associated with OKT3 in patients who are fluid overloaded is flash pulmonary edema.

REFERENCE

Scheve, P., Bendon, P., & Perler, R. (1991). Liver transplantation: The recovery phase. *Critical Care Nursing Quarterly,* 13 (4), 51–61.

11. Answer (**a**). OKT3 blocks the generation of functional T cells and inhibits the activity of mature cytotoxic effector lymphocytes. This prevents the T cells from rejecting the liver.

REFERENCE

Thistlethwaite, J.R., Gaber, A.O., Haag, B.W., et al. (1987). OKT3: Treatment of steroid resistant renal allograft rejection. *Transplantation,* 43 (2), 176–184.

12. Answer (**d**). The most serious first dose reaction (severe pulmonary edema) is potentially fatal. This side effect is seen most frequently in patients who receive OKT3 and are fluid overloaded or are third spacing fluid.

REFERENCE

Ortho Pharmaceuticals. (1987). OKT3 product information sheet. Raritan, NJ: Ortho Pharmaceuticals Corp.

CHAPTER *18*

Toxic Ingestions

NATALIE MADAR, RN, BS, CCRN

CASE 18-1

J., a 22-month-old girl, has just arrived at the emergency center after ingesting crack cocaine. J.'s mother's boyfriend left the cocaine rocks on the table, and J. swallowed an undetermined amount.

1. What clinical manifestations does the nurse anticipate?
   a. Tachycardia and hypertension.
   b. Bradycardia and hypotension.
   c. Hypothermia.
   d. Hypotonia.

2. J.'s pupils are found to be
   a. Unequal.
   b. Constricted.
   c. Dilated.
   d. Normal.

Initial assessment of J. reveals a regular heart rate of 220 beats per minute (bpm), blood pressure of 134/88 mmHg, respiratory rate of 80 breaths per minute, and shallow breathing. Her skin is flushed; she fluctuates between irritable and listless states; and she shows signs of hyperreflexia. Her peripheral pulses are 3+; the capillary refill time is less than 2 seconds; and her rectal temperature is 42.8°C. She vomited 45 mL of green fluid during assessment.

3. Which of the following medications will be used to treat J.'s blood pressure?
   a. Dopamine.
   b. Verapamil.

c. Nitroprusside.
d. Amrinone.

After placing J. on a cooling blanket, the nurse notices clonic-tonic movements. Nursing care includes airway management, safety measures, and intravenous administration of Ativan.

4. Seizures are probably caused by
   a. Cerebral anoxia.
   b. Hyperthermia.
   c. Increased levels of angiotensin II.
   d. Increased potassium levels.

5. What equipment will be critical to have at J.'s bedside after administration of an anticonvulsant?
   a. Syringe and naloxone.
   b. Nasogastric tube.
   c. Bag-valve-mask (BVM) device.
   d. Blood pressure monitor.

Gastric lavage and activated charcoal are ordered by the physician.

6. Activated charcoal works by
   a. Binding readily with toxins.
   b. Propelling ingested material rapidly through the intestines.
   c. Changing the pH of the stomach.
   d. Neutralizing the toxins.

Ten minutes after administration of the activated charcoal, J.'s assessment shows she has a heart rate of 234 bpm, blood pressure of 54 mmHg/palpable, respirations supported with a BVM device, and a capillary refill time of more than 4 seconds.

7. What action is taken to support J.'s hypotension?
   a. Administer dobutamine intravenously.
   b. Administer epinephrine intravenously.
   c. Administer 0.9% sodium chloride intravenously.
   d. Elevate the head of her bed.

8. The nurse anticipates what length of time for J. to exhibit the clinical manifestations related to cocaine ingestion?
   a. 4 hours.
   b. 12 hours.
   c. 24 hours.
   d. 48 hours.

CASE 18-2

A 2-year-old boy is directly admitted to the pediatric intensive care unit (PICU) after transport from another hospital. His mother states, "I found D. in the dumpster by the shed on our farm. He was having trouble breathing, and I couldn't wake him up." D. is being ventilated with a BVM device when he arrives.

Assessment reveals equal chest rise and breath sounds, systolic blood pressure of 68 mmHg by Doppler, heart rate of 150 bpm, and a capillary refill time of more than 4 seconds. His peripheral pulses are weak and thready. The examiner notices excessive salivation and excessive lacrimation. D is incontinent of urine and stool, and there is evidence of emesis on his body. D. gives no response to painful stimuli, and increased bowel sounds are heard during the examination. There is no evidence of head trauma to explain the assessment findings. Because of the sudden onset, a toxic ingestion is suspected. Insecticides were known to be stored in the shed.

1. Insecticides interfere with impulses at the synapses of neurons because of a decrease of which enzyme?
   a. Insulin.
   b. Cholinesterase.
   c. Amylase.
   d. Angiotensin II.

2. Which of the following clinical manifestations provides a definitive clue to making a diagnosis of ingestion?
   a. Bronchial wheezing.
   b. Excessive salivation and lacrimation.
   c. Hypotension and tachycardia.

   d. Respiratory depression and neurologic instability.

3. What initial clinical symptoms are most significant in an insecticide ingestion?
   a. Excessive salivation.
   b. Tachycardia.
   c. Respiratory depression and neurologic instability.
   d. Hypotension.

4. The onset of symptoms would be more rapid if the poisoning resulted from
   a. Transcutaneous absorption.
   b. Ingestion.
   c. Inhalation.
   d. The route of exposure does not determine the severity or onset of symptoms.

5. After the airway, breathing, and circulation are stabilized, what is the most important nursing intervention?
   a. Bathe D.
   b. Rub D.'s skin vigorously with dry towels.
   c. Call the poison control center before initiating any interventions.
   d. Apply Betadine to sterilize the skin.

D. has just vomited a large amount of yellow-green fluid on himself, the nurse, and the floor.

6. What precautions should the nurse take?
   a. Test emesis for pH.
   b. Call housekeeping.
   c. Follow decontamination protocol.
   d. The nurse is not concerned and will clean up the emesis after things calm down.

7. Which of the following medications is anticipated for D.?
   a. Deferoxamine.
   b. Naloxone (Narcan).
   c. N-Acetylcysteine (Mucomyst).
   d. Atropine or pralidoxime (2-PAM).

CASE 18-3

M., a 5-year-old girl, is admitted to the PICU. M.'s mother stated that the girl ingested the medication she takes to treat her attention deficit disorder (ADD). The referring facility called and reported that M. ingested the whole bottle of clonidine, that her clonidine level was 13 mg/mL, and that she was hypotonic, with periods of apnea and bradycardia. Direct stimulation improved her heart and respiratory rates. Her blood pressure initially was 160/96 mmHg. A nitroprusside drip was effective in controlling her hypertension. Before transfer, her blood pressure stabilized, and the nitroprusside drip was discontinued.

1. Clonidine is a medication frequently used to treat adult patients. Which of M.'s assessment findings is most closely linked to the use of this drug?
   a. Bradycardia.
   b. Tachycardia.
   c. Hypotension.
   d. Hypertension.

2. Children who have ingested clonidine may present as a narcotic overdose. What will the nurse anticipate as she assesses M.?
   a. Seizures.
   b. Dilated pupils.
   c. Hyperthermia.
   d. Respiratory depression.

M. has been in the ICU for 8 hours (12 hours after the ingestion). The nurse notices that M.'s blood pressure has been falling steadily. Despite fluid resuscitation, her blood pressure remains low.

3. What intervention is anticipated?
   a. Start a nitroprusside infusion at 2 μg/kg per minute.
   b. Administer 0.4 mg of atropine intravenously.
   c. Administer a 20-mL/kg bolus of an isotonic solution.
   d. Start a dopamine infusion at 10 μg/kg per minute.

CASE 18-4

T., a 15-year-old girl, is admitted to the PICU. She attempted suicide by taking an overdose of acetaminophen. Although her mother states, "She took the whole bottle," there is some question about the exact amount. T. was treated in the emergency room with syrup of ipecac. The ingestion was approximately 6 hours ago, and the acetaminophen level of 213 μg/mL was determined 4 hours after ingestion.

T. opened her eyes only in response to vigorous stimulation. She had a respiratory rate of 34 breaths per minute, clear lungs, and an oxygen saturation of 98%. She had a heart rate of 104 bpm, blood pressure of 100/66 mmHg, capillary refill time of 3 seconds; was diaphoretic; and had peripheral pulses of 1+. A large emesis of clear fluid was evident, and the urinary catheter was intact, draining 1 to 2 mL/kg per hour of clear yellow urine. The laboratory results showed that her electrolyte level, bilirubin concentration, and prothrombin time were normal.

1. Based on T.'s acetaminophen level of 213 μg/mL 4 hours after ingestion, the nurse is concerned about
   a. Renal tubular injury.
   b. The nurse is not concerned, because this is an insignificant value.
   c. Hepatotoxicity.
   d. Respiratory depression.

2. Which of the following information from T.'s history is of most concern?
   a. She has frequent upper respiratory infections.
   b. She has an allergic reaction to fish.
   c. She takes phenobarbital to control a seizure disorder.
   d. She has few friends.

3. What is the treatment of choice for acute acetaminophen overdose?
   a. Deferoxamine.
   b. Methionine.
   c. *N*-Acetylcysteine.
   d. Cysteamine.

Three days after the ingestion, T. demonstrates the following changes: a response to painful stimuli with decorticate activity, jaundiced sclerae, elevated liver enzymes, petechiae over the abdomen, and bleeding from puncture sites.

4. What is causing these clinical manifestations?
   a. Hepatic cellular necrosis.
   b. Hepatic encephalopathy.
   c. Portal hypertension.
   d. Glomerulonephritis.

5. Based on T.'s assessment, what laboratory values are expected?
   a. Prothrombin time of 24 seconds.
   b. Creatinine level of 1.0 mg/dL.
   c. Hematocrit of 23%.
   d. Platelet count 155,000/mm^3.

6. What is causing T.'s altered neurologic status?
   a. Hepatic encephalopathy.
   b. Sedation.
   c. Use of neuromuscular blockers.
   d. Elevated acetaminophen levels.

CASE 18-5

E., an 18-month-old boy, drank a bottle of mouthwash. He presents 1.5 hours after this ingestion and is able to open his eyes only in response to painful stimuli. He has a shallow respiratory rate of 12 breaths per minute, and his breath sounds are clear. He has a heart rate of 186 bpm, blood pressure of 58/34 mmHg by noninvasive monitoring, a capillary refill time of more than 3 seconds, and a peripheral pulse of 1+. With an orogastric tube in place, his stomach is lavaged with normal saline. He has had no urine output since admission.

E. is intubated for airway protection, and the first-year resident orders activated charcoal to be administered through the orogastric tube.

1. The most appropriate intervention is to
   a. Instill the activated charcoal through a large-bore orogastric tube, ensuring correct placement, and place the patient on his left side.
   b. Ask the resident if he wants the activated charcoal to be mixed with sorbitol.
   c. Remind the resident that activated charcoal is not effective with this type of ingestion.
   d. Encourage the resident to order a 12-lead electrocardiogram.

2. Children with ethanol ingestion are prone to develop
   a. Hyperglycemia.
   b. Hypoglycemia.
   c. Hypercalcemia.
   d. Hypocalcemia.

3. Ethanol can be found in which of the following substances?
   a. Lipstick.
   b. Liquid soap.
   c. Liquid makeup.
   d. Perfume.

4. If this were a methanol ingestion, which of the following laboratory tests would be most helpful?
   a. Chloride levels.
   b. Prothrombin time and partial thromboplastin time.
   c. Aspartate aminotransferase.
   d. Osmolar gap.

CASE 18-6

B., a 2-year-old boy, ingested a questionable amount of his mother's prenatal vitamins 1 to 2 hours ago. His mother stated that there were between 6 and 10 tablets in the bottle before B. found the container and that none were left when she discovered the ingestion. B. presents with pale skin color and is sleepy but easy to arouse. He has a respiratory rate of 44 breaths per minute and no retractions. He has a heart rate of 138 bpm and blood pressure of 76/50 mmHg. There is evident emesis of a large amount of dark gray fluid, and B. has moderate to severe abdominal pain.

1. Which of the following treatments is anticipated?
   a. Ipecac syrup.
   b. Activated charcoal.
   c. Insertion of a large-bore nasogastric tube to begin gastric lavage.
   d. Preparation for peritoneal dialysis.

An abdominal x-ray is ordered to rule out the presence of tablets in the stomach or small intestines. The film shows that tablets are present.

2. What interventions are expected now?
   a. Administration of activated charcoal.
   b. Whole bowel irrigation.
   c. Infusion of clotting factors.
   d. Preparation for endoscopy.

3. Patients with severe iron ingestion present with hypotension because of
   a. Increased capillary permeability.
   b. Hypoglycemia.
   c. Increased catecholamines.
   d. Increased stimulation of the baroreceptors.

Within 8 hours, B.'s symptoms diminish, and deferoxamine (i.e., chelation therapy) is administered by a continuous intravenous infusion.

4. The nurse explains to B.'s mother that deferoxamine therapy causes
   a. Alopecia.
   b. Abdominal papular rash.
   c. Reddish orange urine.
   d. Reddish orange skin coloring.

While caring for B. in the ICU 30 hours after the ingestion, the nurse notices that he has developed hypoglycemia, hypotension, metabolic acidosis, abnormal coagulation study results, and an altered level of consciousness.

5. These clinical manifestations are the result of
   a. Portal hypertension.

b. Hepatocyte damage.
c. Disseminated intravascular coagulation.
d. Hypoglycemia.

CASE 18-7

C., a 2-year-old girl, ingested gasoline 24 hours ago. She is mechanically ventilated and is receiving maintenance intravenous fluids through a right jugular central line. She has a sinus tachycardia with a rate of 166, and her oxygen saturation level is 88%.

1. What gastrointestinal manifestations are anticipated?
   a. Constipation.
   b. Severe abdominal pain.
   c. Hematemesis.
   d. Abdominal distension.

Auscultation provides evidence of bilateral rhonchi and diminished breath sounds at the left base.

2. A diagnosis of pneumonitis can be anticipated because
   a. Surfactant has been lost because of the hydrocarbon.
   b. Strictures are present in the mainstem bronchi.
   c. Surfactant has been lost because of increased catecholamines.
   d. It is a common complication of intubation.

3. C. will require
   a. Good pulmonary toilet.
   b. Extracorporeal membrane oxygenation.
   c. Administration of packed cells.
   d. Insertion of a left chest tube.

4. C.'s respiratory status does not improve, and the nurse prepares to
   a. Increase the F_{IO_2}.
   b. Increase the ventilator rate.
   c. Increase the positive end-expiratory pressure (PEEP).
   d. Increase the tidal volume.

Two weeks after the ingestion, C. is being transferred to the pediatric floor later today. Her mother wants to know if C. will have any complications.

5. The best response is
   a. There are no permanent complications.
   b. She will be prone to infections.

c. There may be damage that will result in future respiratory problems.
d. Are you worried about sending her to a different unit?

CASE 18-8

R. is a 13-month-old boy who was found under the bathroom sink after ingesting toilet bowl cleaner. R.'s assessment on admission to the emergency department finds tachypnea, tachycardia, and substernal, clavicular, and intercostal retractions. R. is irritable and restless. He has visible burns on his oral mucosa, and he is drooling.

1. What is the first priority?
   a. Administer syrup of ipecac.
   b. Institute airway management.
   c. Insert a nasogastric tube.
   d. Give activated charcoal.

After a difficult intubation, the nurse notices that R.'s abdomen is distended.

2. Based on this assessment, the nurse will
   a. Insert a nasogastric/orogastric tube.
   b. Manually decompress the abdomen.
   c. Notify the attending physician.
   d. Place the patient on his left side.

3. Children who ingest caustic agents most frequently require long-term follow-up because of
   a. Chronic infections.
   b. Esophageal strictures.
   c. Chronic atelectasis.
   d. Developmental delays.

ANSWERS ■ CASE 18-1

1. Answer (a). Cocaine causes a powerful "fight or flight" response because of stimulation of the sympathetic nervous system. The brain and heart are highly susceptible to the effects of cocaine. Fortunately, except for sudden death and with massive oral ingestion, toxic effects are short lived because of the short serum half-life.

REFERENCES

Longo, C., & Dickenson C. (1996). Toxic ingestions. In M.A.Q. Curley, J.B. Smith, & P.A. Moloney-Harmon (Eds.). *Critical care nursing of infants and children* (pp. 940–962). Philadelphia: W.B. Saunders.

Soloway, R.A. (1993). Street-smart advice on treating drug overdose. *American Journal of Nursing,* 93 (9), 67.

2. Answer (c). Pupil dilation is associated

with the increased catecholamine release that results from central nervous system stimulation.

REFERENCE

Soloway, R.A. (1993). Street-smart advice on treating drug overdose. *American Journal of Nursing, 93* (9), 67.

3. **Answer (c).** Nitroprusside (Nipride) causes systemic and pulmonary artery and venous dilation, which counteracts the catecholamine storm. Nitroprusside is a short-acting agent that lowers blood pressure quickly in hypertensive emergencies. Because nitroprusside is sensitive to light, the solution must be covered with an opaque material. Labetalol or propranolol may also be used.

REFERENCES

Hazinski, M.F. (1992). Cardiovascular disorders. In M.F. Hazinski (Ed.). *Nursing care of the critically ill child* (2nd ed., pp. 117–394). St. Louis: Mosby–Year Book.
Longo, C., & Dickenson, C. (1996). Toxic ingestions. In M.A.Q. Curley, J.B. Smith, & P.A. Moloney-Harmon (Eds.). *Critical care nursing of infants and children* (pp. 940–962). Philadelphia: W.B. Saunders.
Soloway, R.A. (1993). Street-smart advice on treating drug overdose. *American Journal of Nursing, 93* (9), 66.

4. **Answer (a).** Cerebral anoxia results from the severe central vasoconstriction that occurs with overstimulation of the sympathetic nervous system. Seizures can be controlled with short-acting anticonvulsants such as diazepam and lorazepam. Refractory seizures can be treated with phenytoin or phenobarbital.

REFERENCES

Longo, C., & Dickenson, C. (1996). Toxic ingestions. In M.A.Q. Curley, J.B. Smith, & P.A. Moloney-Harmon (Eds.). *Critical care nursing of infants and children* (pp. 940–962). Philadelphia: W.B. Saunders.
Reed, G., & Anderson, R. (1990). Street drugs: Cocaine & PCP. In D.L. Levine & F.C. Morriss (Eds.). *Essentials of pediatric intensive care* (pp. 665–669). St. Louis: Quality Medical Publishers.

5. **Answer (c).** Anticonvulsants are frequently associated with respiratory depression. Measures must be taken to protect J.'s airway and maintain adequate ventilation.

REFERENCE

Reed, G., & Anderson, R. (1990). Street drugs: Cocaine & PCP. In D.L. Levine & F.C. Morriss (Eds.). *Essentials of pediatric intensive care* (pp. 665–669). St. Louis: Quality Medical Publishers.

6. **Answer (a).** Activated charcoal binds with the toxic compounds, and intestinal absorption is decreased. The charcoal should be administered with a cathartic such as sorbitol.

REFERENCE

Reed, M. (1990). Poisoning: General principles. In J. Blumer (Ed.). *The practical guide to pediatric intensive care* (3rd ed., pp. 660–671). St. Louis: Mosby–Year Book.

7. **Answer (c).** Hypotension is usually supported with 0.9% sodium chloride intravenously and Trendelenburg positioning. Vasoactive drugs should be avoided, if possible, because J.'s myocardium is sensitized and susceptible to serious ventricular dysrhythmias.

REFERENCE

Reed, G., & Anderson, R. (1990). Street drugs: Cocaine & PCP. In D.L. Levine & F.C. Morriss (Eds.). *Essentials of pediatric intensive care* (pp. 665–669). St. Louis: Quality Medical Publishers.

8. **Answer (a).** The sympathetic effects of cocaine last for a short period, usually a few hours.

REFERENCE

Soloway, R.A. (1993). Street-smart advice on treating drug overdose. *American Journal of Nursing, 93* (9), 66.

ANSWERS ■ CASE 18–2

1. **Answer (b).** Organophosphates are powerful inhibitors of the enzyme acetylcholinesterase (cholinesterase). Cholinesterase is an enzyme present in nervous tissue, skeletal muscle, and erythrocytes. It is responsible for converting acetylcholine, a neurotransmitter, to acetic acid and choline. Because acetylcholine conversion is inhibited, acetylcholine accumulates at synapses throughout the central and peripheral nervous system. Initially, there is excitation and then depression of neurotransmission at the synapses.

REFERENCES

Berkowitz, I., Banner, W., & Rogers, M. (1992). Poisoning and the critically ill child. In M. Rogers (Ed.). *Textbook of pediatric intensive care* (2nd ed., pp. 1290–1356). Baltimore: Williams & Wilkins.
Zeviener, R., & Ginsburg, C. (1990). Organophosphate and carbamate poisoning. In D.L. Levine & F.C. Morriss (Eds.) *Essentials of pediatric intensive care* (pp. 648–653). St. Louis: Quality Medical Publishers.

2. Answer (**b**). The response to intoxication is complex because of the diverse location and function of cholinergic receptors. A helpful mnemonic used to categorize presenting symptoms of organophosphate poisoning is SLUDGE, which stands for *excessive* **s**alivation, **l**acrimation, **u**rination, **d**efecation, **g**astric emesis, and **e**mesis.

Bradycardia, tachycardia, respiratory depression, hypotension, hypertension, neurologic instability, and hypotonia are also frequently associated symptoms. Some insecticides may have a petroleum base, and the child will present with clinical manifestations of a hydrocarbon and an insecticide ingestion.

REFERENCES

Berkowitz, I., Banner, W., & Rogers, M. (1992). Poisoning and the critically ill child. In M. Rogers (Ed.). *Textbook of pediatric intensive care* (2nd ed., pp. 1290–1356). Baltimore: Williams & Wilkins.
Zeviener, R., & Ginsburg, C. (1990). Organophosphate and carbamate poisoning. In D.L. Levine & F.C. Morriss (Eds.). *Essentials of pediatric intensive care* (pp. 648–653). St. Louis: Quality Medical Publishers.

3. Answer (**c**). Respiratory depression and altered mental status dominate the clinical picture. These patients require emergent care to correct the airway, breathing, and circulatory problems before any other treatment. Respiratory failure is the most common cause of death.

REFERENCE

Berkowitz, I., Banner, W., & Rogers, M. (1992). Poisoning and the critically ill child. In M. Rogers (Ed.). *Textbook of pediatric intensive care* (2nd ed., pp. 1290–1356). Baltimore: Williams & Wilkins.

4. Answer (**b**). The onset of signs and symptoms of organophosphate toxicity depends on the dose, route of exposure, potency, and solubility of the agent. Children are most commonly exposed through ingestion, and clinical manifestations are seen within minutes to hours.

REFERENCES

Berkowitz, I., Banner, W., & Rogers, M. (1992). Poisoning and the critically ill child. In M. Rogers (Ed.). *Textbook of pediatric intensive care* (2nd ed., pp. 1290–1356). Baltimore: Williams & Wilkins.
Zeviener, R., & Ginsburg, C. (1990). Organophosphate and carbamate poisoning. In D.L. Levine & F.C. Morriss (Eds.). *Essentials of pediatric intensive care* (pp. 648–653). St. Louis: Quality Medical Publishers.

5. Answer (**a**). Bathing the patient and decontaminating the skin is imperative to prevent further exposure. Liberal use of water is recommended. Follow self-protection guidelines while caring for these children.

REFERENCES

Berkowitz, I., Banner, W., & Rogers, M. (1992). Poisoning and the critically ill child. In M. Rogers (Ed.). *Textbook of pediatric intensive care* (2nd ed., pp. 1290–1356). Baltimore: Williams & Wilkins.
Mortensen, M. (1990). Organophosphates and carbamates. In J. Blumer (Ed.). *A practical guide to pediatric intensive care* (3rd ed., pp. 713–718). St. Louis: Mosby–Year Book.

6. Answer (**c**). Because the insecticide may still be present in the emesis, it can cause transcutaneous absorption. The patient, any health care providers who have contact, and the floor should be decontaminated.

REFERENCES

Berkowitz, I., Banner, W., & Rogers, M. (1992). Poisoning and the critically ill child. In M. Rogers (Ed.). *Textbook of pediatric intensive care* (2nd ed., pp. 1290–1356). Baltimore: Williams & Wilkins.
Mortensen, M. (1990). Organophosphates and carbamates. In J. Blumer (Ed.). *A practical guide to pediatric intensive care* (3rd ed., pp. 713–718). St. Louis: Mosby–Year Book.

7. Answer (**d**). Atropine is an antagonist of acetylcholine and counteracts the effects of excess acetylcholine at parasympathetic neuroeffector junctions. Because atropine has no effect on cholinergic receptors of the neuromuscular junction, respiratory depression will continue despite therapy. An initial dose of 0.02 mg/kg and up to 0.05 mg/kg may be needed. The maximum dose is 2 to 4 mg. The dose may need to be repeated every 1.5 to 2 hours, and continuous drips may be necessary. The route of administration can be subcutaneous, intramuscular, or intravenous. The goal is to have the patient exhibit signs of "atropinization": dilated pupils, diminished secretions, decreased bowel sounds, and cutaneous flushing. Even though some patients present with tachycardia and hypertension, atropine should not be stopped because of an increased heart rate. The heart rate may reflect the toxins and not the atropinization.

Pralidoxime (2-PAM) reactivates cholinesterase, liberates active acetylcholinesterase, and detoxifies the remaining poison. Skeletal muscle strength (especially respiratory muscles) is restored within minutes after administration. 2-PAM does not cross the blood-brain barrier, and there are few or no changes in central nervous system symptoms. This drug is most effective if started within the first 24 to 48 hours after exposure. Dosage is 25 to 50 mg/kg over 15 or more minutes in a diluted solution, administered each hour. Rapid infusion can cause headache, nausea, vomiting, blurred vision, dizziness, tachycardia, and hyperventilation. Toxic doses of 2-PAM cause neuroblockade, and it is contraindicated in carbamate insecticide ingestion because it can enhance the toxicity. A continuous infusion at 10 to 20 mg/kg can be used, but a loading dose of 10 to 15 mg/kg is recommended.

REFERENCES

Mortensen, M. (1990). Organophosphates and carbamates. In J. Blumer (Ed.). *A practical guide to pediatric intensive care* (3rd ed., pp. 713–718). St. Louis: Mosby–Year Book.

Zeviener, R., & Ginsburg, C. (1990). Organophosphate and carbamate poisoning. In D.L. Levine & F.C. Morriss (Eds.). *Essentials of pediatric intensive care* (pp. 648–653). St. Louis: Quality Medical Publishers.

ANSWERS ■ CASE 18-3

1. Answer (**c**). Clonidine is an antihypertensive agent used to treat adult patients with hypertension and children with ADD. It decreases the release of norepinephrine, inhibits efferent central impulses, and stimulates baroreflexes, which slows the heart rate. An increase in blood pressure is sometimes seen after therapy is begun.

REFERENCES

Longo, C., & Dickenson, C. (1996). Toxic ingestions. In M.A.Q. Curley, J.B. Smith, & P.A. Moloney-Harmon (Eds.). *Critical care nursing of infants and children* (pp. 940–962). Philadelphia: W.B. Saunders.

Mack, R.B. (1988). Clonidine overdose: Kingdom of the temporarily infirm. *Contemporary Pediatrics, 5* (10), 149.

Morriss, F.C. (1990). Antihypertensive agent ingestions. In D.L. Levine & F.C. Morriss (Eds.). *Essentials of pediatric intensive care* (3rd ed., pp. 624–630). St. Louis: Quality Medical Publishers.

Wiley, J., Wiley, C., Torey, S., & Henretig, F. (1990). Clonidine poisoning in young children. *Journal of Pediatrics, 116* (4), 654–658.

2. Answer (**d**). Clonidine overdoses present as narcotic overdoses because of the depletion of norepinephrine. Sedation, indifference to external stimuli, and psychic phenomena (i.e., nightmares and depression) are often seen. The use of naloxone is controversial, and the mechanism of action is unknown. Airway maintenance may need to be initiated, and transient hypertension, lasting less than 1 hour, may be seen in children with massive ingestions.

REFERENCES

Heidemann, S., & Sarnaik, A. (1990). Clonidine poisoning in children. *Critical Care Medicine, 18* (60), 618–620.

Longo, C., & Dickenson, C. (1996). Toxic ingestions. In M.A.Q. Curley, J.B. Smith, & P.A. Moloney-Harmon (Eds.). *Critical care nursing of infants and children* (pp. 940–962). Philadelphia: W.B. Saunders.

3. Answer (**d**). If hypotension is not resolved with fluid therapy, the use of a dopamine infusion at 10 μg/kg per minute may be required. Dopamine infusions at 10 μg/kg per minute stimulate the β-adrenergic receptors, which results in a release of norepinephrine and epinephrine.

REFERENCES

Hazinski, M.F. (1992). Cardiovascular disorders. In M.F. Hazinski (Ed.). *Nursing care of the critically ill child* (2nd ed., pp. 117–356). St. Louis: Mosby–Year Book.

Longo, C., & Dickenson, C. (1996). In M.A.Q. Curley, J.B. Smith, & P.A. Moloney-Harmon (Eds.). *Critical care nursing of infants and children* (pp. 940–962). Philadelphia: W.B. Saunders.

ANSWERS ■ CASE 18-4

1. Answer (**c**). If the plasma acetaminophen level is greater than 200 μg/mL at 4 hours or more than 50 μg/L at 12 hours after ingestion, or if less than 125 mg/kg of acetaminophen was ingested, the patient is at risk for developing hepatotoxicity. Excessive amounts of acetaminophen can produce fatal hepatic, renal, and myocardial necrosis.

REFERENCE

Squires, R. (1990). Acetaminophen poisoning. In D.L. Levine & F.C. Morriss (Eds.). *Essentials of pediatric intensive care* (pp. 612–615). St. Louis: Quality Medical Publishers.

2. Answer (**c**). Toxicity can be potentiated by drugs such as phenobarbital or disease states such as malnutrition, chronic liver failure, and alcohol abuse.

REFERENCE

Squires, R. (1990). Acetaminophen poisoning. In D.L. Levine & F.C. Morriss (Eds.). *Essentials of pediatric intensive care* (pp. 612–615). St. Louis: Quality Medical Publishers.

3. Answer (**c**). Although intravenous cyste-amine and oral methionine have been used to treat acetaminophen toxicity, *N*-acetylcysteine is the drug of choice. It neutralizes the active metabolite and reduces toxic effects. It is most effective when administered within the first 18 hours after ingestion, but it can be started up to 24 hours after ingestion. The loading dose of 140 mg/kg is taken orally, followed by 70 mg/kg taken orally every 4 hours for 17 doses. Intravenous administration is used in other countries but is under investigation in the United States. If the patient vomits within the first hour of administration, the dose must be repeated. Gastric aspiration and lavage should be performed before *N*-acetylcysteine therapy, and activated charcoal should not be given, because it interferes with absorption.

REFERENCES

Jaimovich, D. (1993). Transport management of the patient with acute poisoning. *Pediatric Clinics of North America, 40* (2), 40.
Longo, C., & Dickenson, C. (1996). Toxic ingestions. In M.A.Q. Curley, J.B. Smith, & P.A. Moloney-Harmon (Eds.). *Critical care nursing of infants and children* (pp. 940–962). Philadelphia: W.B. Saunders.
Squires, R. (1990). Acetaminophen poisoning. In D.L. Levine & F.C. Morriss (Eds.). *Essentials of pediatric intensive care* (pp. 612–615). St. Louis: Quality Medical Publishers.

4. Answer (**a**). Acetaminophen toxicity develops over 3 to 7 days. Signs and symptoms of liver dysfunction occur 48 to 96 hours after ingestion as a result of damage to hepatocytes. *Stage one* (12–24 hours after ingestion) is characterized by nausea, vomiting, and anorexia, although the patient may be asymptomatic. Liver study results are normal. In *stage two* (24–48 hours after ingestion), the patient may be "feeling better," but the results of liver studies may be elevated. In *stage three* (72–96 hours after ingestion), the signs and symptoms of liver dysfunction are evident, liver study abnormalities peak, and coagulopathy may require treatment. In *stage four* (7–8 days after ingestion) or the recovery stage, liver study results return to normal. Permanent liver damage is rare in children.

REFERENCES

Jaimovich, D. (1993). Transport management of the patient with acute poisoning. *Pediatric Clinics of North America, 40* (2), 409.

Longo, C., & Dickenson, C. (1996). Toxic ingestions. In M.A.Q. Curley, J.B. Smith, & P.A. Moloney-Harmon (Eds.). *Critical care nursing of infants and children* (pp. 940–962). Philadelphia: W.B. Saunders.

5. Answer (**a**). Bleeding from puncture sites, petechiae, and ecchymosis are the result of a decreased production of serum clotting factors. The normal prothrombin time is 10 to 13 seconds.

REFERENCE

Cahill-Alsip, C., & McDermott, B. (1996). Hematologic critical care problems. In M.A.Q. Curley, J.B. Smith, & P.A. Moloney-Harmon (Eds.). *Critical care nursing of infants and children* (pp. 793–817). Philadelphia: W.B. Saunders.

6. Answer (**a**). Hepatic encephalopathy with increased intracranial pressure can result from liver failure. Astute neurologic assessment and early detection of symptoms are important nursing functions.

REFERENCE

Jakobowski , D.S., Harmon, T.W., Peck, S.N., & Stellar, J.J. (1996). Gastrointestinal critical care problems. In M.A.Q. Curley, J.B. Smith, & P.A. Moloney-Harmon (Eds.). *Critical care nursing of infants and children* (pp. 724–755). Philadelphia: W.B. Saunders.

ANSWERS ■ CASE 18-5

1. Answer (**c**). Charcoal is unable to bind with this substance because of its molecular composition. Ethanol is rapidly absorbed (30–60 minutes), and 90% is metabolized in the liver.

REFERENCES

Haley, N., & Baker, P. (1993). *Emergency nursing pediatric course.* Park Ridge, IL: Emergency Nurses Association.
Longo, C., & Dickenson, C. (1996). Toxic Ingestions. In M.A.Q. Curley, J.B. Smith, & P.A. Moloney-Harmon (Eds.). *Critical care nursing of infants and children* (pp. 940–962). Philadelphia: W.B. Saunders.

2. Answer (**b**). Interruption of gluconeogenesis results in profound hypoglycemia. Coma and seizures may be the result of significant hypoglycemia. Serum glucose levels must be assessed frequently.

REFERENCES

Haley, N., & Baker, P. (1993). *Emergency nursing pediatric course.* Park Ridge, IL: Emergency Nurses Association.
Jaimovich, D. (1993). Transport management of the patient with acute poisoning. *Pediatric Clinics of North America, 40* (2), 418.
Longo, C., & Dickenson, C. (1996). Toxic ingestions. In M.A.Q. Curley, J.B. Smith, & P.A. Moloney-Harmon (Eds.). *Critical care nursing of infants and children* (pp. 940–962). Philadelphia: W.B. Saunders.

3. Answer (**d**). Ethanol is found in alcoholic beverages, perfumes, radiator antifreeze, windshield wiper solutions, and mouthwash.

REFERENCES

Haley, N., & Baker, P. (1993). *Emergency nursing pediatric course.* Park Ridge, IL: Emergency Nurses Association.

Jaimovich, D. (1993). Transport management of the patient with acute poisoning. *Pediatric Clinics of North America,* 40 (2), 418.

Mortensen, M. (1990). Alcohols and glycols. In J. Blumer (Ed.). *A practical guide to pediatric intensive care* (3rd ed., pp. 705–713). St. Louis: Mosby–Year Book.

4. Answer (**d**). Alterations in the osmolar gap reflect changes in the water content of blood. Calculation of the osmolar gap is a rapid method of diagnosing poisoning by alcohols or ethylene glycol. The osmolar gap and the anion gap provide helpful information for treating alcohol ingestions. Metabolic acidosis with an anion gap indicates an elevated plasma concentration of an unknown measured anion. Such anions include the acidic metabolites of methanol, ethylene glycol, paraldehyde, lactate, carbon monoxide, iron, or aspirin. Calculating osmolar gaps is not usually necessary for cases of pure ethanol ingestions, because ethanol levels are readily available.

REFERENCES

Berkowitz, I., Banner, W., & Rogers, M. (1992). Poisoning and the critically ill child. In M. Rogers (Ed.). *Textbook of pediatric intensive care* (2nd ed., pp. 1290–1356). Baltimore: Williams & Williams.

Longo, C., & Dickenson, C. (1996). Toxic ingestions. In M.A.Q. Curley, J.B. Smith, & P.A. Moloney-Harmon (Eds.). *Critical care nursing of infants and children* (pp. 940–962). Philadelphia: W.B. Saunders.

Mortensen, M. (1990). Alcohols and glycols. In J. Blumer (Ed.). *A practical guide to pediatric intensive care* (3rd ed., pp. 705–713). St. Louis: Mosby–Year Book.

ANSWERS ■ CASE 18-6

1. Answer (**c**). Ipecac syrup is not given to any patient with changes in the level of consciousness, and activated charcoal binds inadequately with iron. The best response is to initiate lavage. The solution of choice is sodium bicarbonate, because it creates a less absorbable form of ferrous sulfate. Although lavage is the best option, it is often difficult to retrieve these large tablets through a nasogastric tube.

REFERENCE

Longo, C., & Dickenson, C. (1996). Toxic ingestions. In M.A.Q. Curley, J.B. Smith, & P.A. Moloney-Harmon

(Eds.). *Critical care nursing of infants and children* (pp. 940–962). Philadelphia: W.B. Saunders.

2. Answer (**b**). Whole bowel irrigation augments gastric emptying of iron from the gastrointestinal tract. A polyethylene glycol electrolyte solution is used, and diarrhea is the desired effect. If this treatment is unsuccessful, gastrectomy may be considered to remove the tablets.

REFERENCES

Durbin, D. (1989). Whole bowel irrigation for iron ingestion. *Toxtalk,* 2 (2), 2.

Everson, G.W., Bertaccini, E.J., & O'Leary, J. (1991). Use of whole bowel irrigation in an infant following iron overdose. *American Journal of Emergency Medicine,* 9, 369.

Longo, C., & Dickenson, C. (1996). Toxic ingestions. In M.A.Q. Curley, J.B. Smith, & P.A. Moloney-Harmon (Eds.). *Critical care nursing of infants and children* (pp. 940–962). Philadelphia: W.B. Saunders.

3. Answer (**a**). Increased capillary permeability and vasodilation are the results of free iron circulation, which causes movement of fluids out of the vascular spaces. Free circulating iron results when the total iron-binding capacity is surpassed by the total serum iron in circulation.

REFERENCES

Longo, C., & Dickenson, C. (1996). Toxic ingestions. In M.A.Q. Curley, J.B. Smith, & P.A. Moloney-Harmon (Eds.). *Critical care nursing of infants and children* (pp. 940–962). Philadelphia: W.B. Saunders.

Steinhart, C., & Pearson-Shaver, A. (1988). Poisoning. *Critical Care Clinics of North America,* 4 (4), 845–872.

4. Answer (**c**). After chelation begins, the patient's urine turns a reddish orange to pink (classically referred to as vin rosa) color. This color change is the result of the deferoxamine's binding to the iron and producing feroxamine, which is excreted by the kidneys.

REFERENCE

Longo, C., & Dickenson, C. (1996). Toxic ingestions. In M.A.Q. Curley, J.B. Smith, & P.A. Moloney-Harmon (Eds.). *Critical care nursing of infants and children* (pp. 940–962). Philadelphia: W.B. Saunders.

5. Answer (**b**). Hepatic involvement is related to the damage of hepatocytes, resulting in coagulopathies, level of consciousness changes, and hypoglycemia. Treatment includes blood products, dextrose infusions, and supportive measures based on symptoms. Cellular dysfunction causes metabolic acidosis, which requires large amounts of sodium bicarbonate for correction.

REFERENCE

Longo, C., & Dickenson, C. (1996). Toxic ingestions. In M.A.Q. Curley, J.B. Smith, & P.A. Moloney-Harmon (Eds.). *Critical care nursing of infants and children* (pp. 940–962). Philadelphia: W.B. Saunders.

ANSWERS ■ CASE 18-7

1. Answer (**c**). Gasoline is a petroleum-based hydrocarbon, and significant amounts can be absorbed. Nausea, diarrhea, and hematemesis are clinical manifestations of the gastrointestinal irritability seen with any hydrocarbon ingestion.

REFERENCE

Longo, C., & Dickenson, C. (1996). Toxic ingestions. In M.A.Q. Curley, J.B. Smith, & P.A. Moloney-Harmon (Eds.). *Critical care nursing of infants and children* (pp. 940–962). Philadelphia: W.B. Saunders.

2. Answer (**a**). The pneumonitis produced by hydrocarbons is the result of the loss of surfactant. Without surfactant, alveoli collapse, causing respiratory dysfunction.

REFERENCE

Longo, C., & Dickenson, C. (1996). Toxic ingestions. In M.A.Q. Curley, J.B. Smith, & P.A. Moloney-Harmon (Eds.). *Critical care nursing of infants and children* (pp. 940–962). Philadelphia: W.B. Saunders.

3. Answer (**a**). Pulmonary toilet is an essential part of good pulmonary hygiene and helps in maintaining normal airway function.

REFERENCE

Longo, C., & Dickenson, C. (1996). Toxic Ingestions. In M.A.Q. Curley, J.B. Smith, & P.A. Moloney-Harmon (Eds.). *Critical care nursing of infants and children* (pp. 940–962). Philadelphia: W.B. Saunders.

4. Answer (**c**). Intubation and the use of PEEP help to maintain adequate oxygenation. PEEP helps stabilize airways, mobilize areas of atelectasis, and redistribute lung fluid from the alveoli to peribronchial areas. PEEP should not be withdrawn until 48 to 72 hours into the course of treatment, when the lungs begin to heal.

REFERENCES

Amoroso, K., & Ginsburg, C. (1990). Hydrocarbon ingestions. In D.L. Levine & F.C. Morriss (Eds.). *Essentials of pediatric intensive care* (pp. 639–643). St. Louis: Quality Medical Publishers.

Jaimovich, D. (1993). Transport management of the patient with acute poisoning. *Pediatric Clinics of North America,* 40 (2), 422.

5. Answer (**c**). Permanent damage is possible. Children can have abnormal pulmonary function test results for years.

REFERENCE

Longo, C., & Dickenson, C. (1996). Toxic ingestions. In M.A.Q. Curley, J.B. Smith, & P.A. Moloney-Harmon (Eds.). *Critical care nursing of infants and children* (pp. 940–962). Philadelphia: W.B. Saunders.

ANSWERS ■ CASE 18-8

1. Answer (**b**). Airway management is always the first priority. Syrup of ipecac and activated charcoal are contraindicated in treating any caustic ingestion, because they reintroduce the agent into the esophagus, and aspiration may result.

REFERENCE

Haley, K., & Baker, P. (1993). *Emergency nursing pediatric course.* Park Ridge, IL: Emergency Nurses Association.

2. Answer (**c**). The nurse should not attempt to insert an orogastric or nasogastric tube without a consultation with the physician. Insertion of an orogastric or nasogastric tube may cause a perforation.

REFERENCE

Mortensen, M. (1990). Household cleaning agents. In J. Blumer (Ed.). *A practical guide to pediatric intensive care* (3rd ed., pp. 725–731). St. Louis: Mosby–Year Book.

3. Answer (**b**). Esophageal constriction is a common complication. As many as 80% of esophageal strictures occur within 10 weeks after injury. Children with such ingestions should be referred for immediate medical evaluation any time dysphagia develops.

REFERENCE

Mortensen, M. (1990). Household cleaning agents. In J. Blumer (Ed.). *A practical guide to pediatric intensive care* (3rd ed., pp. 725–731) St. Louis: Mosby–Year Book.

ACKNOWLEDGMENT

The author wishes to acknowledge Sven A. Normann, Pharm.D., American Board of Applied Toxicology (ABAT), Director of the Florida Poison Information Center, for his contribution to the development of this manuscript.

CHAPTER *19*

Thermal Injuries

ELIZABETH I. HELVIG, RN, MS
PATRICIA DIMICK, RN, BSN

CASE 19-1

M., a 9-year-old boy, was asleep at 1:00 A.M., when his 7-year-old brother ignited their shared bedroom with a lighter. M. was conscious when pulled from the fire. He was transported directly to the local community hospital. M. arrives in the emergency department restless, agitated, and climbing off the stretcher.

1. The best treatment at this time is to
   a. Administer oxygen.
   b. Administer pain medication.
   c. Apply restraints.
   d. Wrap him in a blanket.

M.'s agitation and confusion are possibly caused by carbon monoxide exposure.

2. In the emergency department, the best way to assess for carbon monoxide poisoning is to
   a. Attach a pulse oximeter.
   b. Look for cherry red color.
   c. Request carboxyhemoglobin level on blood sent for arterial blood gas determinations.
   d. Send venous blood for a carboxyhemoglobin measurement.

3. Based on M.'s carboxyhemoglobin level of 20%, appropriate treatment is to
   a. Administer 100% F_{IO_2}.
   b. Administer oxygen based on P_{O_2}.
   c. Cough and deep breathe hourly.
   d. Intubate.

4. The nurse places a non-rebreathing face mask on the child, and constantly assesses for signs that his condition is deteriorating. The nurse should prepare for intubation if she notices
   a. A 50% or greater burn.
   b. Confusion or short-term memory loss.
   c. Hoarseness and burns about the mouth and tongue.
   d. The eyes swelling shut.

When M.'s respiratory status is stabilized, his wounds are assessed to determine the degree of skin involvement. On admission to the pediatric intensive care unit (PICU), the burns appear pearly white, dry, leathery to the touch, cool, and of normal contour, with thrombosed veins. The sheets are saturated with fluid.

5. What depth of injury is this?
   a. First degree.
   b. Superficial partial thickness.
   c. Deep partial thickness.
   d. Full thickness.

M.'s burns are determined to be a 60% full-thickness injury.

6. Which statement is true of full-thickness burns?
   a. It is unusual to see them result from a flame injury.
   b. They are usually very painful.
   c. They may extend into the subcutaneous tissue.

d. They extend to the middle layers of the dermis.

On admission to the PICU, M.'s weight is determined to be 35 kg without dressings.

7. According to the *Advanced Burn Life Support* guidelines, his fluid needs are calculated for the first 24 hours after the burn based on which formula?
   a. $(2–4 \text{ mL } D_5W) \times (\text{kg}) \times (\%\text{burn})$
   b. $(2–4 \text{ mL } D_5W) \times (\text{lb}) \times (\%\text{burn})$
   c. $(2–4 \text{ mL RL}) \times (\text{kg}) \times (\%\text{burn})$
   d. $(2–4 \text{ mL RL}) \times (\text{lb}) \times (\%\text{burn})$

8. If it is calculated that the patient should receive 8400 mL in the first 24 hours, the nurse should begin the intravenous fluids (30 minutes after injury) at
   a. 275 mL/hour.
   b. 350 mL/hour.
   c. 420 mL/hour.
   d. 525 mL/hour.

9. The nurse should anticipate that the presence of which of the following will increase fluid resuscitation needs?
   a. Burns of the hands and feet.
   b. Burns of the head.
   c. More full-thickness burns than partial-thickness burns.
   d. Smoke inhalation.

10. The best indicator of the adequacy of fluid resuscitation is
    a. Capillary refill in burned hands.
    b. Central venous pressure of 12 mmHg.
    c. Laboratory values.
    d. Urine output of 1.0 mL/kg per hour.

The physician has completed the admission orders on M., and the nurse is reviewing them and trying to determine her nursing care priorities.

11. The lowest priority in stabilizing a seriously burned patient is
    a. Fluid resuscitation.
    b. Monitoring urine output.
    c. Prevention of hypothermia.
    d. Wound care.

12. Which medication order should M.'s nurse question?
    a. Intramuscular morphine sulfate.
    b. Intramuscular tetanus toxoid.
    c. Intravenous Ativan.
    d. Intravenous morphine sulfate.

M.'s urine output has remained marginal since admission. At 6 hours after the injury, his laboratory values are reassessed.

13. For a patient with a large burn, the nurse would expect to see
    a. Decreased colloid osmotic pressure.
    b. Fall in hematocrit.
    c. Hypernatremia.
    d. Metabolic alkalosis.

M. has circumferential, full-thickness burns of his leg, and the distal pulses become progressively weaker, until the nurse is unable to detect with Doppler the pedal pulses. The surgeon arrives to perform an escharotomy.

14. An escharotomy
    a. Is a surgical procedure and requires written consent.
    b. May be safely performed in the emergency room, ICU, or burn unit.
    c. Will be done in the operating room under general anesthesia.
    d. Will leave a longitudinal scar for life.

M. is successfully stabilized by 24 hours after the injury.

15. M.'s 60% full-thickness burns will heal secondary to
    a. Contracture of wound margins.
    b. Regeneration of epithelial cells from within the wound.
    c. Transplantation of another person's skin to the burn wound.
    d. Transplantation of the patient's own skin to the burn wound.

M. is scheduled for surgery for debridement and grafting of his wounds. At the first surgery, the burn wounds are excised, and autografts from available donor sites are placed over the entire back. The excised wounds on the legs are covered with allograft (homograft).

16. Allograft
    a. Is preferably taken from a close relative of the patient.
    b. Is selected based on tissue typing.
    c. Is used as a permanent wound covering for burns.
    d. May become vascularized and lead to a rejection reaction.

17. The excised anterior trunk is covered with "artificial skin," an experimental wound covering that is
    a. A plastic that resembles real skin.
    b. A synthetic dermis, which must be grafted with epidermis.
    c. A temporary wound covering.
    d. Skin grown in a test tube.

M. has minimal donor site availability, and other treatment options are explored.

18. If tissue culture cells are applied to the wound, the nurse must recognize that these cells
   a. Are a temporary wound covering.
   b. Need to be covered with a strong antibiotic.
   c. Should be protected from pressure and shearing.
   d. Should be washed daily.

M. is very hypermetabolic secondary to his massive burn injury.

19. To meet his high protein and caloric needs, the nurse expects to
   a. Encourage the patient to eat as many calories as needed to meet caloric requirements.
   b. Insert a small feeding tube for enteral feedings.
   c. Make the patient take nothing orally to prevent paralytic ileus.
   d. Initiate total parenteral nutrition immediately.

M. undergoes five operations to obtain wound closure. He is released from the hospital 2 months after the injury, but he continues to undergo daily physical therapy after discharge.

CASE 19-2

Eight-month-old A. presents with a 25% scald burn that she received in the tub when her 21-month-old sister turned on the hot water.

1. The leading cause of burn morbidity in children between birth and 4 years of age is
   a. Contact burns.
   b. Electrical.
   c. Fires.
   d. Scalds.

A. is taken to the local community hospital and presents in the emergency department within 30 minutes of the time of injury.

2. The initial management of her burn wound is to
   a. Cover with clean dry sheet.
   b. Lavage with iced solution.
   c. Wash with iodine or other strong solution.
   d. Wrap with wet sheets.

The nurse assigned to A. assesses her burn size and severity as soon as the child's respiratory status is determined to be normal.

3. In estimating burn size in an infant, it is important to recall that
   a. Each leg is 18% of the body.
   b. One surface of the patient's hand is about 2.5%.
   c. The head is 18% of the body.
   d. The trunk and arms are about half of the proportion of an adult's.

4. In assessing the severity of the burn in this infant, it is important to consider that
   a. Children have fewer pain sensors in their skin.
   b. Children heal more slowly than adults.
   c. Children scar less than adults.
   d. The child's skin is thin.

The burn size is calculated at 25%, and the nurse determines A.'s fluid requirements.

5. In prescribing fluid resuscitation for a seriously burned infant, it is important to consider that
   a. Colloids are usually added in the first 8 hours.
   b. Pediatric patients rarely need more than 75% of the Parkland formula fluid.
   c. The Parkland formula may need to be supplemented with additional volume.
   d. The resuscitation rate is altered, with volume evenly divided over 24 hours.

6. A. is transferred to the regional burn center, where she is determined to have a large partial-thickness injury, which heals by
   a. Migration of epithelial cells across the wound surface from wound edges.
   b. Primary closure.
   c. Growth of epithelial cells from wound margins and within the dermis.
   d. Skin grafting.

The wound heals within 2.5 weeks.

7. The nurse manager looks for documentation of discharge teaching and is confused to find which of the following instructions?
   a. Apply lotion to healed burns to decrease itching.
   b. Drink high-calorie and high-protein supplements.
   c. Apply pressure wraps to healed wounds 23 hours/day.
   d. Shield healed burns from sunlight.

At A.'s first visit to the clinic after discharge, the dietary supplements are discontinued, and the nutritionist talks to A.'s mother regarding the child's caloric needs. All wounds appear fine, and the mother is instructed to continue healed skin care as she has been doing.

CASE 19-3

K. is a 14-year-old boy who was on his parents' front lawn when he extended a pole and struck a high-tension wire. He immediately fell to the ground.

1. The assessment priority after an electrical injury is
   a. Assessment for associated trauma.
   b. Cardiac function.
   c. Computed tomography (CT) scan of the head.
   d. Wound management, because these wounds are often deep.

K. is taken to the nearby medical center. On admission, intravenous fluids are started, and a Foley catheter is inserted.

2. The nurse recognizes that there is a high incidence of renal failure after electrical injury secondary to
   a. Aminoglycoside administration.
   b. Application of mafenide (Sulfamylon) to wounds.
   c. Pyelonephritis.
   d. Myoglobinuria.

3. The treatment for myoglobinuria is
   a. Provision of cranberry juice.
   b. Administration of Lasix.
   c. Maintenance of urine output at 1 to 2 mL/kg per hour.
   d. Maintenance of urine output at 30 mL/hr.

K.'s mother is concerned that the boy has decreased movement in his hand and that its color is mottled.

4. The nurse needs to tell K.'s mother that
   a. It often takes several days before viability status can be fully determined.
   b. K.'s fingers are not viable.
   c. Such extremities usually require amputation.
   d. Such extremity wounds usually improve over the first couple of days.

ANSWERS ■ CASE 19-1

1. Answer (**a**). Administer oxygen, and the

patient often becomes less agitated. It is important to look beyond the burn wounds and pain in the initial assessment of the burn patient. It is easy for priorities to become side-tracked by the visibility of burn wounds and the nurse's gut response of "this must be horrible and painful." It is important for the nurse to do a rapid but complete head-to-toe assessment of the patient, treating the priorities such as hypoxia and shock and identifying associated injuries before sedating the patient.

REFERENCES
Burgess, M.C. (1991). Initial management of a patient with extensive burn injury. *Critical Care Nursing Clinics of North America,* 3 (2), 165–179.
Helvig, E.I., & Herndon, D.N. (1989). Airway and pulmonary management of burn patients. *Trauma Quarterly,* 5 (4), 19–32.

2. Answer (**c**). Carbon monoxide levels may be assessed by evaluating arterial blood for carboxyhemoglobin level; a normal level is less than 5%. The pulse oximeter cannot differentiate between oxygen and carbon monoxide because of similarities in light refraction. Cherry red color is usually associated with very high levels of carbon monoxide and is not commonly seen in the health care setting.

REFERENCE
Helvig, E.I., & Herndon, D.N. (1989). Airway and pulmonary management of burn patients. *Trauma Quarterly,* 5 (4), 19–33.

3. Answer (**a**). Carbon monoxide is treated with 100% oxygen by means of a non-rebreathing face mask and started as soon as possible. Carbon monoxide levels are reduced by one half every 60 to 90 minutes that the patient receives 100% oxygen, because high levels of oxygen displace the carbon monoxide on the hemoglobin. Patients may have a normal PaO_2 despite lethal carbon monoxide levels, because the PaO_2 reflects oxygen dissolved in the plasma, not oxygen associated with the hemoglobin. If oxygen can be delivered by mask, it may not be necessary to intubate.

REFERENCES
Carrougher, G.J. (1993). Inhalation injury. *AACN Clinical Issues in Critical Care Nursing,* 4 (2), 367–377.
Reynolds, E.M., Ryan, D.P., & Doody, D.P. (1993). Mortality and respiratory failure in a pediatric burn population. *Journal of Pediatric Surgery,* 28 (10), 1326–1331.

4. Answer (c). Large burns alone are not an indication for intubating the patient. Confusion may be indicative of carbon monoxide poisoning and can be treated with oxygen delivered by a face mask. When there are even minor burns of the face, it is common for the eyes to swell shut, and this in itself does not indicate airway swelling. However, if the patient has burns about the mouth and tongue, soot in his sputum, and develops hoarseness or stridor, he may require intubation. Many burn centers base the decision to intubate a patient on the results of bronchoscopy when swelling of the airway is visualized.

REFERENCES
Barone, C.M. (1992). Management of pediatric burns. *Trauma Quarterly,* 8 (3), 35–43.
Carrougher, G.J. (1993). Inhalation injury. *AACN Clinical Issues in Critical Care Nursing,* 4 (2), 367–377.
Herndon, D.N., Rutan, R.L., & Rutan, T.C. (1993). Management of the pediatric patient with burns. *Journal of Burn Care and Rehabilitation,* 14 (1), 3–8.

5. Answer (d). The deep, full-thickness wound is usually dry and leathery to the touch, and it often appears pearly white, brown, or black. Thrombosed veins are always indicative of full-thickness injuries. Despite the dry appearance, these wounds leak fluid through the damaged tissue.

REFERENCES
Burgess, M.C. (1991). Initial management of a patient with extensive burn injury. *Critical Care Nursing Clinics of North America,* 3 (2), 165–179.
Finkelstein, J.L., Schwartz, S.B., & Madden, M.R. (1992). Pediatric burns: A overview. *Pediatric Clinics of North America,* 39 (5), 1145–1163.
Lyebarger, P., & Daly, W. (1996). Thermal injury. In M.A.Q. Curley, J.B. Smith, & P.A. Moloney-Harmon (Eds.). *Critical care nursing of infants and children* (pp. 924–939). Philadelphia: W.B. Saunders.

6. Answer (c). Full-thickness burns often result from contact with concentrated chemicals, hot objects, high-voltage electricity, or flames. They extend through the entire epidermis and dermis into the subcutaneous tissue beneath. They usually have minimal pain, because most pain receptor nerve endings (located in the dermis) have been destroyed. However, many full-thickness burns have partial-thickness margins that may be very painful.

REFERENCES
Finkelstein, J.L., Schwartz, S.B., & Madden M.R. (1992). Pediatric burns: An overview. *Pediatric Clinics of North America,* 39 (5), 1145–1163.

Heimbach, D., Engrav, L., Grube, B., et al. (1992). Burn depth: A review. *World Journal of Surgery,* 16 (1), 10–15.
Lyebarger, P., & Daly, W. (1996). Thermal injuries. In M.A.Q. Curley, J.B. Smith, & P.A. Moloney-Harmon (Eds.). *Critical care nursing of infants and children* (pp. 924–939). Philadelphia: W.B. Saunders.

7. Answer (c). Fluid needs of the burned patient are calculated by the formula of 2 to 4 mL of Ringer's lactate per kilogram, multiplied by the percentage of total body surface area that is burned. Lactated Ringer's most closely resembles the fluid lost from intravascular spaces. Dextrose and water is contraindicated, because it dilutes electrolytes and can lead to hyponatremia and hyperglycemia.

REFERENCES
Lyebarger, P., & Daly, W. Thermal injuries. In M.A.Q. Curley, J.B. Smith, & P.A. Moloney-Harmon (Eds.). *Critical care nursing of infants and children* (pp. 924–939). Philadelphia: W.B. Saunders.
Nebraska Burn Institute (1990) Pediatric thermal injuries. In *Advanced burn life support course.* Lincoln: Nebraska Burn Institute.
Rieg, L.S., & Jenkins, M. (1991). Burn injuries in children. *Critical Care Nursing Clinics of North America,* 3 (3), 457–470.

8. Answer (d). The patient requiring 8400 mL in the first 24 hours should receive one half of this volume in the first 8 hours after injury, a fourth of the volume in the second 8 hours, and a fourth in the third 8 hours. This patient would require 4200 mL in the first 8 hours, and intravenous fluids should be started at 525 mL/hour.

REFERENCE
Nebraska Burn Institute. (1990). Pediatric thermal injuries. In *Advanced Burn Life Support Course.* Lincoln: Nebraska Burn Institute.

9. Answer (d). Severe smoke inhalation in addition to burn injuries can increase fluid requirements by as much as 50%. Fluid resuscitation formulas are based on the percentage of total body surface area (% TBSA) burned, regardless of whether the burns are partial thickness or full thickness; however, first-degree burns are not included in burn size calculations.

REFERENCE
Herndon, D.N., Barrow, R.E., Linares, H.A., et al. (1988). Inhalation injury in burn patients: Effects and treatment. *Burns,* 14, 349–356.

10. Answer (**d**). Fluid administration should maintain urine output of at least 1.0 mL/kg per hour in children, reflecting end-organ perfusion. Central venous pressure is often low, and capillary refill may be obscured by deep burns of the hands.

REFERENCES

Nebraska Burn Institute. (1990). Pediatric thermal injuries. In *Advanced burn life support course*. Lincoln: Nebraska Burn Institute.
Warden, G.D. (1992). Burn shock resuscitation. *World Journal of Surgery*, 16, 16–23.

11. Answer (**d**). As with any type of trauma, hemodynamic and pulmonary stabilization should precede any attention to wound management.

REFERENCES

Burgess, M.C. (1991). Initial management of a patient with extensive burn injury. *Critical Care Nursing Clinics of North America*, 3 (2), 165–179.
Walter, P.H. (1993). Burn wound management. *AACN Clinical Issues in Critical Care Nursing*, 4, 2, 378–387.

12. Answer (**a**). Morphine is commonly given to relieve burn pain. In any burned patient with large burns (>20% TBSA), opiates must be administered intravenously in the emergent phase, when edema and stasis can lead to inadequate or sluggish absorption of intramuscular or subcutaneously administered medications. Intravenous anxiolytics are also sometimes given. The only medication given intramuscularly in the resuscitation phase of burn care is tetanus toxoid, because slow absorption does not affect its effectiveness.

REFERENCES

Rieg, L.S., & Jenkins, M. (1991). Burn injuries in children. *Critical Care Nursing Clinics of North America*, 3 (3), 457–470.
Watkins, P.N. (1993). This one's for Billy. *Journal of Burn Care and Rehabilitation*, 14 (1), 58–64.

13. Answer (**a**). The capillary leak associated with burn injuries permits the leaking of water, electrolytes, and proteins from the vasculature to the extravascular space. Erythrocytes do not leak, because they are too large to leak from the capillaries. This defect results in the reduction of intravascular proteins and colloid osmotic pressure, hypovolemia, and a rising hematocrit. Cellular changes result in decreased cell transmembrane potential and increased intracellular sodium concentration, with extracellular sodium depletion. The decreased cardiac output and circulatory compromise induced by hypovolemia causes a metabolic acidosis, which is often combined with a respiratory alkalosis resulting from hyperventilation associated with pain and fear.

REFERENCES

Faldmo, L., & Kravitz, M. (1993). Acute burn care/burn shock resuscitation. *AACN Clinical Issues in Critical Care Nursing*, 4, 2, 351–366.
Rieg, L.S., & Jenkins, M. (1991). Burn injuries in children. *Critical Care Nursing Clinics of North America*, 3 (3), 457–470.
Warden, G.D. (1992). Burn shock resuscitation. *World Journal of Surgery*, 16, 16–23.

14. Answer (**b**). An escharotomy is an emergency intervention used to salvage tissue distal to the circumferential full-thickness eschar by surgical release of the eschar along the lateral and medial aspects of the affected extremity. The surgeon cuts the constricting eschar with a scalpel or electrocautery unit, releasing the pressure on the edematous, viable tissue underneath. It is safely performed in the patient's bed with opiate analgesia. Because all the dead tissue will ultimately be removed and the extremity grafted, the escharotomy will not leave permanent longitudinal scars.

REFERENCE

Mann, R., & Heimbach, D.M. (1994). Wound management. *Trauma Quarterly*, 11 (2), 127–136.

15. Answer (**d**). The full-thickness wound extends through all layers of the dermis, destroying all epithelial elements. This makes it impossible for such a wound to heal from within. Although small full-thickness wounds are capable of healing by contracture, this is not possible with a 60% TBSA burn. Full-thickness wounds are grafted with the patient's own skin (autograft), taken from an uninjured area or from a healed partial-thickness wound.

REFERENCE

Mann, R., & Heimbach, D.M. (1994). Wound management. *Trauma Quarterly*, 11 (2), 127–136.

16. Answer (**d**). Allograft or homograft is skin taken from another human being, usually cadaver skin. Because it is foreign tissue, it will be rejected if it stays on the wound long enough, unless the patient is immunosuppressed. It is

therefore placed on the wound as a temporary biologic dressing. As the patient's own skin becomes available, the allograft will be replaced. Because it is used for temporary wound coverage, efforts to find a close match are normally not done.

REFERENCES
Alsbjorn, B.F. (1992). Biologic wound coverings in burn treatment. *World Journal of Surgery,* 16, 43–46.
Duncan, D.J., & Driscoll, D.M. (1991). Burn wound management. *Critical Care Nursing Clinics of North America,* 3 (2), 199–220.

17. Answer (**b**). Artificial skin is a composite dermis (of collagen and chondroitin 6-sulfate) with a Silastic covering. It is placed on a full-thickness wound after all dead material has been carefully removed. The patient's own connective tissue and capillaries grow into the scaffolding of this synthetic material, creating a new dermis (i.e., neodermis) before the components of the artificial skin are degraded and absorbed. Once vascularized, the Silastic covering is removed, and a thin graft of the patient's own epidermis is placed on the artificial skin to close the wound. This technique is being used in some burn centers, but it is still in its research phase.

REFERENCES
Lyebarger, P., & Daly, W. (1996). Thermal injuries. In M.A.Q. Curley, J.B. Smith, & P.A. Moloney-Harmon (Eds.). *Critical care nursing of infants and children* (pp. 924–939). Philadelphia: W.B. Saunders.
Tompkins, R.G., & Burke, J.F. (1990). Progress in burn treatment and the use of artificial skin. *World Journal of Surgery,* 14, 819–824.

18. Answer (**c**). Cultured epithelial autografts are created by growing the patient's own epidermal cells in a culture medium and then transplanting the sheet of cells to the patient's wounds after removal of all dead tissue. This procedure is being done on an experimental level. The greatest concern about the use of these cells is their fragility and lack of shear strength. They need to be protected from harsh chemicals, drying, and shearing for weeks after their application, making the percentage of "take" or adherence a challenge that researchers are still trying to overcome.

REFERENCES
Clugston, P.A., Snelling, C.F.T., & Macdonald, I.B. (1991). Cultured epithelial autografts: Three years of clinical experience with eighteen patients. *Journal of Burn Care and Rehabilitation,* 12 (6), 533–539.

Lyebarger, P., & Daly, W. Thermal injuries. In M.A.Q. Curley, J.B. Smith, & P.A. Moloney-Harmon (Eds.). *Critical care nursing of infants and children* (pp. 924–939). Philadelphia: W.B. Saunders.
McAree, K.G., Klein, R.L., & Boeckman, C.R. (1993). The use of cultured epithelial autografts in the wound care of severely burned patients. *Journal of Pediatric Surgery,* 28 (2), 166–168.

19. Answer (**b**). The nutritional support of the hypermetabolic burn patient is achieved through the delivery of a high-protein, high-calorie diet. This is accomplished in almost all burn care settings by the administration of enteral nutrition through a small feeding tube. Gastric feeding is important because it helps to maintain the integrity of gastrointestinal mucosa in addition to meeting caloric requirements. Parenteral nutrition is not done if other options are available because of complications of sepsis, thrombosis, greater elevations of serum insulin levels, elevations of tumor necrosis factor in response to endotoxin exposure, lower helper-suppressor T-lymphocyte ratio in patients, and a higher mortality rate among patients with severe burns compared to those receiving enteral nutrition. Burned patients need nutritional support, which is usually started at a low volume within hours of injury. Large-burn patients are not encouraged to "eat" the numbers of calories required, because such a practice encourages eating practices that are not healthy or advantageous after discharge.

REFERENCE
Waymack, J.P., & Herndon, D.N. (1992). Nutritional support of the burned patient. *World Journal of Surgery,* 16 (1), 80–86.

ANSWERS ■ CASE 19-2

1. Answer (**d**). Flames and smoke inhalation result in the greatest numbers of deaths, but the leading cause of burn morbidity is scalding. Factors contributing to the high incidence of pediatric burns in the birth to 4-year age group are increasing mobility and curiosity, inability to escape life-threatening situations, and lack of experience and cognitive development. Peclet (1990) reports that the median age for children with burns is 1 year.

REFERENCES

Hazinski, M.F., Francescutti, L.H., & Lapidus, G.D. (1993). Pediatric injury prevention. *Annals of Emergency Medicine,* 22 (2, part 2), 456–467.

Peclet, M.H., Newman, K.D., Eichelberger, M.R., et al. (1990). Patterns of injury in children. *Journal of Pediatric Surgery,* 25 (1), 85–91.

2. Answer (**a**). At the scene, burns that are warm to touch should be cooled with water to stop the burning process. Most are already cool to touch by the time a first responder arrives on the scene. In that situation, cool water is no longer therapeutic. Greases hold in the heat, and ice can cause vasoconstriction and freeze damage to injured tissue; both of these treatments are contraindicated. After stopping the burning process, burns should be wrapped in a clean dry sheet and blanket to protect the wound and prevent hypothermia. Wounds should be cleaned with a mild soap and water solution, with care taken to maintain patient warmth.

REFERENCES

Lyebarger, P., & Daly, W. (1996). Thermal injuries. In M.A.Q. Curley, J.B. Smith, & P.A. Moloney-Harmon (Eds.). *Critical care nursing of infants and children* (pp. 924–939). Philadelphia: W.B. Saunders.

Mozingo, D.W., Barillo, D.J., & Pruitt, B.A., Jr. (1994). Acute resuscitation and transfer management of burned and electrically injured patients. *Trauma Quarterly,* 11 (2), 94–113.

3. Answer (**c**). In calculating the percentage of burn in infants, it is important to recognize that the head is 18% of an infant's total body surface area. Infants with head burns have a more severe injury than may be immediately appreciated. Infants have legs that are about 14% of their body surface area; as the infant grows, the proportion of the head decreases, and the percentage of each leg increases. Like an adult, the infant's torso is 36% of his body surface area, and one surface of each hand is about 1% of his body surface area.

REFERENCES

Lyebarger, P., & Daly, W. (1996). Thermal injuries. In M.A.Q. Curley, J.B. Smith, & P.A. Moloney-Harmon (Eds.). *Critical care nursing of infants and children* (pp. 924–939). Philadelphia: W.B. Saunders.

Mozingo, D.W., Barillo, D.J., & Pruitt, B.A. (1994). Acute resuscitation and transfer management of burned and electrically injured patients. *Trauma Quarterly,* 11 (2), 94–113.

4. Answer (**d**). Because of the thinness of the child's skin, the amount of heat that creates a partial-thickness burn in an adult may produce a full-thickness burn in an infant. Although a scald burn is usually partial thickness in an adult, it may require grafting in this infant. Children tend to heal more quickly than adults, and they often seem to scar more. Pediatric patients may report pain in partial-thickness and full-thickness burns.

REFERENCES

Atchison, N.E., Osgood, P.F., Carr, D.B., et al. (1991). Pain during burn dressing change in children: Relationship to burn area, depth and analgesic regimens. *Pain,* 47, 41–45.

Heimbach, D., Engrav, L., & Grube, B. (1992). Burn depth: A review. *World Journal of Surgery,* 16, 10–15.

5. Answer (**c**). An infant has a relatively larger body surface area in relation to weight than an adult, resulting in a larger degree of evaporative water loss per kilogram. According to the Parkland formula, a 10-kg child with a 25% burn would require 1000 mL of resuscitation solution ($10 \times 25 \times 4 = 1000$ mL). Fluid maintenance requirement for a 10-kg child is 1000 mL/24 hours (100 mL per each of the first 10 kg). If only 1000 mL was administered in a 24-hour period, maintenance needs would be reached, without any additional fluid for the 25% burn injury. For very young children, the Parkland formula needs to be supplemented with additional volume. Specific fluid resuscitation formulas based on total body surface area and body surface area burned are used in some burn units.

REFERENCES

Helvig E. (1993). Pediatric burn injuries. *AACN Clinical Issues in Critical Care Nursing,* 4 (2), 433–442.

Herndon, D.N., Tompson, P.B., Desai, M.H., et al. (1985). Treatment of burns in children. *Pediatric Clinics of North America,* 32, 1311–1332.

Warden, G.D. (1992). Burn shock resuscitation. *World Journal of Surgery,* 16, 16–23.

6. Answer (**c**). Partial-thickness wounds extend partially through the dermis, sparing the deepest epithelial appendages that are at the base of the hair follicles. The epithelial cells grow out of the deep dermal appendages, creating islands (or buds) of healing tissue throughout the partial-thickness wound. Epithelial cells then divide and grow from the edges of the wound and from the epithelial islands within the wound until the wound has been totally re-epithelialized.

REFERENCES
Bayley, E.W. (1987). The three degrees of burn care. *Nursing 87, 17* (3), 34–41.
Knoop, D.J. (1991) General local treatment. In R. Trofine (Ed.). *Nursing care of the burn injured patient* (pp. 42–67). Philadelphia: F.A. Davis.

7. Answer (**b**). Partial-thickness wounds can develop significant hypertrophic scarring. Pressure is often placed on healed wounds through the use of elastic wraps; stretchable tubular stockings, sleeves, and body suits; or custom-made pressure garments to decrease scarring and support the vasculature. Patients may experience itching in their healed wounds, which is often relieved by moisturizers and medications such as diphenhydramine HCl, hydroxazine, or cyproheptadine HCl. Patients should be cautioned to avoid direct sun exposure through the use of clothing, hats, umbrellas, and sunscreens because of the chance of severe sunburn and the development of hyperpigmentation of the scars. After wounds are healed, the hypermetabolism of burns resolves. Patients who continue to take in excess calories over those needed for normal growth and maintenance may have a problem with significant weight gain.

REFERENCES
Finkelstein, J.L., Schwartz, S.B., & Madden, M.R. (1992). Pediatric burns: An overview. *Pediatric Emergency Medicine, 39* (5), 1145–1163.
Robson, R.C., Barnett, R.A., Leitch, I.O.W., et al. (1992). Prevention and treatment of postburn scars and contracture. *World Journal of Surgery, 16,* 87–96.
Walter, P.H. (1993). Burn wound management. *AACN Clinical Issues in Critical Care Nursing, 4* (2), 378–387.

ANSWERS ■ CASE 19-3

1. Answer (**b**). The primary survey always begins with assessing airway, breathing, and circulation. Cardiopulmonary arrest (i.e., ventricular fibrillation or asystole) may occur with high-voltage injuries, and resuscitation efforts need to be directed toward restoring cardiac function.

REFERENCES
Gillespie, R.W. (1989). Prehospital care and evaluation of the burn patient. *Trauma Quarterly, 5* (4), 1–5.
Nebraska Burn Institute. (1990). Electrical burns. In *Advanced burn life support course.* Lincoln: Nebraska Burn Institute.

2. Answer (**d**). Electrical injuries often result in damage to muscle, and there is a high risk for compartment syndrome. Damaged muscle releases myoglobin, which can accumulate in the kidneys and result in acute tubular necrosis. Myoglobinuria is recognized by the red or sometimes brownish pigmentation in the urine.

REFERENCE
Faldmo, L., & Kravitz, M. (1993). Acute brain care/burn shock resuscitation. *AACN Clinical Issues in Critical Care Nursing, 4* (2), 351–366.

3. Answer (**c**). Maintain urine output at more than 100 mL/hour in an adult and 1 to 2 mL/kg per hour in a child to flush the myoglobin through the kidneys. This high rate of urine output is necessary until the red pigment has cleared.

REFERENCE
Faldmo, L., & Kravitz, M. (1993) Acute burn care/burn shock resuscitation. *AACN Clinical Issues in Critical Care Nursing, 4* (2), 351–366.

4. Answer (**a**). Electrical injuries are associated with wounds that are often progressive in nature secondary to microvascular damage proximal to the injury. Although electrical injuries do result in a high number of amputations, it is prudent to be conservative about conveying the prognosis for an extremity at the time of admission, unless the extremity is clearly dead.

REFERENCES
Luce, E.A., & Gottlieb, S.E. (1984). "True" high-tension electrical injuries. *Annals of Plastic Surgery, 12* (4), 321–325.
Zelt, R.G., Daniel, R.K., Ballard, P.A., et al. (1988). High voltage electrical injury: Chronic wound evolution. *Plastic and Reconstructive Surgery, 82* (6), 1027–1041.

CHAPTER *20*

Human Immunodeficiency Virus

NANCY M. KRAUS, RN, MSN, CCRN

CASE 20-1

M., a 4-month-old girl, was seen 2 weeks ago in the outpatient clinic. She had a 1-week history of cough, clear rhinorrhea, and oral and diaper candidal rash. Examination revealed that she also had otitis media. M. was started on amoxicillin, nystatin oral suspension, and nystatin cream.

At her 2-week follow-up visit, she presents with persistent otitis media and persistent oral and diaper candidal infections. She also has hepatomegaly (i.e., the liver is palpable 6 to 7 cm below the right costal margin) and left lower lobe pneumonia.

The family history at the second visit reveals that M.'s mother has a history of intravenous drug use. The mother states that M. was tested previously for virus-induced immunodeficiency at 1.5 months of age. The test was done at another facility, and the results are unknown. A diagnosis of human immunodeficiency virus (HIV) infection is considered.

1. Based on the mother's history, the most likely route of viral transmission to M. is
   a. Casual contact.
   b. Direct inoculation.
   c. Perinatal transmission.
   d. Sexual contact.

2. This case is considered a part of the Centers for Disease Control and Prevention (CDC) pediatric HIV and acquired immunodeficiency syndrome (AIDS) data.

Cases of pediatric HIV or AIDS include affected children of what age?
   a. Those younger than 1 year of age.
   b. Those younger than 8 years of age.
   c. Those younger than 13 years of age.
   d. Those younger than 18 years of age.

M. is admitted to the medical floor and is started on cefotaxime for the pneumonia and fluconazole for a fungal or yeast infection. The laboratory results reveal elevated levels of liver enzymes, a negative hepatitis profile, and decreased concentrations of immunoglobulins G, A, and M. Twenty-four hours later, M. demonstrates increasing respiratory distress and is transferred to the pediatric intensive care unit (PICU) with acute respiratory failure. Vital signs at this time include a heart rate of 158 beats per minute (bpm), respiratory rate of 72 breaths per minute, and temperature of 38.3°C. Additional laboratory studies reveal a positive enzyme-linked immunoabsorbent assay (ELISA) result, a positive p24 antigen test result, an abnormally depressed T4 cell count, and a low T4 to T8 ratio.

3. The pathophysiologic changes in M. that require her admission to the PICU are related to
   a. Acute infection.
   b. Lymphadenopathy.
   c. Pulmonary complications.
   d. Hepatomegaly.

4. The positive ELISA test results indicate that

a. M. definitely has virus-induced immunodeficiency.
b. M.'s results are inconclusive regarding virus-induced immunodeficiency.
c. M. does not have virus-induced immunodeficiency.
d. M.'s mother has virus-induced immunodeficiency.

5. The length of time that maternal antibodies remain in the baby's system is
a. 6 months.
b. 12 months.
c. 15 months.
d. 18 months.

6. M.'s mother questions the nurse about the chances of M. developing HIV disease. The nurse explains to M.'s mother that
a. Approximately 25% to 35% of babies born to HIV-positive women develop HIV disease.
b. Approximately 50% of babies born to HIV-positive women develop HIV disease.
c. Almost 100% of babies born to HIV-positive women develop HIV disease.
d. It is difficult to determine M.'s chances at this time.

7. M.'s abnormally depressed number of T4 cells is a significant finding within the pathophysiology of the immune system. The lowered number of T4 cells results in
a. Diminished ability to directly attack the invading virus.
b. Decreased production of antibodies for protection against bacteria and viruses.
c. Absence of the production of antibodies for humoral immunity.
d. Minimal release of lymphokines, which activate the other cells of the immune system.

8. Another laboratory finding of concern is M.'s low T4 to T8 cell ratio. What is the significance of a low T4 to T8 ratio?
a. Depletion of T4 cells and a low T4 to T8 ratio leaves the host with less cellular immunity.
b. The low T4 to T8 cell ratio correlates with an increased release of lymphokines.
c. Decreased T4 to T8 ratio directly affects the replication ability of the HIV virus.
d. When the number of T4 cells is less

than the number of T8 cells, the patient requires extensive pharmacologic support.

9. The p24 antigen test is sometimes used as a determinant of active or latent HIV. How does the amount of p24 antigen in the blood change as the virus becomes active?
a. It becomes detectable.
b. It becomes undetectable.
c. It is less reliable.
d. It decreases.

In the PICU, M. is started on supplemental oxygen, placed on oximetry monitoring, and observed closely for potential deterioration or complications of her acute respiratory failure. Based on the positive p24 antigen test result, she is treated with intravenous zidovudine (AZT) and gradually shows some improvement. After her course is stabilized, prophylactic administration of trimethoprim-sulfamethoxazole (TMP-SMX) three times each week and administration of intravenous immunoglobulin are initiated. Ultimately, all antibiotics other than prophylactic TMP-SMX are stopped. M. is transferred to the medical floor and later is discharged. On discharge, her condition is markedly improved, and she will be followed closely by the outpatient HIV team.

10. M. is started on TMP-SMX three times each week rather than daily because
a. Better patient or family compliance occurs.
b. Less neutropenia occurs.
c. Less gastric upset occurs.
d. More therapeutic drug levels are achieved.

11. M. is started on antiretroviral therapy with AZT based on her positive p24 results and low T4 cell count. The nurse monitors M. for
a. Dry mucous membranes and mouth sores.
b. Rash, redness, and urticaria.
c. Nausea, headache, and vomiting.
d. Tachycardia and hypotension.

12. The major long-term side effect of AZT is
a. Bone marrow suppression with anemia.
b. Neurologic impairment and dementia.
c. Peripheral neuropathy.
d. Pancreatitis.

CASE 20-2

R., a 2.5-year-old boy, has a medical history of congenital immunodeficiency and a positive HIV status. His mother died 4 months earlier of complications from her immunodeficient condition. R.'s father is an intravenous drug abuser, also with immunodeficiency.

R. presents with a several-day history of nasal and chest congestion. He is progressing to tachypnea, with retractions, grunting, irritability, and decreased feeding. Pulse oximetry on room air demonstrates an oxygen saturation of 70%. When placed on 3 L of oxygen by nasal cannula, his oxygen saturation level improves to 90%. A chest x-ray film shows air trapping and diffuse bilateral interstitial infiltrates suggestive of *Pneumocystis carinii* pneumonia (PCP). R. is admitted to the PICU for monitoring and observation. He is being treated with AZT and TMP-SMX.

1. According to the CDC classification system for pediatric HIV, R. would be in what clinical category if he has PCP?
   a. Category N.
   b. Category A.
   c. Category B.
   d. Category C.

2. The nurse knows that the most likely procedure to confirm R.'s diagnosis of PCP is
   a. Bronchopulmonary lavage.
   b. Chest radiograph.
   c. Sputum analysis.
   d. Transbronchial biopsy.

3. Because R. shows signs of deterioration despite being treated with AZT, the second antiretroviral drug of choice to be considered for use in his treatment is
   a. ddI.
   b. ddC.
   c. D4T.
   d. 3TC.

R.'s condition worsens. He becomes more tachypneic, with further hypoxia, hypercapnia, and wheezing. A diagnosis of lymphoid interstitial pneumonitis (LIP), the other common pulmonary disease associated with HIV and AIDS is suspected. Mechanical ventilation for his worsening respiratory failure is required, with a fraction of inspired oxygen of 70% and a positive end-expiratory pressure of 8 cmH_2O.

4. The basic physiologic changes associated with LIP are
   a. Airway narrowing and hyperinflation.
   b. Patchy infiltrates and hilar lymphadenopathy.
   c. Lymphocytic infiltrates and restrictive lung disease.
   d. Pulmonary infiltrates with consolidation.

5. Critical care management for R. includes
   a. Antibiotics and mechanical ventilation.
   b. Oxygen, bronchodilators, and steroids.
   c. Aerosolized or intravenous pentamidine.
   d. Rifampin and isoniazid.

R. has been maintained on mechanical ventilation for 2 weeks, producing only minor improvement in his respiratory status. He is unresponsive and comatose. During the last 24 hours, he has experienced fever as high as 39.5°C and appears to be developing the clinical picture of septic shock. His blood pressure is 65/30 mmHg. He has weak pulses, a prolonged capillary refill time, and decreased cardiac output.

6. At this point, the nurse considers that R. requires
   a. Afterload reduction and antiarrhythmics.
   b. Antimicrobial therapy and increased doses of antiretrovirals.
   c. Preload reduction and digoxin administration.
   d. Volume expansion, inotropic support, and antimicrobial therapy.

7. R.'s sudden neurologic deterioration may be a result of HIV infection of the brain and HIV encephalopathy. Other acute neurologic diagnoses seen in children such as R. are
   a. Central nervous system (CNS) tumors and coma.
   b. CNS infections, lymphomas, and stroke.
   c. Seizures and neurologic deficits.
   d. Impaired brain growth and ataxia.

After maximal PICU support for an additional 2 weeks, R.'s status continues to deteriorate, and he dies after a sudden full arrest. This family's battle with HIV infection brings with it several psychosocial issues that R.'s father begins to verbalize to the nurse.

8. The nurse considers that the most significant sources of psychosocial stress for this family during R.'s hospitalization were
   a. The recent death of his mother, critical

status of R., and HIV status of his father.

b. The mounting financial burdens of this hospitalization and a lack of outside support.

c. The stressors of the PICU environment, including R.'s appearance and multiple procedures.

d. R.'s father's history of substance abuse and the death of R.'s mother.

ANSWERS ■ CASE 20-1

1. Answer (**c**). Perinatal transmission is the most likely mode of transmission for M. Approximately 80% of all children with HIV infection acquire the disease through perinatal transmission from HIV-infected mothers. The primary risk behavior of the mother is intravenous drug use.

REFERENCES
Caldwell, M.B., & Rogers, M.F. (1991). Epidemiology of pediatric HIV infection. *Pediatric Clinics of North America*, 38(1), 1–16.
Centers for Disease Control and Prevention (1994). *HIV/AIDS surveillance report. Fourth quarter edition.* 6 (4).

2. Answer (**c**). According to the guidelines outlined by the CDC, pediatric AIDS refers to cases that have been reported of children younger than 13 years of age.

REFERENCE
Centers for Disease Control and Prevention (1993). *HIV/AIDS surveillance report. First quarter edition.* 5 (1), 1–19.

3. Answer (**c**). M.'s pulmonary complications are the reason she is admitted to the PICU. Pulmonary complications, including infectious and noninfectious pulmonary diseases, are the most common reasons pediatric HIV or AIDS patients are admitted to the PICU. These complications often lead to acute respiratory failure.

REFERENCES
Hoyt, L.G., & Oleske, J.M. (1992). The clinical spectrum of HIV infection in infants and children: An overview. In R. Yogev & E. Connor (Eds.). *Management of HIV infection in infants and children* (pp. 227–246). St. Louis: Mosby–Year Book.
Jones, K., LeBeouf, M., & Dillman, P. (1996). HIV in the critically ill child. In M.A.Q. Curley, J.B. Smith, & P.A. Moloney-Harmon (Eds.). *Critical care nursing of infants and children* (pp. 861–873). Philadelphia: W.B. Saunders.

4. Answer (**b**). These results are inconclusive, because babies born to infected women test positive as a result of maternal antibody transmission to the fetus in utero. In this instance the infant's positive ELISA result mirrors the mother's HIV-positive and antibody status. It is impossible to determine the true HIV status of the baby at this time.

REFERENCE
Tinkle, M.B., Amaya, M.A., & Tamayo, O.W. (1992). HIV disease and pregnancy. Part 1: Epidemiology, pathogenesis, and natural history. *Journal of Obstetric, Gynecologic and Neonatal Nursing*, 21 (2), 86–93.

5. Answer (**c**). Research has demonstrated that maternal antibodies remain in the babies system for as long as 15 months. During this time, a baby may have a positive antibody test result that does not necessarily reflect the baby's true HIV status.

REFERENCE
Lewis, K.D., & Thompson, H.B. (1989). Infants, children and adolescents. In J.H. Flaskerud (Ed.). *AIDS/HIV infection: A reference guide for nursing professionals* (pp. 111–127). Philadelphia: W.B. Saunders.

6. Answer (**a**). Statistics indicate that 25% to 35% of the babies born to HIV-positive women will develop HIV disease themselves. Researchers are unsure why 100% of the babies do not become HIV positive and are unable to determine which infants will or will not progress to HIV disease.

REFERENCES
Ellerbrook, T.V., Bush, T.J., Chamberland, M.E., & Oxtoby, M.T. (1991). Epidemiology of women with AIDS in the United States, 1981 through 1990. *Journal of the American Medical Association*, 265 (22), 2971–2975.
Smeltzer, S.C., & Whipple, B. (1991). Women and HIV infection. *Image: Journal of Nursing Scholarship*, 23 (4), 249–256.

7. Answer (**d**). T4 cells, also called inducer or helper T cells, are often referred to as the conductor of the immune system. Their primary function is to release lymphokines, which stimulate or activate the other cells of the immune system. The other cells would not know that invasion by the virus has occurred without lymphokines being released.

REFERENCE
Grady, C. (1989). The immune system and AIDS/HIV infection. In J.H. Flaskerud (Ed.). *AIDS/HIV infec-*

tion: *A reference guide for nursing professionals* (pp. 37–57). Philadelphia: W.B. Saunders.

8. Answer (**a**). Normally, there are twice as many T4 cells as T8 cells within a healthy immune system. As the disease progresses, the percentage and absolute number of T4 cells decrease. Because the primary function of T4 cells is to release lymphokines and stimulate the other cells of the immune system (including T8 cells); a low T4 to T8 ratio indicates disease progression and overall decreased cellular immunity. This leaves the host more susceptible to infections and malignancies and ultimately leads to death.

REFERENCES
Grady, C. (1989). The immune system and AIDS/HIV infection. In J.H. Flaskerud (Ed.). *AIDS / HIV infection: A reference guide for nursing professionals* (pp. 37–57). Philadelphia: W.B. Saunders.
Wade, N. (1991). Immunologic considerations in pediatric HIV infection. *Journal of Pediatrics,* 119 (1S), S5–S6.

9. Answer (**a**). The p24 antigen is the core protein found inside HIV. When an individual initially becomes infected with HIV, p24 is detected in the blood. The p24 antigen then becomes undetectable as the person develops antibodies and HIV enters its latent phase. When the virus again becomes active, the amount of p24 antigen in the blood becomes detectable.

REFERENCES
Grady, C., & Vogel, S. (1993). Laboratory methods for diagnosing and monitoring HIV infection. *Journal of the Association of Nurses in AIDS Care,* 4 (2), 11–21.
Michael, N.L., & Burke, D.S. (1991). Natural history of human immunodeficiency virus infection. *Dermatologic Clinics of North America,* 9 (3), 429–441.

10. Answer (**b**). Because many patients become neutropenic when treated daily with TMP-SMX, administration three times each week is often used. This dosing has been found to be equally effective and causes less neutropenia.

REFERENCE
Wasserman, R. (1990). AIDS. In D.L. Levine & F.C. Morriss (Eds) *Essentials of pediatric intensive care* (pp. 378–382). St. Louis: Quality Medical Publishing.

11. Answer (**c**). The most commonly reported short-term side effects of AZT therapy include nausea, headache, insomnia, myalgia, and vomiting. Resolution of these side effects usually occurs as the individual continues with therapy.

REFERENCE
Fischl, M.A. (1990). Treatment of HIV infection. In M.A. Sande & P.A. Volberding (Eds.). *The medical management of AIDS* (2nd ed., pp. 103–113). Philadelphia: W.B. Saunders.

12. Answer (**a**). AZT has the potential to interfere with red blood cell production, causing the major long-term side effects of bone marrow suppression and anemia. If this complication does occur, the dose of AZT is decreased, and red blood cell transfusions are considered. Persistent bone marrow suppression is the reason to consider discontinuing AZT and placing the patient on a different antiretroviral medication.

REFERENCE
Fischl, M.A. (1990). Treatment of HIV infection. In M.A. Sande & P.A. Volberding (Eds.). *The medical management of AIDS* (2nd ed., pp. 103–113). Philadelphia: W.B. Saunders.

ANSWERS ■ CASE 20-2

1. Answer (**d**). The CDC pediatric classification system developed in 1987 and revised in 1994 classifies infected children into mutually exclusive clinical categories according to infection status, immunologic status, and clinical status. Children are classified into clinical categories based on signs, symptoms, or diagnoses related to HIV infection. Category N is not symptomatic; Category A is mildly symptomatic; Category B is moderately symptomatic; and Category C is severely symptomatic. Based on the information given in this case to this point, R. fits into Category C because of a suggested diagnosis of PCP. A diagnosis of LIP will place him in Category B since several reports have indicated a better prognosis for children with LIP compared to children with other AIDS-defining conditions.

REFERENCE
Centers for Disease Control and Prevention. (1994). 1994 revised classification system for human deficiency virus infection in children less than 13 years of age. *Morbidity and Mortality Weekly Review,* 43(RR-12), 1–10.

2. Answer (**c**). PCP can be diagnosed with

noninvasive or invasive techniques. Noninvasive techniques such as sputum analysis, gastric washings or endotracheal secretions to show evidence of the organism are usually attempted first. At times, more invasive methods may be necessary.

REFERENCE

Tribett, D. (1993). The patient with human immunodeficiency virus (HIV). In M.R. Kinney, D.R. Packa, & S.B. Dunbar (Eds.). *AACN's clinical reference for critical care nursing* (pp. 1059–1067). St. Louis: Mosby–Year Book.

3. Answer (**a**). Didanosine or ddI (Videx) is the alternative drug to AZT that is used to slow the progression of HIV disease. It is indicated for children with AIDS who have AZT intolerance or progression of disease while on AZT.

REFERENCE

Volberling, P.A. (1994). Strategies for antiretroviral therapy in adult HIV disease: The San Francisco perspective. In S. Broder, T.C. Merigan, & D. Bulogness (Eds.). *Textbook of AIDS medicine* (pp. 773–787). Baltimore: Williams & Wilkins.

4. Answer (**c**). LIP is identified by diffuse interstitial infiltration of the alveolar septa with lymphocytes and plasma cells. The results of this infiltration include restrictive lung disease, and the child demonstrates hypoxia and hypercapnia.

REFERENCE

Joshi, V. (1991). Pathology of children with AIDS. *Pediatric Clinics of North America,* 38 (1), 97–120.

5. Answer (**b**). The clinical management of LIP is largely supportive because there is no specific therapy. Oxygen and bronchodilators are often the initial treatment of choice, followed by corticosteroids for children with disease progression and chronic hypoxemia.

REFERENCE

Scott, G.B., & Mastrucci, M. T. (1992). Pulmonary complications of HIV-1 infection in children. In R. Yogev & E. Connor (Eds.). *Management of HIV infection in infants and children* (pp. 323–356). St. Louis: Mosby–Year Book.

6. Answer (**d**). Critical care management for the child with AIDS experiencing sepsis and low cardiac output is the same as for any child with a "shock state" and includes inotropic support, volume expansion, afterload reduction, and appropriate antimicrobial therapy.

REFERENCE

Stewart, J.M., Kaul, A., Gromisch, D.S., et al. (1989). Symptomatic cardiac dysfunction in children with HIV infection. *American Heart Journal,* 117, 140–144.

7. Answer (**b**). The most common neurologic diagnoses for in HIV-infected children hospitalized in the PICU include CNS infection, such as meningitis and encephalitis, and primary CNS lymphoma. Although infrequent, strokes may occur and are often devastating.

REFERENCE

Wilkinson, J.D., & Greenwald, B.M. (1988). The acquired immunodeficiency syndrome: Impact on the pediatric intensive care unit. *Critical Care Clinics,* 4 (4), 831–843.

8. Answer (**a**). The stress produced by HIV disease is most evident in the simultaneous illnesses of R. and his parents and the recent death of his mother. Although several other psychosocial issues may have arisen during the course of their illnesses, the stress related to severe illness and death is likely to be the most significant issue.

REFERENCE

Spiegel, L., & Mayers, A. (1991). Psychosocial aspects of AIDS in children and adolescents. *Pediatric Clinics of North America,* 38 (1), 153–167.

CHAPTER *21*

Resuscitation

KERRI OATES, RN, MSN, CCRN

CASE 21-1

A., a 1-month-old girl, was found unresponsive in her crib by her parents. She had been sleeping on her stomach, and when turned over, she was limp and cyanotic. Her parents were familiar with cardiopulmonary resuscitation (CPR), which they initiated before calling 911. The ambulance arrived at the house within 15 minutes. A quick assessment revealed a cold female infant with a pulse of less than 60 and an unobtainable blood pressure. Intubation was unsuccessful. Mask ventilation was initiated and continued during transport.

In the emergency department, ventilation and chest compressions continue. A. has a heart rate of 60 beats per minute (bpm), blood pressure of 70 by palpation, and is apneic. Her distal pulses are nonpalpable, and her capillary refill time is 4 seconds.

1. The initial assessment of the pediatric patient in distress includes
   a. Airway size, breathing, and circulation.
   b. Airway patency, breathing, and circulation.
   c. Airway patency, capillary refill, and breathing.
   d. Central nervous system perfusion, aeration, and breathing.

2. The resuscitation priorities for A. are
   a. Ventilation and circulation.
   b. Ventilation and volume replacement.
   c. Ventilation and oxygenation.
   d. Ventilation and medication administration.

Endotracheal intubation is performed with the placement of a 3.5-mm uncuffed endotracheal tube (ETT). The child is hyperventilated, and 100% oxygen is administered. Vital signs are reassessed after endotracheal intubation, revealing a heart rate of 70 bpm, blood pressure 50/30 mmHg, and no spontaneous respirations. Her lips and nailbeds are pale pink, the capillary refill time is 4 seconds, extremities are cool, and distal pulses are weak. Peripheral access is unobtainable.

3. The treatment of choice for A. at this time is
   a. A 1:10,000 epinephrine solution administered at 0.1 mL/kg through the ETT and crystalloid solution administered at 20 mL/kg over 20 minutes.
   b. A 1:1000 epinephrine solution administered at 0.1 mL/kg through the ETT, placement of an intraosseous line, and crystalloid solution administered at 20 mL/kg over 40 minutes.
   c. A 1:10,000 epinephrine solution administered at 0.1 mL/kg through the ETT, placement of an intraosseous line, CPR, and crystalloid solution administered at 20 mL/kg over 20 minutes.
   d. A 1:1000 epinephrine solution administered at 0.1 mL/kg through the ETT, placement of an intraosseous line,

CPR, and crystalloid solution administered at 20 mL/kg over 20 minutes.

Intraosseous access is obtained, and epinephrine is repeated at the same dose and concentration given through the endotracheal route. CPR is stopped to reassess the situation. At this time, A. has a heart rate of 100 bpm, blood pressure of 88/40 mmHg, and respiratory rate of 10 breaths per minute. A fluid bolus of 20 mL/kg is given, and the vital signs are stabilized. The team transfers the infant to the pediatric intensive care unit (PICU).

4. What is the absolute contraindication to the placement of an intraosseous line?
   a. Child younger than 6 years of age.
   b. Recently fractured bone.
   c. Presence of infection.
   d. Bleeding disorder.

5. The priority interventions after CPR for A. are to
   a. Discontinue intravenous access, provide adequate oxygenation and ventilation, and consider enteral nutrition.
   b. Assess the adequacy of oxygenation, ventilation, cardiac output, and tissue perfusion and initiate antibiotic therapy.
   c. Perform a neurologic examination, obtain vital signs, assess cardiac output and tissue perfusion, and maintain hypothermia.
   d. Assess airway, breathing, and circulation; evaluate vascular access; and perform a thorough neurologic examination.

On arrival at the PICU, a chest radiograph is obtained to verify ETT and nasogastric tube placements. Once verified, arterial and central lines are placed while maintaining the intraosseous line. A. has a rectal temperature of 36°C, heart rate of 110 bpm, and blood pressure of 68/40 mmHg. She is being mechanically ventilated at a rate of 20 breaths per minute. Her extremities are cool, her capillary refill time is 3 seconds, and her urine output is 0.3 mL/kg per hour. Inotropic support is begun to aid in renal perfusion and to stabilize the blood pressure.

6. The nurse caring for this child knows that many inotropes can be considered for A., but the ideal inotrope in this situation is
   a. Dobutamine administered at 5 μg/kg per minute by a central route.
   b. Dopamine administered at 15 μg/kg per minute by a central route.
   c. Isoproterenol administered at 0.05 μg/kg per minute by a central route.
   d. Dopamine administered at 5 μg/kg per minute by a central or peripheral route.

A. responds well to inotropic support and stabilizes with maintenance fluids, dopamine administered at 5 μg/kg per minute, and mechanical ventilation. Ventilator settings include the fraction of inspired oxygen of 0.6, positive end-expiratory pressure of 5 cmH$_2$O, tidal volume of 70 mL, and intermittent mandatory ventilation of 20 breaths per minute.

A neurologic examination reveals that A. is flaccid, with absent corneal, cough, and gag reflexes. Her pupils are dilated and nonreactive.

A.'s parents are waiting in the parent's room located outside the unit. They have not seen their child for more than an hour. The father comes to the desk to ask for information.

7. The nurse can meet the family's needs in this situation by
   a. Keeping the family in the waiting room until the child is stable and linen is changed.
   b. Informing the family that everything is being done to save their child and that they will be kept informed.
   c. Encouraging the parents to be at the bedside, providing information and giving the option to touch and hold their child.
   d. Providing a private place for the parents and keeping them informed of their child's condition.

A.'s parents express their concerns and fears to the nurse. They do not want A. to suffer and wish to end life support if there is no hope. After the neurologic examination, it is decided that support will be terminated. A.'s parents' spend private time with A. to say their good-byes.

CASE 21-2

M., a 4-year-old boy, is brought to the emergency department in respiratory distress by his mother. His mother states that he has a history of asthma. He had a runny nose and cough for the past few days, and his mother noticed today that he had increased difficulty with breathing.

He is sitting on his mother's lap and leaning forward. He is alert but irritable. The findings of the physical examination are significant for his use of intercostal, shoulder, and abdominal muscles and for tachypnea and tachycardia. His expiratory phase is prolonged, and wheezes are audible with a stethoscope. A non-rebreathing mask with 100% humidified oxygen is placed. His oxygen saturation level monitored by pulse oximeter is 87%. Despite several albuterol treatments, his respiratory status worsens. A chest film reveals air trapping, atelectasis, and a flattened diaphragm.

The arterial blood gas determinations include hydrogen ion concentration (pH), partial pressures of oxygen (Po_2) and carbon dioxide (Pco_2), bicarbonate (HCO_3^-) level, and base excess (BE). The following values are the results for M.:

pH: 7.32 HCO_3^-: 18 mEq/L
Po_2: 60 mmHg   BE: −6.4
Pco_2: 55 mmHg

M. becomes lethargic, and he remains tachycardic and tachypneic with poor aeration; wheezes are no longer audible. His skin color is dusky, and he no longer interacts with his parents.

1. Respiratory failure is recognized in M. by which of the following signs?
   a. Prolonged capillary refill, tachycardia, tachypnea, and pulse oximeter reading of 95%.
   b. Interactive and playful manner, minimal oxygen requirement, and a good appetite.
   c. Oxygen requirement, tachypnea, and an irritable manner but responds and recognizes his parents.
   d. Lethargic manner, tachypneic pattern, dusky skin color, and a change in breath sounds with increased use of accessory muscles.

2. The priority in managing M.'s airway is to
   a. Raise the head of his bed and repeat the albuterol treatment.
   b. Repeat the arterial blood gas.
   c. Bag-mask ventilate and prepare for endotracheal intubation.
   d. Notify PICU staff that they will be getting an admission.

3. The nurse obtains which size laryngoscope blade and ETT?

   a. Miller 2 blade with a 5.0-mm uncuffed ETT; a 4.5-mm and a 5.5-mm uncuffed ETT.
   b. Miller 2 blade with a 5.0-mm ETT; a 4.0-mm and a 5.5-mm ETT.
   c. Macintosh 1 blade with a 3.5-mm cuffed ETT; a 3.0-mm and a 4.0-mm cuffed ETT.
   d. Miller 3 blade with a 7.5-mm cuffed ETT; a 6.5-mm and a 7.5-mm ETT.

M. is successfully intubated with a 5.0 uncuffed ETT. A chest film shows that the ETT is in the proper position.

4. The nurse listens to which area of the chest to determine placement of the ETT?
   a. Midaxillary line bilaterally.
   b. Midaxillary line bilaterally and over the stomach.
   c. Anterior chest bilaterally.
   d. Anterior chest bilaterally and over the stomach.

5. What is the landmark to determine correct position of the ETT on the chest film?
   a. Level of the 4th rib.
   b. Between 1 and 2 cm above the carina.
   c. At the carina.
   d. Just above the opening of the right mainstem bronchus.

The ETT is secured in place with tape. Before transfer to the PICU, M. is placed on 100% oxygen and hyperventilated.

6. Hyperventilation and oxygenation with 100% oxygen is indicated for M. to
   a. Prevent atelectasis and replenish oxygen stores.
   b. Replenish carbon dioxide and oxygen stores.
   c. Remove carbon dioxide and improve systemic oxygenation.
   d. Decrease the oxygen and carbon dioxide level.

CASE 21-3

K., a 14-year-old girl, presents to the emergency department with complaints of palpitations and shortness of breath. Her medical history is significant for corrective surgery for transposition of the great arteries.

K. is admitted to the PICU for observation. On admission, she has a heart rate of 210 bpm, blood pressure of 110/64 mmHg, and respiratory rate of 24 breaths per minute. Her weight is 46 kg. Physical examination reveals that she is alert with pink mucous membranes and nail beds and a capillary refill time of less than 2 seconds. Approximately 1 hour after admission, K.'s blood pressure drops to 70/34 mmHg. Her heart rate remains at 210 bpm, and her respiratory rate is 28 breaths per minute. Her capillary refill time is prolonged.

1. Based on the progression of the tachyarrhythmia, what is the immediate intervention required?
   a. Give adenosine at a dose of 0.1 mg/kg by slow intravenous push; may increase the dose by 0.05 mg/kg every 2 minutes to a maximum dose of 0.25 mg/kg.
   b. Defibrillate at 0.5 joules/kg; give lidocaine at a dose of 1 mg/kg by intravenous push, followed by a lidocaine infusion of 20 μg/kg per minute; and maintain airway, breathing, and circulation.
   c. Maintain airway, breathing, and circulation; cardiovert at 0.5 joules/kg; and give lidocaine at a dose of 1 mg/kg by intravenous push, followed by a lidocaine infusion of 20 μg/kg per minute.
   d. Maintain airway, breathing, and circulation. Administer digoxin; one half of the total digitalizing dose is given initially, followed in 8 hours with one fourth of the total digitalizing dose for two doses.

2. Supraventricular tachycardia is identified by which of the following signs?
   a. Ventricular rate of 120 bpm, wide QRS, indistinguishable P waves, and inverted T waves.
   b. High ventricular rate, regular rhythm with normal P waves, and normal QRS duration.
   c. Rapid heart rate (240 bpm), paroxysmal and regular rhythm, indistinguishable P waves, and a narrow QRS complex.
   d. Chaotic heart rate, disorganized complexes, and no identifiable P, QRS, or T waves.

K. is given 100% oxygen, intravenous access is established, and a sedative and analgesic are given. Cardioversion with 0.5 joules/kg is attempted unsuccessfully.

3. What is the next step in treating K.?
   a. Give adenosine at 0.1 mg/kg by rapid intravenous push.
   b. Repeat cardioversion at 1.0 joule/kg.
   c. Give lidocaine at 1 mg/kg by intravenous push.
   d. Check the defibrillator to ensure that it is working.

4. What is the major advantage of adenosine in the treatment of supraventricular tachycardia?
   a. Adenosine produces a transient atrioventricular block, has a short half-life, does not interfere with other cardiac drugs, and has a rapid intravenous absorption.
   b. Adenosine inhibits sodium and potassium exchange, is inotropic and chronotropic, and slows heart rate and improves contractility.
   c. Adenosine exerts negative inotropic and chronotropic actions, and it increases the refractory period of the atrioventricular node, slowing the ventricular response to rapid atrial arrhythmias.
   d. Adenosine improves left ventricular diastolic relaxation and filling, and it prolongs atrioventricular junctional conduction time.

K. converts to a normal sinus rhythm with a heart rate of 100 bpm after the second cardioversion. She remains in the PICU for 2 days until she is digitalized and is able to maintain a heart rate appropriate for her age. She is discharged home after 5 days.

ANSWERS ■ CASE 21-1

1. Answer (**b**). Airway patency, breathing, and circulation are the basic steps of assessment in basic and advanced pediatric life support. These are sequential steps designed to support or restore effective ventilation and circulation to the child in respiratory or cardiorespiratory arrest. Establishment and maintenance of a patent airway and support of ventilation are the most important components of pediatric CPR.

REFERENCE
Hazinski, M., & Chameides, L. (Eds.) (1994). Pediatric basic life support. In *Pediatric advanced life support* (pp. 3.1–3.13). Dallas: American Heart Association.

2. Answer (**c**). Priorities for resuscitation are addressed by the ABCs: airway patency, breathing, and circulation. Establishment of ventilation and oxygenation

is critical in maximizing a successful outcome. Reestablishing a patent airway is usually the treatment necessary to restore adequate ventilation and oxygenation.

REFERENCE

Curley, M.A.Q., & Ead, N. (1996). Resuscitation of infants and children. In M.A.Q. Curley, J.B. Smith, & P.A. Moloney-Harmon (Eds.). *Critical care nursing of infants and children* (pp. 963–988). Philadelphia: W.B. Saunders.

3. Answer (**d**). When intravenous access is not available, certain medications can be administered through the ETT. These include lidocaine, atropine, Narcan, and epinephrine (mnemonic: LANE). The recommended *endotracheal* epinephrine dose is 0.1 mg/kg (0.1 mL/kg) of the 1 : 1000 solution. All endotracheal medications are flushed with 3 to 5 mL of normal saline after instillation. This method of administration is effective because epinephrine is readily absorbed by the mucosa of the tracheobronchial tree. The *intravenous* or *intraosseous* dose is 0.1 mg/kg (0.1 mL/kg) of the 1 : 10,000 solution for the first dose. If this does not produce a response, 0.1 mg/kg of the 1 : 1000 dose is given.

REFERENCES

Gorodischer, R., & Koren, G. (1992). Cardiac drugs. In S. Yaffe & J. Aranda (Eds.). *Pediatric pharmacology therapeutic principles in practice* (pp. 345–354). Philadelphia: W.B. Saunders.
Hazinski, M., & Chameides, L. (Eds.) (1994). Fluid therapy and medications. In *Pediatric advanced life support* (pp. 6.1–6.11). Dallas: American Heart Association.

4. Answer (**b**). The contraindication to placement of an intraosseous device is a fracture in that bone. Placement also is contraindicated when a pelvic fracture exists. The fracture would allow the fluid or medications instilled to extravasate into local tissue.

REFERENCE

Hazinski, M., & Chameides, L. (Eds.) (1994). Vascular access. In *Pediatric advanced life support* (pp. 5.1–5.6). Dallas: American Heart Association.

5. Answer (**d**). Postresuscitation interventions are done to further stabilize the airway and to maintain oxygenation, ventilation, cardiac output, and tissue perfusion. These interventions are important to preserve neurologic function. A thorough neurologic examination is performed to detect any detrimental effects of resuscitation. During the immediate postresuscitation period, the ABCs of resuscitation are continually assessed because of the recurrent nature of hypoxemia, hypercapnia, hemodynamic instability, and altered sensorium until the patient is stabilized.

REFERENCES

Curley, M.A.Q., & Ead, N. (1996). Resuscitation of infants and children. In M.A.Q. Curley, J.B. Smith, & P.A. Moloney-Harmon (Eds.). *Critical care nursing of infants and children* (pp. 963–988). Philadelphia: W.B. Saunders.
Hazinski, M., & Chameides, L. (Eds.) (1994). Immediate postarrest stabilization and secondary transport. In *Pediatric advanced life support* (pp. 10.1–10.4). Dallas: American Heart Association.

6. Answer (**d**). Dopamine has a positive inotropic effect on the myocardium, resulting in direct stimulation of β_1-adrenergic receptors. At doses of 2 to 5 μg/kg per minute, the predominant effects are β_1-adrenergic actions. These include increased heart rate and systolic blood pressure, renal vasodilation, and promotion of diuresis by stimulation of the dopaminergic receptors. Dobutamine does not stimulate renal receptors. Epinephrine increases vascular resistance and decreases plasma flow, which may decrease renal blood flow. Isuprel does increase renal blood flow, but it also increases myocardial oxygen demand and is therefore not recommended.

REFERENCE

Gorodischer, R., & Koren, G. (1992). Cardiac drugs. In S. Yaffe & J. Aranda (Eds.). *Pediatric pharmacology therapeutic principles in practice* (pp. 345–354). Philadelphia: W.B. Saunders.

7. Answer (**c**). When a child is critically ill, parents require information and support. Providing a private place for the parents is essential. Allowing parents to touch and hold their child is an important measure to remember. Whether the resuscitation is successful or not, studies have revealed that family members would choose to witness the resuscitation again. By remaining at the place of resuscitation, family members are able to see and understand that everything possible has been done for their child.

REFERENCE

Curley, M.A.Q., & Ead, N. (1996). Resuscitation of infants and children. In M.A.Q. Curley, J.B. Smith, & P.A. Moloney-Harmon (Eds.). *Critical care nursing of infants and children* (pp. 963–988). Philadelphia: W.B. Saunders.

ANSWERS ■ CASE 21-2

1. Answer (**d**). Respiratory failure occurs when the lungs are no longer able to adequately oxygenate the arterial blood and fail to remove carbon dioxide from the bloodstream. Children are able to compensate initially by increasing the respiratory rate in an attempt to overcome a compromised tidal volume. As chest compliance decreases, the use of accessory muscles becomes more pronounced in an attempt to compensate. Breath sounds change as the airway becomes increasingly obstructed. Because children position themselves to maximize the airway, it is important not to change their positions. As hypoxia worsens, children become restless, agitated, and irritable. The skin color changes to a dusky or cyanotic color, most notably affecting the oral mucosa. All of the signs and symptoms are "red flags" at various stages of compromise that the bedside practitioner should be aware of and that should prompt intervention as appropriate.

REFERENCES
Curley, M.A.Q., & Ead, N. (1996). Resuscitation. In M.A.Q. Curley, J.B. Smith, & P.A. Moloney-Harmon (Eds.). *Critical care nursing of infants and children* (pp. 963–988). Philadelphia: W.B. Saunders.
West, J. (1992). Respiratory failure. In J. West (Ed.). *Pulmonary pathophysiology—The essentials* (4th ed., p. 151). Baltimore: Williams & Wilkins.

2. Answer (**c**). The priority is to maintain adequate oxygenation and ventilation. This child is in respiratory distress, as evidenced by the use of accessory muscles, his position, and an oxygen saturation level of 87%. Despite supplemental oxygen and several albuterol treatments, his condition worsens. The absence of wheezing is a sign of severe airway obstruction and warrants immediate intervention.

REFERENCE
Eigen, H., & Gerberding, K. (1993). Lower airway disease. In P. Holbrook (Ed.). *Textbook of pediatric critical care* (pp. 517–522). Philadelphia: W.B. Saunders.

3. Answer (**a**). A Miller 2 blade is the appropriate size laryngoscope blade. The equation (**age + 16)/4** can be used to determine the correct ETT size. For example, 4 years old + 16/4 = 5; the appropriate-size ETT

is 5.0 mm. An ETT that is 0.5 mm smaller and larger should also be selected in the event that the child's airway is smaller or larger than determined.

REFERENCE
Hazinski, M., & Chameides, L. (Eds.) (1994). Airway and ventilation. In *Pediatric advanced life support* (pp. 4.1–4.20). Dallas: American Heart Association.

4. Answer (**a**). After intubation, breath sounds are auscultated high along the midaxillary line. Because children have thin chest walls, referred breath sounds are common. A slight change in breath sounds from the right lung to the left may indicate right mainstem bronchus intubation.

REFERENCE
Curley, M.A.Q., & Ead, N. (1996). Resuscitation of infants and children. In M.A.Q. Curley, J.B. Smith, & P.A. Moloney-Harmon (Eds.). *Critical care nursing of infants and children* (pp. 963–988). Philadelphia: W.B. Saunders.

5. Answer (**b**). The ETT should be positioned 1 to 2 cm above the carina to provide equal aeration to the right and left lungs. If positioned lower, right mainstem bronchus intubation is likely, resulting in hyperinflation of the right lung and hypoventilation of the left lung.

REFERENCE
Hazinski, M. (1992). Chest X-ray interpretation. In M. Hazinski (Ed.). *Nursing care of the critically ill child* (pp. 499–519). St. Louis: Mosby–Year Book.

6. Answer (**c**). The priority is to establish a patent airway and provide supplemental oxygen to improve systemic arterial oxygenation. In addition, hyperventilation will aid in the removal of carbon dioxide.

REFERENCE
Hazinski, M., & Chameides, L. (Eds.) (1994). Fluid therapy and medications. In *Pediatric advanced life support* (pp. 6.1–6.11). Dallas: American Heart Association.

ANSWERS ■ CASE 21-3

1. Answer (**c**). After airway patency, breathing, and circulation have been assessed, the unstable tachyarrhythmia requires intervention. Synchronized cardioversion is the treatment of choice for patients who show evidence of cardiovascular compromise. The dose is 0.5 joules/kg. If this dose is unsuccessful, the dose is doubled, and

cardioversion repeated. Lidocaine may be given before cardioversion if intravenous access is available. If unavailable, treatment should proceed with cardioversion. Lidocaine raises the threshold for ventricular fibrillation and suppresses postcardioversion ventricular ectopy.

REFERENCE

Hazinski, M., & Chameides, L. (Eds.) (1994). Cardiac rhythm disturbance. In *Pediatric advanced life support* (pp. 7.1–7.11). Dallas: American Heart Association.

2. Answer (**c**). Supraventricular tachycardia is a rapid, paroxysmal, regular rhythm. The rate is usually greater than 220 bpm with narrow QRS complexes. It is one of the most common arrhythmias seen in children.

REFERENCE

Hazinski, M., & Chameides, L. (Eds.) (1994). Cardiac rhythm disturbance. In *Pediatric advanced life sup-* *port* (pp. 7.1–7.11). Dallas: American Heart Association.

3. Answer (**b**). If the initial attempt at cardioversion is not successful, the dose is doubled to 1.0 joules/kg for subsequent attempts. The dosage may be continually doubled to a maximum dosage of 10 joules/kg.

REFERENCE

Vetter, V. (1993). Arrhythmias. In P. Holbrook (Ed.). *Textbook of pediatric critical care* (pp. 384–412). Philadelphia: W.B. Saunders.

4. Answer (**a**). Adenosine has a rapid onset of action and a short half-life. It is administered by rapid intravenous push. Adenosine can be used in the acutely ill patient but should not delay cardioversion.

REFERENCE

Vetter, V. (1993). Arrhythmias. In P. Holbrook (Ed.). *Textbook of pediatric critical care* (pp. 384–412). Philadelphia: W.B. Saunders.

CHAPTER *22*

Nutrition

NORMA L. LIBURD, RN,C, MN

CASE 22-1

B., a malnourished-appearing 8-year-old boy, is brought to the emergency department by his maternal grandmother. He was diagnosed with perinatally acquired human immunodeficiency virus infection at 6.5 years of age. Two months ago, B. was hospitalized for *Pneumocystis carinii* pneumonia and dehydration. The family relocated to this state 1 month ago. B. has been coughing and "breathing hard" since yesterday. He has a history of failure to thrive with poor appetite and has vomited several times in the last 2 days.

B. presented with a heart rate of 160 beats per minute (bpm), respiratory rate of 80 breaths per minute, diminished breath sounds, blood pressure of 60/42 mmHg, and poor skin turgor. He has mild intercostal retractions. His oxygen saturation is 91% on room air.

1. Based on this information, which is the first priority for B.'s care?
   a. Start an intravenous line and fluid resuscitation at 20 mL/kg.
   b. Obtain a chest film to rule out pneumonia.
   c. Administer a high flow rate of oxygen by face mask.
   d. Obtain blood gases to determine the effectiveness of oxygenation.

B. is placed on a pulse oximeter, which shows an oxygen saturation of 95% on 6 L of oxygen by face mask. Vascular access is obtained using a 24-gauge catheter, and 5% dextrose in normal saline is infusing at 50 mL/hour. A chest x-ray indicates bilateral pneumonia. B. is transferred to the pediatric intensive care unit (PICU). His orders include a complete nutritional assessment by the dietitian.

B.'s weight is 12.3 kg, which is below the fifth percentile. His height is 115 cm, which is also below the fifth percentile. His serum albumin is 2.2 g/dL. His grandmother tells the nurse that B.'s mother refused placement of a gastrostomy tube last year.

2. Based on this information, the nurse determines that
   a. B.'s malnutrition has been a chronic process.
   b. B.'s malnutrition is an acute process.
   c. Other laboratory work must be completed to identify the type of malnutrition.
   d. Midarm circumference and height are needed to evaluate the status of malnutrition.

3. Which of the following biochemical indices is the most sensitive to acute visceral protein changes and is helpful in determining the presence of malnutrition?
   a. Albumin.
   b. Transferrin.
   c. Prealbumin.
   d. Somatomedin C.

The dietitian recommends that parenteral nutrition be initiated at a very low rate and then increased slowly.

4. Treatment of long-term growth failure requires an increase in calories of
   a. 10% to 20% above the resting energy expenditure.
   b. 50% to 100% above the resting energy expenditure.
   c. 110% to 150% above the resting energy expenditure.
   d. 160% to 200% above the resting energy expenditure.

5. What is the most important thing the nurse should do before hanging a new bag of parenteral nutrition solution?
   a. Check the intravenous site for patency and presence of inflammation.
   b. Confirm that she or he is hanging the appropriate solution by checking the content with the physician's original order.
   c. Check the most recent glucose levels to ensure that hypoglycemia or hyperglycemia have not developed.
   d. Change the intravenous tubing and the dressing over the catheter insertion site.

6. Many factors must be taken into consideration when deciding between enteral and parenteral nutrition. One reason to choose parenteral over enteral is that the child
   a. Is hemodynamically unstable.
   b. Is having mild diarrhea.
   c. Has a stress ulcer.
   d. Has a resolved ileus.

On the third day in the PICU, B. is started on enteral tube feeding. His weight is down to 11.86 kg, and his albumin level is 1.95 g/dL.

7. What is an important nursing responsibility when placing a nasogastric tube in a child?
   a. The head of the bed should be elevated 30 degrees.
   b. The patient's head should be slightly extended to ensure smoother passage of the tube.
   c. A decompression tube is used to decrease the risk of aspiration.
   d. The correct size is ensured by measuring from the tip of the nose to the ear and then to the xiphoid process.

8. After inserting the nasogastric tube, the most appropriate method of checking for placement is
   a. Obtaining an abdominal radiograph.
   b. Putting air into the tube and auscultating for a "whooshing" sound over the upper left quadrant of the abdomen.
   c. Aspirating fluid.
   d. Checking the aspirate's pH with pH paper.

B. is started on one-half strength Pedia-Sure at 20 mL/hour. This half rate will be gradually increased to the full rate over the next 48 hours.

9. The nursing care includes
   a. Routine mouth care with saline or an antimicrobial mouth wash.
   b. Checking for tube placement every 6 to 8 hours.
   c. Checking specific gravity twice each day to evaluate for fluid imbalance.
   d. Hanging no more than 12 hours' worth of formula at one time.

10. The priority nursing concern for B. at this time is
    a. Pain management.
    b. Prevention of decubiti.
    c. Fluid administration.
    d. Prevention of pulmonary aspiration.

On day 4 of B.'s hospital stay in the PICU, his respiratory rate is 26 breaths per minute, and he continues to have diminished lung sounds bilaterally. He is transferred to the medical pediatric floor, where he will continue to receive enteral and parenteral nutrition. After his pneumonia resolves, a gastrostomy tube for long-term nutritional support will be placed.

CASE 22-2

S. is a 3-year-old girl who sustained second degree burns over her chest and arms. The total body surface area (TBSA) involved was 18%. The accident occurred at home when she pulled a large pot of boiling soup off the stove. Her mother called 911, and she was transported to the hospital and admitted to the PICU.

S. weighs 15 kg. The nurse is unable to obtain S.'s upright height. Her recumbent length is 100 cm.

1. An upright height for S. would be approximately
   a. 92 cm.
   b. 96 cm.
   c. 98 cm.
   d. 100 cm (the same).

Although oral feeding is the preferred route of nutrition, S. has been able to take in only 45% of her caloric requirements during the first 24 hours in the PICU. An order for continuous enteral feedings is written.

2. What is the goal of early nutritional support in the critically ill child?
   a. To improve patient recovery and survival.
   b. To treat protein-energy malnutrition.
   c. To meet the child's higher energy requirements.
   d. To improve ventilatory drive and respiratory efficiency.

3. S. will require a diet high in protein to meet her increased energy needs and facilitate wound healing. What is the danger associated with giving large amounts of protein?
   a. Amino acid deficiencies will result.
   b. Plasma protein imbalances will occur.
   c. The development of metabolic acidosis.
   d. The development of metabolic alkalosis.

4. What is the primary advantage of enteral feedings over parenteral nutrition in critically ill children?
   a. Enteral nutrition is a safer and less expensive mode of providing nutrient delivery.
   b. Enteral feedings are advantageous for patients with severe shock, upper gastrointestinal bleeding, and necrotizing enterocolitis.
   c. With enteral feedings, there are significantly fewer side effects than when nutrition is provided through parenteral feedings.
   d. Overall gut function is promoted, which reduces the potential for bacterial translocation and sepsis.

5. Nursing interventions include
   a. Measuring abdominal girth every hour during the duration of the feeding.
   b. Checking feeding residual volume every 4 hours.
   c. Maintaining no oral intake during enteral feedings.
   d. Restraining S.'s arms to prevent her from pulling out the tube.

Management of the fluid intake of a child with burns includes monitoring for specific signs and symptoms of third spacing of fluid.

6. The goal of initial fluid resuscitation and replacement in a burned child is to
   a. Restore adequate intravascular volume.
   b. Restore adequate extravascular volume.
   c. Prevent pulmonary edema from occurring.
   d. Prevent shock from occurring.

S. is eating only small amounts of food orally while receiving the continuous enteral feedings. S.'s mother is very upset about the nasogastric tube and points out that S. "has always been a picky eater." She assures the nurse that she can get S. to eat better if the nasogastric tube is removed.

7. The nurse's response is based on the knowledge that
   a. Basal metabolic rate significantly increases when a TBSA burn of 15% or more occurs.
   b. Basal metabolic rate significantly decreases when a TBSA burn of 15% or more occurs.
   c. Nutrition is important to wound healing and in preventing decreased resistance to infection.
   d. If adequate nutritional intake is not provided to meet the body's needs, there will be a loss of lean body mass.

Three days after starting the enteral feedings, the nurse notices that S. has lost 1.2 kg of weight from the previous morning. Despite a wide selection of food, her oral intake continues to be poor. She has had no nausea or vomiting. Her skin is supple.

8. The next intervention is to
   a. Begin parenteral nutrition.
   b. Increase the enteral feeding rate.
   c. Stop the enteral feeding and re-evaluate the nutritional status.
   d. Obtain an abdominal x-ray.

9. If S. develops diarrhea, the most important intervention is to
   a. Administer antidiarrheals.
   b. Keep her skin clean and dry.
   c. Obtain a stool culture.
   d. Hold her enteral feedings.

10. Realizing that gastric distention and constipation are also complications of enteral feedings, the nurse attempts to minimize these issues for S. She
    a. Recommends a fiber-containing feeding.
    b. Adds fat to the feeding.

c. Increases S.'s activity as much as possible.

d. Stops all pain medications.

CASE 22-3

M. is a 10-month-old girl who is transported to the hospital by ambulance after having a generalized seizure lasting 3 minutes at home. Her mother reports that M. has been sick for 2 days with fever and diarrhea. She was examined by her pediatrician that morning and an antibiotic was ordered, but before the mother could administer it, M. had the seizure. According to the mother, her child turned blue around the lips and stopped breathing. The mother performed cardiopulmonary resuscitation and called 911.

On admission to the emergency department, M. has a temperature of 40.3°C, regular pulse of 120 bpm, respiratory rate of 30 breaths per minute, and blood pressure of 88/50 mmHg. Her skin color is pink on 100% oxygen. Oxygen saturation is 99%. Her skin turgor is poor, peripheral pulses are weak, and the capillary refill time is 3 to 4 seconds. She does not cry when the phlebotomist draws blood for a complete blood count and blood chemistry tests.

1. Based on M.'s presenting symptoms, the nurse suspects
   a. Respiratory distress.
   b. A postictal state.
   c. Septic shock.
   d. Cardiopulmonary failure.

2. What is the first priority for M.'s care?
   a. Obtain an electroencephalogram and chest x-ray.
   b. Start an intravenous line and fluid resuscitation at 20 mL/kg.
   c. Start an intravenous line and fluid resuscitation at 10 mL/kg.
   d. Intubate the infant and provide artificial ventilation.

M. is admitted to the PICU. Her electroencephalogram is normal. She has a temperature of 39.9°C, pulse of 116 bpm, respiratory rate of 32 breaths per minute, and blood pressure of 96/60 mmHg. Her intravenous solution is infusing well after she received an intravenous bolus of lactated Ringer's solution. She is alert but irritable. She has had no urine output but has had two watery stools since her admission. Her admission weight is 2 kg less than her weight obtained

3 days earlier at the pediatrician's office. She has had no further seizures.

3. What is the primary nursing diagnosis at this time?
   a. Diarrhea.
   b. Fluid volume deficit.
   c. High risk for altered body temperature.
   d. High risk for impaired skin integrity.

Twenty-four hours after M.'s admission to the PICU, she continues to have diarrhea, and her weight has remained unchanged. She is receiving nothing orally, and her urine output has increased to 2 mL/kg per hour.

4. What type of nutrition would be most appropriate for M. at this time?
   a. Total parenteral nutrition.
   b. Enteral feedings.
   c. Enteral feedings with supplemental oral formula feedings.
   d. Oral formula feedings.

5. What is the highest glucose content for parenteral nutrition that can safely be administered by the peripheral intravenous route?
   a. 5% dextrose.
   b. 12.5% dextrose.
   c. 15% dextrose.
   d. 20% dextrose.

6. Excessive delivery of dextrose in infants and children is associated with
   a. Hypercapnia.
   b. Hyperkalemia.
   c. Hypocalcemia.
   d. Intraventricular hemorrhage.

7. A fat emulsion is added to M.'s parenteral nutrition, which can be associated with
   a. Increased CO_2 production.
   b. Enhanced immune function.
   c. Platelet dysfunction.
   d. Renal dysfunction.

8. If M. develops renal dysfunction as the result of her septic shock, her parenteral nutrition would be adjusted by
   a. Increasing sodium.
   b. Decreasing potassium.
   c. Increasing magnesium.
   d. Increasing phosphorus.

Forty-eight hours after her admission, M.'s stool culture reveals *Salmonella*. Her temperature is 38.7°C, and she has had no additional seizures. She is on ampicillin intravenously, and if she remains stable, she will be transferred to the pediatric floor this afternoon.

ANSWERS ■ CASE 22-1

1. **Answer (c).** The first priority for the pediatric patient is to maintain a patent airway. In an emergency, the cause of the respiratory problem may not be evident or necessary to initiate the steps of emergency airway management. The child should be assessed for signs of respiratory distress, including tachypnea, retractions, nasal flaring, stridor, diminished level of consciousness, and decreased air movement on auscultation. Although vascular access is important and occurs simultaneously with securing the airway, the airway is the primary focus.

REFERENCES

Chameides, L., & Hazinski, M.F. (1994). *Textbook of pediatric advanced life support* (pp. 4–5). Dallas: American Heart Association.
Thomas, D.O. (1991). Pediatric physical assessment in the emergency department. In D.O. Thomas (Ed.). *Quick reference to pediatric emergency nursing* (pp. 31–37). Gaithersburg, MD: Aspen Publications.

2. **Answer (a).** B.'s malnutrition has been a chronic process. A low level of serum albumin is associated with low dietary protein intake. It is also associated with increased morbidity and mortality. Severe protein depletion is seen in children with serum protein levels less than 2.1 g/dL. His poor growth in both height and weight also indicate a chronic malnutrition process.

REFERENCE

Benjamin, D. (1989). Laboratory tests and nutritional assessment, protein-energy status. *Pediatric Clinics of North America, 36*, 139–161.

3. **Answer (c).** Prealbumin is the most helpful biochemical measurement in identifying nutritional deficiencies. It has a half life of 2 days and a smaller body pool than transferrin and albumin. It also decreases quickly with lower than normal protein intake.

REFERENCES

Benjamin, D. (1989). Laboratory tests and nutritional assessment, protein-energy status. *Pediatric Clinics of North America, 36*, 139–161.
Figueroa-Colon, R. (1992). Clinical and laboratory assessment of the malnourished child. In R.M. Suskind & L. Lewinter-Suskind (Eds.). *Textbook of pediatric nutrition* (2nd ed., pp. 191–205). New York: Raven Press.

4. **Answer (b).** Routine activities that are common to the intensive care unit increase oxygen consumption. Most critically ill children with moderate stress require a 50% increase above the resting energy expenditure. Those with a protein-energy malnutrition due to chronic disease experience increases between 50% and 100% above the resting energy expenditure. Adjustment of calories to compensate for the degree of stress is important.

REFERENCE

Pollack, M. (1993). Nutritional support of children in the intensive care unit. In R.M. Suskind & L. Lewinter-Suskind (Eds.). *Textbook of pediatric nutrition* (2nd ed., pp. 207–215). New York: Raven Press.

5. **Answer (b).** An important nursing responsibility is to verify that the appropriate total parenteral nutrition solution has been prepared. Initial daily laboratory monitoring of electrolytes is necessary, but as they become stable, monitoring is not required as regularly. Although the intravenous tubing is changed when the new solution is hung, the dressing is changed at least three times each week or when it becomes soiled. Catheter-related infection is a complication of parenteral nutrition therapy. The child should be assessed for the systemic signs of infection, such as fever and chills, in addition to the local signs of infection, such as redness, pain, swelling, and exudate at the site.

REFERENCES

Barnard, J.A., & Hazinski, M.F. (1992). Pediatric gastrointestinal disorders. In M.F. Hazinski (Ed.). *Nursing care of the critically ill child* (2nd ed.). St. Louis: Mosby–Year Book.
Robertson, J. (1991). Changing central venous catheter lines: Evaluation of a modification to clinical practice. *Journal of Pediatric Oncology Nursing, 4*, 173–179.
Verger, J. (1996). Nutrition. In M.A.Q. Curley, J.B. Smith, & P.A. Moloney-Harmon (Eds.). *Critical care nursing of infants and children* (pp. 410–448). Philadelphia: W.B. Saunders.

6. **Answer (a).** Parenteral nutrition is preferable in patients who are significantly unstable hemodynamically. In these patients, blood flow to the intestine may not be sufficient to support digestion,

and intestinal ischemia could result. Enteral feedings may be beneficial for patients with mild diarrhea and stress ulcers. Parenteral nutrition is preferred in patients with severe diarrhea. The gastrointestinal tract cannot be used if the child has an ileus.

REFERENCE
Evans, N. (1994). The role of total parenteral nutrition in critical illness: Guidelines and recommendations. *AACN Clinical Issues in Critical Care Nursing, 5* (4), 476–484.

7. Answer (**d**). Placement of a feeding tube is best accomplished using an appropriate-size tube, lubricating jelly, gloves, syringe, hypoallergenic tape, and a stethoscope. The length of the nasogastric tube insertion is determined by measuring from the tip of the nose to the ear and then from the ear to the xiphoid process. Decompression tubes should not be used in children because of the risk of aspiration.

REFERENCES
A.S.P.E.N. Board of Directors. (1993). Guidelines for the use of parenteral and enteral nutrition in adult and pediatric patients. *Journal of Parenteral and Enteral Nutrition, 17,* (Suppl. 4).
Verger, J. (1996). Nutrition. In M.A.Q. Curley, J.B. Smith, & P.A. Moloney-Harmon (Eds.). *Critical care nursing of infants and children* (pp. 410–448). Philadelphia: W.B. Saunders.

8. Answer (**a**). There have been questions regarding the reliability of the traditional methods for checking nasogastric tube placement. The method of air insufflation and auscultation of the "whooshing" sound has been found to be unreliable. Aspiration of fluid is also not reliable, because fluid may be aspirated from the pleural space or lung. The fluid's pH can be checked, and an acidic pH of 1.0 to 5.5 indicates that the tube is in the stomach. However, when gastric inhibitors are used, this method is not reliable. The most definitive method of checking correct tube placement is an abdominal radiograph.

REFERENCES
Metheny, N. (1988). Measures to test placement of nasogastric and nasointestinal feeding tubes and review. *Nursing Research, 37* (6), 324–329.
Verger, J. (1996). Nutrition. In M.A.Q. Curley, J.B. Smith, & P.A. Moloney-Harmon (Eds.). *Critical care nursing of infants and children* (pp. 410–448). Philadelphia: W.B. Saunders.

9. Answer (**a**). Routine mouth care is important in providing comfort and preventing oral cavity infection. Feeding bags and delivery sets should be changed every 24 to 48 hours, and no more than 4 to 8 hours of formula should be hung at one time. Tube placement should be checked every 3 to 4 hours. The specific gravity is checked every 4 to 8 hours initially. If a fluid imbalance is detected, the formula rate or concentration is adjusted.

REFERENCES
Anderson, K., Norris, D., Godfrey, L., Avent, C., & Butterworth, C. (1984). Bacterial contamination of tube feeding formulas. *Journal of Parenteral and Enteral Nutrition, 8,* 673–678.
Hendricks, R., & Walker, W.A. (1990). *Manual of pediatric nutrition* (2nd ed.). Philadelphia: B.C. Decker.

10. Answer (**d**). Pulmonary aspiration is the most serious complication of enteral tube feedings. B. should be monitored for nausea and vomiting, which may be a direct result of large volumes, rapid infusion rates, or hyperosmolar formulas. The other concerns will be addressed as B. stabilizes.

REFERENCES
Gaedeke Norris, M.K., & Steinhorn, D.M. (1994). Nutritional management during critical illness in infants and children. *AACN Clinical Issues in Critical Care Nursing, 5* (4), 485–494.
Verger, J. (1996). Nutrition. In M.A.Q. Curley, J.B. Smith, & P.A. Moloney-Harmon (Eds.). *Critical care nursing of infants and children* (pp. 410–448). Philadelphia: W.B. Saunders.

ANSWERS ■ CASE 22-2

1. Answer (**c**). Measurement of the recumbent length of a child up to age 5 is approximately 2 cm greater than the upright height measurement. After the child is 5 years of age, this variation tends to decline.

REFERENCE
Hamill, P., Drizd, T., Johnson, C., Reed, R., Roche, A., & Moore, W. (1979). Physical growth: National Center for Health Statistics percentiles. *American Journal of Clinical Nutrition, 32* (3), 607–629.

2. Answer (**a**). Acute protein-energy malnutrition in the early phase of a critically ill child's hospital course has been associated with higher mortality and physiologic instability. Protein and calo-

rie depletion compromise the immune system, which results in increased risk of infection. Malnutrition alters cell-mediated immunity, alters antibody responses, and impairs wound healing. Although early nutritional support is necessary for all of the responses, the ultimate goal is to improve recovery and survival of the critically ill child.

REFERENCES

Lehmann, S. (1993). Nutrition support of the hypermetabolic patient. *Critical Care Nursing Clinics of North America*, 5 (1), 97–103.
Pollack, M., Ruttiman, U., & Wiley, J. (1985). Nutritional depletion in critically ill children: Association with physiologic instability and increased quality of care. *Journal of Parenteral and Enteral Nutrition*, 6, 20–24.
Sorenson, R., Leiva, L., & Kuvibidila, S. (1993). Malnutrition and the immune response. In R.M. Suskind & L. Lewinter-Suskind (Eds.). *Textbook of pediatric nutrition* (pp. 141–160). New York: Raven Press.

3. Answer (**c**). Protein is crucial to healing after critical illness. Infants and children have even greater needs than adults because of their additional growth and developmental demands. Giving protein in greater amounts than required can cause metabolic acidosis and usually should be avoided. Patients with burns, however, have greatly increased protein needs, and high-protein replacements are required.

REFERENCES

Gaedeke Norris, M.K., & Steinhorn, D. (1994). Nutritional management during critical illness in infants and children. *AACN Clinical Issues in Critical Care Nursing*, 5 (4), 485–492.
Rieg, L., & Jenkins, M. (1991). Burn injuries in children. *Critical Care Nursing Clinics*, 3 (3), 457–470.

4. Answer (**d**). Although enteral nutrition is less costly and safer to administer, its primary advantage is that it is associated with reduced morbidity and mortality, along with a decreased potential for bacterial translocation and sepsis. Even small amounts of nutrients administered enterally can benefit the function and integrity of the gastrointestinal tract. Enteral feedings are contraindicated in patients who are in severe shock, have upper gastrointestinal bleeding, or have necrotizing enterocolitis.

REFERENCES

Dunn, L., Hulman, S., Weiner, J., & Kliegman, R. (1988). Beneficial effects of early hypocaloric enteral feeding on neonatal gastrointestinal function: Preliminary report of a randomized trial. *Journal of Pediatrics*, 112, 622–629.
Gaedeke Norris, M.K., & Steinhorn, D.M. (1994). Nutritional management during critical illness in infants and children. *AACN Clinical Issues in Critical Care Nursing*, 5 (4), 485–494.

5. Answer (**b**). Residual volume is checked every 4 hours and as needed. If the residual equals more than one half of the previous 2 hours' feeding, changing the concentration or feeding volume may be necessary. After S. begins to tolerate oral feedings, she can be gradually weaned from the tube feeding.

Abdominal girth is measured hourly at the initiation of feeding and when the rate is increased. During feedings, it is measured every 2 to 4 hours. Regurgitation and aspiration may occur if gastric distention develops.

REFERENCES

Sadowski, D.A. (1992). Care of the child with burns. In M.F. Hazinski (Ed.). *Nursing care of the critically ill child* (pp. 875–927). St. Louis: Mosby–Year Book.
Verger, J. (1996). Nutrition. In M.A.Q. Curley, J.B. Smith, & P.A. Moloney-Harmon (Eds.). *Critical care nursing of infants and children* (pp. 410–448). Philadelphia: W.B. Saunders.

6. Answer (**a**). The initial fluid resuscitation is intended to restore adequate intravascular volume and maintain tissue and organ perfusion. During the first few hours after a significant burn, there is an increase in capillary permeability that produces third spacing of fluid. If this volume loss is not replaced, cardiac output will fall, with a resultant compromise in systemic perfusion.

REFERENCES

Carvajal, H.F. (1993). Energy and protein metabolism in the pediatric burn patient. In R.M. Suskind & L. Lewinter-Suskind (Eds.). *Textbook of pediatric nutrition* (2nd ed., pp. 217–223). New York: Raven Press.
Sadowski, D.A. (1992) Care of the child with burns. In M.F. Hazinski. *Nursing care of the critically ill child* (pp. 875–927). St. Louis: Mosby–Year Book.

7. Answer (**a**). The basal metabolic rate increases significantly. Adjustment for the degree of stress should be made. For example, the stress factor can be as much as 2.0, depending on the size and severity of the burn. Other factors include the increased oxygen consumption for specific activities in the PICU, such as dressing changes (25%). Severe burns or major stress may increase the resting energy expenditures 80% to 100%. Although responses **c** and **d** are true, they provide supportive information to the statement in **a**. Every effort should be made to minimize energy demands by reducing stresses such as pain, anxiety, fear, and lowered temperatures. These stimulate the release of catecholamines and increase the body's energy requirements.

REFERENCE

Carvajal, H.F. (1993). Energy and protein metabolism in the pediatric burn patient. In R.M. Suskind & L. Lewinter-Suskind (Eds.). *Textbook of pediatric nutrition* (2nd ed., pp. 217–223). New York: Raven Press.

8. Answer (**b**). Because S. is not experiencing nausea or vomiting, the enteral feeding rate or concentration should be increased. A weight loss indicates that she is not receiving adequate nutrition for her daily caloric needs. An abdominal radiograph is not helpful in determining the cause of the weight loss.

REFERENCE

Sadowski, D.A. (1992). Care of the child with burns. In M.F. Hazinski (Ed.). *Nursing care of the critically ill child* (pp. 875–927). St. Louis: Mosby–Year Book.

9. Answer (**c**). A stool culture must be obtained so that an antibiotic specific to the microbe can be chosen. Treatment with antidiarrheal agents without appropriate antimicrobial therapy could be catastrophic. Keeping the skin clean and dry is important and can be a challenge if severe diarrhea results. Feedings should not be held or changed to parenteral therapy unless obstruction or perforation is imminent.

REFERENCE

Shuster, M. (1994). Enteral feeding of the critically ill. *AACN Clinical Issues in Critical Care Nursing, 5* (4), 459–475.

10. Answer (**c**). Any activity that promotes gut motility is encouraged. Fiber-containing products help with constipation, but they increase the bloating. Increasing the fat content can delay gastric emptying and add to the constipation and bloating. Narcotics contribute to decreased gastric motility, but it is not possible to discontinue them.

REFERENCE

Shuster, M. (1994). Enteral feedings of the critically ill. *AACN Clinical Issues in Critical Care Nursing, 5* (4), 459–475.

ANSWERS ■ CASE 22-3

1. Answer (**c**). M. has septic shock. Children between the ages of 3 months and 5 years usually present with high fever, tachycardia, tachypnea, and poor perfusion. Other common symptoms include petechial rash, altered level of consciousness, and seizures.

REFERENCE

Quigley, R.P., & Alexander, S.R. (1990). Acute renal failure. In D.L. Levine & F.C. Morris (Eds.). *Essentials of pediatric intensive care* (pp. 106–118). St. Louis: Quality Medical Publishing.

2. Answer (**b**). An intravenous line should be started. When signs of hypovolemic shock are detected, a fluid bolus should be administered. Careful assessment of the child's response is important. Additional fluid should be administered until the systemic perfusion improves and the signs and symptoms of shock are corrected.

REFERENCE

Chameides, L., & Hazinski, M.F. (1994). *Textbook of pediatric advanced life support.* Dallas: American Heart Association.

3. Answer (**b**). M.'s primary problem at this time is fluid volume deficit. She has received one bolus of intravenous fluid but remains dehydrated. Accurate intake and output evaluation is essential and should include diaper weights. After an initial bolus of fluid is administered, the child is reassessed. If signs of shock persist, a second bolus should be administered. Gastrointestinal infection and diarrhea can result in dehydration and severe fluid loss. The end result is hypovolemic shock. Gastroenteritis with dehydration is the primary cause of shock in children. Signs of dehydration include weight loss, irritability, absence of tears, dry mucous membranes, sunken fontanelles, and dry skin. Signs of shock include tachycardia, diminished peripheral pulses, oliguria, irritability or lethargy, and acidosis. Rapid volume replacement is necessary to prevent cardiovascular collapse.

REFERENCE

Chameides, L., & Hazinski, M.F. (1994). *Textbook of pediatric advanced life support.* Dallas: American Heart Association.

4. Answer (**a**). Enteral feeding is not appropriate for critically ill infants or children who have persistent or unresolved diar-

rhea. Parenteral feedings would be the best alternative for providing adequate nutritional therapy. It is also important to provide a pacifier for non-nutritive sucking. In the stressed infant or toddler, sucking a thumb or pacifier may provide important comfort.

REFERENCE

Gaedeke Norris, M.K., & Steinhorn, D.M. (1994). Nutritional management during critical illness in infants and children. *AACN Clinical Issues in Critical Care Nursing, 5* (4), 485–494.

5. Answer (**b**). The peripheral route is used to meet short-term nutritional needs without high nutritional requirements. However, this route is restricted to 10% to 12.5% dextrose and 2% amino acid solutions.

REFERENCE

Verger, J. (1996). Nutrition. In M.A.Q. Curley, J.B. Smith, & P.A. Moloney-Harmon (Eds.). *Critical care nursing of infants and children* (pp. 410–448). Philadelphia: W.B. Saunders.

6. Answer (**a**). Excessive delivery of dextrose in infants and children is associated with hepatic steatosis, hypercapnia, and hypokalemia because of intravascular shifting of electrolytes. Neonates are very susceptible to the intraventricular hemorrhage resulting from the administration of excessive amounts of glucose.

REFERENCE

Gaedeke Norris, M.K., & Steinhorn, D. (1994). Nutritional management during critical illness in infants and children. *AACN Clinical Issues in Critical Care Nursing, 5* (4), 457–470.

7. Answer (**c**). Excessive fat infusion can be associated with compromised immune function, hypertriglyceridemia, and platelet dysfunction. Metabolism of fat results in less carbon dioxide production than carbohydrate metabolism, which can be a definite advantage for patients with pulmonary dysfunction.

REFERENCE

Gaedeke Norris, M.K., & Steinhorn, D. (1994). Nutritional management during critical illness in infants and children. *AACN Clinical Issues in Critical Care Nursing, 5* (4).

8. Answer (**b**). Daily electrolyte requirements are affected by renal dysfunction. Sodium, potassium, magnesium, and phosphorus should all be decreased.

REFERENCE

Zaloga, G., & Ackerman, M. (1994). A review of disease-specific formulas. *AACN Clinical Issues in Critical Care Nursing, 5* (4), 421–435.

CHAPTER *23*

Thermoregulation

CATHY HAUT, RN, MS, CCRN

CASE 23-1

L., a 3-year-old girl, is brought into the emergency department after a near-drowning incident. She wandered through an open backyard gate and fell through the cover of the family's in-ground swimming pool. Within about 10 minutes, L.'s mother noticed she was missing from the backyard. L. was removed from the cold water, and emergency help arrived. L. was unconscious, very cold, and wet. On-site assessment revealed a heart rate of 30 beats per minute (bpm), no respiratory effort, and a blood pressure of 80/42 mmHg.

1. Based on this assessment, what is the first priority in providing emergency care for L.?
   a. Remove the wet clothing and cover with warm blankets.
   b. Establish an airway and begin ventilation.
   c. Obtain a rectal temperature.
   d. Transport L. to the emergency room.

Artificial ventilation was begun, and L.'s wet clothing was removed at the site. A peripheral infusion of lactated Ringer's solution was initiated, and L. was then transported to the emergency room. On arrival in the emergency room, L. is covered with warm blankets, and ventilation is continued with a heated humidity circuit. A rectal thermometer reveals a temperature of 33°C.

2. L.'s primary mechanism of heat loss in cold water submersion is through
   a. Conduction.
   b. Convection.
   c. Radiation.
   d. Evaporation.

3. L.'s potential neurologic outcome, based on the clinical picture, is considered
   a. Very poor, because of the length of hypoxia during submersion.
   b. Poor, based on negative respiratory effort and the need for artificial ventilation.
   c. Good, based on the cool temperature of the water, in which vasoconstriction occurs but cerebral blood flow is maintained.
   d. Good, based on adequate circulation as evidenced by heart rate and blood pressure.

4. Mild hypothermia, as in L.'s case often manifests with
   a. Tachypnea, tachycardia, and irritability.
   b. Tachypnea, tachycardia, and lethargy.
   c. Bradycardia, bradypnea, and lethargy.
   d. Ventricular fibrillation, hypotension, and coma.

L. is stabilized quickly in the emergency room. One hour later, her heart rate is 120 bpm, and her blood pressure is

96/54 mmHg. She remains intubated and ventilated. Her rectal temperature is 34°C. She is transported to the pediatric intensive care unit (PICU), where she remains covered with warm blankets. An overbed warming light is used to continue the warming process.

5. On admission to the PICU, what intervention is a first priority for L.?
   a. Computed tomography (CT) scan of the head.
   b. Initiation of a radial arterial line with continuous blood pressure monitoring.
   c. Initiation of core temperature monitoring.
   d. Chest x-ray film to determine fluid infiltrates.

6. Continuous cardiac monitoring is another priority for the patient who is hypothermic as a result of cold water submersion because of the
   a. Cardiac ischemia related to vasodilatation during submersion.
   b. Potential for development of complete heart block.
   c. Potential for life-threatening arrhythmias, including ventricular fibrillation and asystole.
   d. Potential for congestive heart failure related to fluid aspiration.

During the rewarming process, L. begins to shiver and awakens. However, she remains lethargic. On synchronized intermittent mandatory ventilation (SIMV), her respiratory rate is 62 breaths per minute. L. has a peripheral arterial line inserted.

7. The nurse can anticipate the following intervention as the next priority:
   a. Chest x-ray film to assess tachypnea.
   b. Arterial blood gas and serum electrolyte determinations.
   c. CT scan of the head to assess edema.
   d. Liver function tests.

8. Early assessment for shivering includes
   a. Inspection for raised areas on the skin surface called fasciculations.
   b. Palpation of the mandible and close inspection of the neck and chest muscles.
   c. Inspection for "shaking" of the trunk and long muscle groups.
   d. Palpation of the long muscle groups and trunk for generalized tremors.

9. Shivering is a mechanism used by the body to increase temperature through
   a. Inhibition of the primary motor center located in the posterior hypothalamus.
   b. Stimulation of the primary motor center located in the hypothalamus.
   c. Increasing muscle tone and irritability initiated by the cortex.
   d. Stimulation of thermogenesis.

Blood is drawn from L.'s peripheral arterial line for laboratory tests. The arterial blood gas determinations include the hydrogen ion concentration (pH), bicarbonate (HCO_3^-) level, and the partial pressures of oxygen (Po_2) and carbon dioxide (Pco_2):

$$pH: 7.52 \qquad Po_2: 156 \text{ mmHg}$$
$$HCO_3^-: 30 \text{ mEq/L} \quad Pco_2: 28 \text{ mmHg}$$

Levels also are determined for sodium (Na^+), potassium (K^+), chloride (Cl^-), carbon dioxide (CO_2), and glucose (Glu):

$$Na^+: 130 \text{ mEq/L} \qquad CO_2: 45 \text{ mEq/L}$$
$$K^+: 5.2 \text{ mEq/L} \qquad Glu: 158 \text{ mg/dL}$$
$$Cl^-: 98 \text{ mEq/L}$$

Ventilator settings are adjusted, and a Foley catheter is inserted.

10. Expected urine output in a child who experiences a submersion injury is
    a. Excessive or "cold diuresis" as the renal response to hypothermia.
    b. Diminished as a result of the hypothermic effect on renal tubular absorption of water.
    c. Diminished because of decreased blood flow to vital organs.
    d. Initially diminished and then adequate as body temperature begins to regulate.

11. Anticipated alteration in electrolytes during hypothermia include
    a. Increased glucose, increased blood urea nitrogen (BUN), and creatinine.
    b. Decreased glucose, decreased K^+, and Na^+.
    c. Increased or decreased glucose, increased K^+, and decreased Na^+.
    d. Increased BUN and creatinine, decreased K^+, and Na^+.

On day 3, L. is weaned from mechanical ventilation but continues to require 40% oxygen by mask. She is awake and responsive, although still somewhat lethargic. Her temperature has stabilized, and electrolyte levels are also stable. A recent chest x-ray film indicates a left lower lobe infiltrate.

12. L.'s clinical status probably indicates
    a. Aspiration pneumonia caused by prolonged hypothermia and hypoxia during the submersion.
    b. Pneumonia due to bronchorrhea and intrapulmonary leukocytosis associated with hypothermia and the aspiration of contaminated water.
    c. Lower respiratory tract contamination by water, with decreased metabolic rate and resulting stasis caused by hypothermia.
    d. Aspiration of contaminated water, necessitating prolonged mechanical ventilation.

L. is treated with intravenous antibiotics and is weaned to room air by day 5. She is transferred to a regular pediatric unit to continue her course of therapy and plan for discharge.

CASE 23-2

J., a 6-week-old boy, was born at term by spontaneous vaginal delivery and weighed 4130 g. J.'s mother's cervical culture was positive for group B streptococcus before delivery. A complete blood count and cultures of blood drawn from J. 2 hours after birth were negative for infection.

J.'s parents brought him to the emergency room with complaints of lethargy, poor feeding, and fever during the past 3 days. On examination, J.'s extremities are very cool to touch, and his axillary temperature is 35.2°C. His extremities are flaccid, and petechiae are present over his trunk area. His anterior fontanelle is full and bulging. He has a heart rate of 195 bpm, blood pressure of 60/25 mmHg, and respiratory rate of 68 breaths per minute, with shallow breathing.

1. Based on the history and emergency room presentation, the nurse suspects J. has
   a. Cold septic shock.
   b. Warm septic shock.
   c. Hemorrhagic shock.
   d. Hypovolemic shock.

2. After J.'s respiratory status is stable, his treatment plan should follow what sequence?
   a. Obtain blood cultures and a lumbar

puncture, administer intravenous antibiotics, and transfer to the PICU.
   b. Transfer quickly to the PICU, obtain blood cultures and a lumbar puncture, and administer antibiotics.
   c. Administer intravenous fluids; obtain blood cultures, a complete blood count, and a lumbar puncture; administer intravenous antibiotics; use a warming bed; and transfer to the PICU.
   d. Transfer quickly to PICU, place on warming bed, administer intravenous antibiotics, and obtain blood cultures, a complete blood count, and a lumbar puncture.

J.'s preliminary diagnosis is group B streptococcus meningitis and septic shock. He is tachypneic and tachycardiac, and he appears very pale. His extremities remain cool to touch, and his temperature remains subnormal. After a sepsis workup and administration of antibiotics, he is transferred to the PICU. He is placed on a radiant warmer bed with servocontrol temperature regulation. A radial arterial line is inserted.

3. To support thermoregulation, admission to the PICU for J. should include
   a. Placement of arterial line.
   b. Use of a heating light or radiant warming bed to provide heat.
   c. Measurement of serum glucose levels.
   d. Tightly swaddling and covering the infant with blanket layers.

4. An infant's response to cold stress depends on
   a. Shivering, which is initiated in the hypothalamus.
   b. Nonshivering or chemical thermogenesis, using brown fat stores.
   c. Thermogenesis resulting from glycolysis to provide energy.
   d. A decreased metabolic rate and shivering thermogenesis.

5. The most serious source of heat loss in infants is through
   a. Convection.
   b. Conduction.
   c. Radiation.
   d. Evaporation.

6. J.'s tachypnea could contribute to further heat loss through
   a. Radiative losses from the pulmonary system.

b. Presence of environmental humidity.
c. Evaporative losses through the pulmonary tract.
d. Presence of a lower room temperature.

J. is treated with penicillin and ceftriaxone. After an initial fluid bolus without a response in blood pressure, a dopamine drip is initiated. J. is receiving oxygen by mask. Within 12 hours of PICU admission, J.'s rectal temperature climbs to 39.4°C. His color is flushed, and his heart rate remains elevated. His hands and feet remain cool to touch. He has an episode of apnea.

7. To support J.'s temperature regulation, the first nursing intervention should be to
   a. Turn off the radiant warmer bed.
   b. Check a temperature using the tympanic thermometer.
   c. Check placement of the warmer temperature probe.
   d. Administer a fluid bolus of 10 to 20 mL/kg.

8. If J.'s temperature remains elevated without an external heat source, treatment of the hyperthermia should include
   a. Antipyretics, continuation of antibiotics, and tepid sponge baths.
   b. Antipyretics only.
   c. Antipyretics, continuation of antibiotics, and alcohol and cold water baths.
   d. Antipyretics, continuation of antibiotics, and ice water sponge baths.

9. A significant point regarding fever is that
   a. Fever is considered a type of hyperthermia in which body temperatures increase to greater than 37.8°C orally or 38.8°C rectally.
   b. Fever is a symptom, not a disease entity, for which an underlying causative factor must be considered.
   c. Fever is an elevation of the body's "set point."
   d. Treating the fever is just as important as treating the underlying cause.

10. Which facts should be considered in selecting the type of thermometer and mode of temperature assessment for J.?
    a. Consistency and safety.
    b. Accuracy, consistency, and safety.
    c. Choice of electronic or tympanic over mercury thermometer.

d. Combination of techniques based on accuracy and safety.

J.'s warmer is found to be working accurately and is turned off. He is treated with Tylenol suppositories and continues on antibiotics. His temperature remains unstable for the next 24 hours. Glucose values are also unstable as measured by bedside glucose monitoring, dropping to less than 40 mg/dL twice in same period. J. continues to have episodes of apnea, consequently requiring intubation and an increased fraction of inspired oxygen (F_{IO_2}).

11. An explanation for J.'s unstable glucose level and increasing need for O_2 is
    a. The process of thermogenesis in the infant requires oxygen consumption and calorie or glucose expenditure for energy.
    b. The process of shivering requires oxygen consumption and glycogenolysis.
    c. Brown fat metabolism depends entirely on the presence of glucose.
    d. Temperature regulation is controlled by the hypothalamus and is triggered by a decrease in circulating oxygen.

On day 4 of PICU hospitalization, J.'s status begins to stabilize. His axillary temperature ranges from 36.8°C to 37.2°C without heating or cooling interventions. He still requires mechanical ventilation but is beginning to wean and continues on a full course of antibiotics.

CASE 23-3

R., a 10-month-old boy, has just had cardiac surgery for aortic stenosis. He is transferred from the operating room to the PICU for recovery and monitoring. He is intubated and ventilated. A Swan-Ganz catheter is in place to measure pulmonary artery pressures and central temperature. R. has a heart rate of 128 bpm, respiratory rate of 30 breaths per minute, core temperature of 35.4°C, end-tidal CO_2 of 48, and blood pressure of 110/56 mmHg. Pulmonary artery pressures include a systolic pressure of 28 mmHg, diastolic pressure of 8 mmHg, and wedge pressure of 10 mmHg.

1. Measuring the core temperature and peripheral temperature assists in determining
   a. Metabolic dysfunction.

   b. The difference between temperature taking methods.

   c. Compromised cardiac output.

   d. Pulmonary insufficiency.

2. Factors that contribute to hypothermia in the postoperative cardiac patient include which of the following?

   a. Length of the procedure and the environmental temperature of the operating room.

   b. Use of muscle paralytics during anesthesia, environmental temperature of the operating room, and exposure of the thoracic cavity.

   c. Weight of the patient, preoperative temperature stability, and exposure of the thoracic cavity during procedure.

   d. Environmental temperature of the operating room, cardiopulmonary bypass process, and the use of warm humidification with ventilation.

3. A basic nursing intervention for maintaining a stable thermal zone for R. is

   a. Using a blood warmer to administer intravenous fluids.

   b. Maintaining dry linens and keeping the patient covered consistently.

   c. Increasing the heat in the humidity circuit of the ventilator.

   d. Continuous use of a heating pad placed under the patient.

4. Anesthesia can contribute to hypothermia by

   a. Causing muscle paralysis, which prevents shivering and depression of the hypothalamic thermoregulatory center.

   b. Causing general vasoconstriction and muscle paralysis, preventing shivering.

   c. Causing vasodilation and an increase in metabolic rate, reducing heat production.

   d. Obliterating muscle activity, preventing shivering and stimulation of the hypothalamic thermoregulatory center.

An overbed warmer is used to assist in providing heat for R. postoperatively. He is also covered lightly, and linens are kept dry. Arterial blood gas and electrolyte values are obtained. Paralysis is beginning to diminish, but R. remains sedated and on 100% oxygen.

5. In addition to temperature measurement, it is most important to monitor which parameter for the infant receiving heat by a warmer bed or light?

   a. Pulse oximeter readings.

   b. Intake and output.

   c. Blood pressure.

   d. Pulse and respirations.

6. Based on the admission assessment of hypothermia, the nurse can expect the arterial blood gas results to reflect

   a. Metabolic alkalosis and respiratory acidosis.

   b. Metabolic acidosis and respiratory alkalosis.

   c. Normal pH and HCO_3^- levels.

   d. Metabolic acidosis alone.

7. An infant has a much greater capacity to lose heat than an older child because of

   a. Immature hypothalamic function.

   b. Large body surface area in relation to weight.

   c. Increased metabolism of glucose and calories.

   d. Ability to metabolize brown fat to heat production.

Reviewing R.'s history from his chart, the nurse finds that R.'s father has muscular dystrophy. The anesthesiologist has documented an interview with R.'s family regarding past surgical experiences and responses to anesthesia. R. has received succinylcholine and inhalation anesthesia for his cardiac procedure.

8. Concern about the development of malignant hyperthermia in this infant derives from the

   a. Combination use of local anesthetics and MAO inhibitors.

   b. Combination use of succinylcholine and inhalation anesthetics.

   c. Temperature elevation resulting from traumatized body tissue.

   d. Induction of anesthesia with inhalation agents.

9. Signs and symptoms of malignant hyperthermia include

   a. Tachycardia, tachypnea, and combined respiratory and metabolic acidosis.

   b. Slow increase in temperature, tachycardia, tachypnea, and metabolic acidosis.

   c. Excessive temperature, bradycardia, and increase in P_{CO_2}.

   d. Sudden increase in temperature,

tachycardia, and respiratory alkalosis.

10. Dantrolene treatment for suspected malignant hyperthermia is administered intravenously and is considered

   a. An anesthesia reversal agent that diminishes the muscle relaxant qualities of succinylcholine.

   b. A calcium stimulant useful for increasing myoplasmic calcium ions.

   c. A calcium antagonist useful for stimulating muscle contraction.

   d. A skeletal muscle relaxant that prevents the release of calcium from storage sites in muscle tissue.

As R. begins to move and awaken, his heart rate and respirations increase. He grimaces and frowns. His rectal temperature increases to 36.2°C, and analgesics are administered in the form of a fentanyl drip and intravenous morphine given as needed for pain management. He progresses rapidly and is transferred to the floor 5 days later.

ANSWERS ■ CASE 23-1

1. Answer (**b**). The first priority for the victim of a submersion injury is establishing an airway and initiating ventilation. Inadequate cardiopulmonary function prevents effective treatment of other organ systems, including the central nervous system. Any resuscitative effort includes airway and breathing as first priorities.

REFERENCES

Christensen, D.W., Dean, J.M., & Setzer, N.A. (1992). Near drowning. In M. Rogers (Ed.). *Textbook of pediatric intensive care* (2nd ed., pp. 877–901). Baltimore: Williams & Wilkins.
Corneli, H.M. (1992). Accidental hypothermia. *The Journal of Pediatrics,* 120 (5), 672–673.
Schleien, C.L., & Nichols, D.G. (1991). Environmental injuries. In D.G. Nichols, et al. (Eds.). *Golden hour: The handbook of advanced pediatric life support* (pp. 258–260). St. Louis: Mosby–Year Book.

2. Answer (**a**). Conduction is the primary mechanism of heat loss in cold water submersion. Conduction, the transfer of heat by direct contact with a stationary medium, is a common mode of heat loss. Conduction of heat in water is 24 times faster than in air, and hypothermia therefore occurs at a rapid rate in cold water.

REFERENCES

Corneli, H.M. (1992). Accidental hypothermia. *The Journal of Pediatrics,* 120 (5), 672–673.
Engler, A., & Rushton, C. (1996). Thermal regulation. In M.A.Q. Curley, J.B. Smith, & P.A. Moloney-Harmon (Eds.). *Critical care nursing of infants and children* (pp. 449–467). Philadelphia: W.B. Saunders.
Schleien, C.L., & Nichols, D.G. (1991). Environmental injuries. In D.G. Nichols, et al. (Eds.). *Golden hour: The handbook of advanced pediatric life support* (pp. 254–260). St. Louis: Mosby–Year Book.

3. Answer (**c**). Potential neurologic outcome is considered relatively good for cold water submersion victims. Children, because of their greater body surface area and decreased subcutaneous fat, are susceptible to the rapid cooling and preserved circulation that results in a protective effect. The "diving reflex" associated with respiratory cessation and decreased heart rate results in a normalized blood pressure. This effect increases blood flow to heart and brain, protecting these organs. Hypothermia, defined as a core temperature less than 35°C, causes generalized vasoconstriction in peripheral tissues, which assists this process.

REFERENCES

Christensen, D.W., Dean, J.M., & Setzer, N.A., (1992). Near drowning. In M. Rogers (Ed.). *Textbook of pediatric intensive care* (2nd ed., pp. 877–901). Baltimore: Williams & Wilkins.
Quan, L., Wentz, K.R., Gore, E.J., & Copass, M.K. (1990). Outcome and predictors of outcome in pediatric submersion victims receiving prehospital care in King County, Washington. *Pediatrics,* 86, 587–591.

4. Answer (**b**). Mild hypothermia, defined as a core temperatures of 32°C to 35°C, often manifests with symptoms of tachycardia, tachypnea, and lethargy, as well as incoordination, slurred speech, and polyuria.

REFERENCE

Shleien, C.L., & Nichols, D.G. (1991). Environmental injuries. In D.G. Nichols, et al. (Eds.). *Golden hour: The handbook of advanced pediatric intensive care* (pp. 252–260). St. Louis: Mosby–Year Book.

5. Answer (**c**). On admission to the PICU, core temperature monitoring should be included as a first priority for the hypothermic patient. Core or central temperature reflects the temperature of the blood flowing through the arterial system to the hypothalamus. Core measurements, compared with a regional or peripheral temperature, provide an accurate indication of body temperature.

Core temperature may decline before rewarming begins, because many factors affect temperature regulation. It is imperative to measure core temperature continuously, because rapid rewarming ($>1°C$/hour) can result in circulatory failure and death.

REFERENCES
Corneli, H.M. (1992). Accidental hypothermia. *The Journal of Pediatrics,* 120 (5), 671–674.
Engler, A., & Rushton, C. (1996). Thermal regulation. In M.A.Q. Curley, J.B. Smith, & P.A. Moloney-Harmon (Eds.). *Critical care nursing of infants and children* (pp. 449–467). Philadelphia: W.B. Saunders.
Witte, M.K. (1990). Near drowning. In J.L. Blumer (Ed.). *Textbook of pediatric intensive care* (3rd ed., pp. 315–316). St. Louis: Mosby–Year Book.

6. **Answer (c).** Continuous cardiac monitoring is a priority for the patient who is hypothermic as a result of cold water submersion because of the potential for life-threatening arrhythmias, including ventricular ectopy, fibrillation, and asystole. Arrhythmias result from depressed myocardial contractility and irritability caused by hypothermia.

REFERENCES
Elder, P.T. (1989). Accidental hypothermia. In W.C. Shoemaker, et al. (Eds.). *Textbook of critical care* (2nd ed., pp. 101–109). Philadelphia: W.B. Saunders.
Schleien, C.L., & Nichols, D.G. (1991). Environmental injuries. In D.G. Nichols, et al. (Eds.). *Golden hour: The handbook of advanced pediatric life support* (pp. 255–257). St. Louis: Mosby–Year Book.

7. **Answer (b).** Monitoring blood gas values and serum electrolytes is important during the rewarming process. Even though aspiration of fluid may cause hemodilution with a resulting decrease in sodium and potassium levels, the primary concern is the unpredictability of these values. Hypoglycemia or hyperglycemia, hypokalemia or hyperkalemia, and alkalosis or acidosis may exist. The arterial blood gas results can assist in determining ventilation needs and indicating metabolic disturbances.

REFERENCES
Christensen, D.W., Dean, J.M., & Setzer, N.A. (1992). Near drowning. In M. Rogers (Ed.). *Textbook of pediatric intensive care* (2nd ed., pp. 877–901). Baltimore: Williams & Wilkins.
Corneli, H.M. (1992). Accidental hypothermia. *The Journal of Pediatrics,* 120 (5), 671–674.
Schleien, C.L., & Nichols, D.G. (1991). Environmental injuries. In D.G. Nichols, et al. (Eds.). *Golden hour: The handbook of advanced pediatric life support* (pp. 257–259). St. Louis: Mosby–Year Book.

8. **Answer (b).** Early assessment for shivering includes palpation of the mandible and close inspection of the facial, neck, and chest muscles. Shivering, a mechanism for heat production, develops in a predictable fashion, beginning with small muscle group contractions, proceeding with contractions of the trunk and long muscle groups, and culminating with generalized body shaking and teeth chattering. Assessment for shivering continues until central and peripheral temperatures are normal.

REFERENCE
Engler, A., & Rushton, C. (1996). Thermal regulation. In M.A.Q. Curley, J.B. Smith, & P. A. Moloney-Harmon (Eds.). *Critical care nursing of infants and children* (pp. 449–467). Philadelphia: W.B. Saunders.

9. **Answer (b).** When body temperature falls below 37°C, the primary motor center located in the posterior hypothalamus is stimulated to initiate shivering. When muscle tone increases and shivering begins, heat production can increase four to five times the normal amount.

REFERENCE
Engler, A., & Rushton, C. (1996). Thermal regulation. In M.A.Q. Curley, J.B. Smith, & P.A. Moloney-Harmon (Eds.). *Critical care nursing of infants and children* (pp. 449–467). Philadelphia: W.B. Saunders.

10. **Answer (a).** Urine output in a child who experiences hypothermia as a result of submersion injury is usually excessive. The renal response, a "cold diuresis," results partially from decreased tubular reabsorption in the kidneys. Decreased production of the antidiuretic hormone also results from the early phase of vasoconstriction, which senses an increased blood volume.

REFERENCES
Corneli, H.M. (1992). Accidental hypothermia. *The Journal of Pediatrics,* 120 (5), 672–673.
Schleien, C.L., & Nichols, D.G. (1991). Environmental injuries. In D.G. Nichols, et al. (Eds.). *Golden hour: The handbook of advanced pediatric life support* (pp. 257–259). St. Louis: Mosby–Year Book.

11. **Answer (c).** Anticipated alteration in electrolytes during hypothermia includes increased or decreased glucose levels, increased potassium levels, and decreased sodium levels. Glucose metabolism is unpredictable in hypothermia. In some instances, hypoglycemia may cause hypothermia related to a slow-

down in metabolism. Decreased sodium levels result from diuresis and decreased tubular reabsorption of water, as well as dilution resulting from submersion. Decreased production of antidiuretic hormone also allows the loss of free water and sodium. Elevated potassium levels result from acidosis, a condition in which intracellular potassium moves to the extracellular spaces.

REFERENCES

Corneli, H.M. (1992). Accidental hypothermia. *The Journal of Pediatrics,* 120 (5), 671–677.

Schleien, C.L., & Nichols, D.G. (1991). Environmental injuries. In D.G. Nichols, et al. (Eds.). *Golden hour: The handbook of advanced pediatric life support* (pp. 257–260). St. Louis: Mosby–Year Book.

12. Answer (**b**). New infiltrates recognized on the x-ray film after the acute submersion experience often indicate pulmonary infection. The pattern results from bronchorrhea and intrapulmonary leukostasis associated with hypothermia and aspirated contaminated water.

REFERENCES

Corneli, H.M. (1992). Accidental hypothermia. *The Journal of Pediatrics,* 120 (5), 674–677.

Witte, M.K. (1990). Near drowning. In J.L. Blumer (Ed.). *A practical guide to pediatric intensive care* (3rd ed., pp. 314–315). St. Louis: Mosby–Year Book.

ANSWERS ■ CASE 23-2

1. Answer (**a**). Symptoms of septic shock include temperature instability, tachycardia, tachypnea, and a widened pulse pressure. "Warm" and "cold" septic shock are terms used to identify phases of distributive shock, a condition resulting in maldistribution of blood volume caused by circulating bacteria. Cold septic shock occurs when the extremities are cold and "clamped down" or vasoconstricted. The blood pressure is usually low, and perfusion is poor. Warm septic shock refers to the symptoms of fever and warm extremities. It is not unusual for a child to move between warm and cold shock states.

REFERENCES

Berro, E.A., & Bechler-Karsh, A. (1993). A closer look at septic shock. *Pediatric Nursing,* 19 (3), 289–297.

Wetzel, R.C. (1991). Shock. In D.G. Nichols, et al. (Eds.). *Golden hour: The handbook of advanced pediatric life support* (pp. 97–100). St. Louis: Mosby–Year Book.

2. Answer (**c**). After respiratory stability is established, it is most important to treat sepsis symptomatically. This is accomplished by providing fluids and volume expansion; obtaining cultures, a complete blood count, and lumbar puncture for diagnostic purposes; and administering antibiotics as quickly as possible. Management of hypothermia in this case should include warming, because infants have a large body surface area to weight ratio and no shivering mechanism. Thermoregulation uses glucose and oxygen supplies to provide energy for heat production.

REFERENCES

Goldfarb, J. (1990). Infections of the central nervous system. In J.L. Blumer (Ed.). *A practical guide to pediatric intensive care* (3rd ed., pp. 463–467). St. Louis: Mosby–Year Book.

Lott, J.W., Nelson, K., Fahrner, R., & Kenner, C. (1993). Assessment and management of immunologic dysfunction. In C. Kenner, A. Brueggemeyer, & L.P. Gunderson (Eds.). *Comprehensive neonatal nursing: A physiologic perspective* (pp. 573–575). Philadelphia: W.B. Saunders.

3. Answer (**b**). Techniques to support thermoregulation for an infant include the use of heat lamps, warming bed, and circulating water mattresses. It is also important to provide a warming device for any type of transport either within or outside of the hospital.

REFERENCES

Brueggemeyer, A. (1993). Neonatal thermoregulation. In C. Kenner, A. Brueggemeyer, & L.P. Gunderson (Eds.). *Comprehensive neonatal nursing: A physiologic perspective* (pp. 255–259). Philadelphia: W.B. Saunders.

Engler, A., & Rushton, C. (1996). Thermal regulation. In M.A.Q. Curley, J.B. Smith, & P.A. Moloney-Harmon (Eds.). *Critical care nursing of infants and children* (pp. 449–467). Philadelphia: W.B. Saunders.

4. Answer (**b**). An infant's response to cold stress depends on nonshivering or chemical thermogenesis. This response involves the use of brown fat stores, along with some voluntary muscle activity such as positioning to conserve heat loss. Thermogenesis involves a chemical reaction within brown fat, which contains triglycerides. The triglycerides are broken down into fatty acids by the release of noradrenaline. The fatty acids are oxidized, resulting in the production of heat. Thermogenesis is a limited process, because it increases the consumption of oxygen and glucose.

REFERENCES

Brueggemeyer, A. (1993). Neonatal thermoregulation. In C. Kenner, A. Brueggemeyer, & L.P. Gunderson (Eds.). *Comprehensive neonatal nursing: A physiologic perspective* (pp. 249–252). Philadelphia: W.B. Saunders.

Williams, J.K., & Lancaster, J. (1976). Thermoregulation of the newborn. *Maternal-Child Nursing,* Nov.–Dec., 355–358.

5. Answer (c). The most significant source of heat loss in infants is through radiation. Radiation involves the transfer of heat between two objects in a nonparticulate means independent of environmental temperature. Crib or warmer bed walls and any unwarmed objects placed near the infant can serve as routes for heat loss from the infant. Any warm objects, such as a radiant warmer bed or a heating pad, can radiate heat to the infant.

REFERENCES

Brueggemeyer, A. (1993). Neonatal thermoregulation. In C. Kenner, A. Brueggemeyer, & L.P. Gunderson (Eds.). *Comprehensive neonatal nursing: A physiologic perspective* (pp. 250–258). Philadelphia: W.B. Saunders.

Engler, A., & Rushton, C. (1996). Thermal regulation. In M.A.Q. Curley, J.B. Smith, & P.A. Moloney-Harmon (Eds.). *Critical care nursing of infants and children* (pp. 449–467). Philadelphia: W.B. Saunders.

6. Answer (c). Tachypnea can contribute to further heat loss through evaporation from the pulmonary tract. Heat is lost during evaporation, which is the conversion of a liquid to a vapor. A rapid respiratory rate increases the movement of warm, moistened air, which is exhaled through breathing.

REFERENCE

Merenstain, G.B., Gardner, S.L., & Blake, W.W. (1989). Heat balance. In G.B. Merenstain & S. L. Gardner (Eds.). *Handbook of neonatal intensive care* (pp. 88–102). St. Louis: Mosby–Year Book.

7. Answer (c). A priority nursing intervention in assessing the degree of hyperthermia and supporting infant thermoregulation is to ensure the accuracy of equipment. This is accomplished by checking the servocontrol temperature probe attached to the infant, followed by turning off the heat source or warmer as the infant's temperature warrants.

REFERENCE

Brueggemeyer, A. (1993). Neonatal thermoregulation. In C. Kenner, A. Brueggemeyer, & L.P. Gunderson (Eds.). *Comprehensive neonatal nursing: A physiologic perspective* (pp. 250–258). Philadelphia: W.B. Saunders.

8. Answer (a). Treatment of hyperthermia should include the use of antipyretics, antibiotics if the fever is considered to be sepsis related, and external cooling such as tepid sponge baths. Acetaminophen is relatively free of side effects and appears to be the pharmacologic choice for fever reduction. In addition to reducing the body temperature, antipyretics are used to readjust the hypothalamic set point, the temperature around which body temperature is regulated. Fever is an elevation of the set point, so that body temperature is regulated at a higher level. Sponge bathing with tepid water, a useful adjunct for fever reduction, alone is not effective in reducing the set point. The use of alcohol or cold water sponging is prohibitive, because it induces vasoconstriction and shivering and promotes heat retention.

REFERENCES

Allen, E. (1990). Abnormalities in temperature regulation. In J.L. Blumer (Ed.). *A practical guide to pediatric intensive care* (3rd ed., pp. 126–128). St. Louis: Mosby–Year Book.

Engler, A., & Rushton, C. (1996). Thermal regulation. In M.A.Q. Curley, J.B. Smith, & P.A. Moloney-Harmon (Eds.). *Critical care nursing of infants and children* (pp. 449–467). Philadelphia: W.B. Saunders.

Holter-Gildea, J. (1992). When fever becomes an enemy. *Pediatric Nursing,* 18 (2), 165–167.

9. Answer (b). Fever is a symptom, not a disease entity. Identifying the cause of fever mandates a systematic assessment involving physical data, laboratory analysis (including viral and bacterial blood cultures), urine and cerebrospinal fluid examinations, serum electrolytes and a complete blood count, and other diagnostic studies such as radiographs, ultrasound, CT scans, and magnetic resonance imaging. Treatment must take into account the potential outcome of the hyperthermia, such as febrile seizures and the oxygen and energy consumption associated with shivering and chills.

REFERENCES

Engler, A., & Rushton, C. (1996). Thermal regulation. In M.A.Q. Curley, J.B. Smith, & P.A. Moloney-Harmon (Eds.). *Critical care nursing of infants and children* (pp. 449–467). Philadelphia: W.B. Saunders.

Kluger, M.J. (1992). Fever revisited. *Pediatrics,* 90 (6), 846–850.

10. Answer (d). In selecting the type of thermometer and mode of temperature assessment, it is most advantageous to use a combination of techniques, based on safety and accuracy. Speed and convenience also play a part in decision making. Other important factors related to temperature assessment include the disease process and presence of hypothermia or hyperthermia. Any condition that causes vasoconstriction and decreased skin blood flow, such as shock or hypothermia, can cause inaccurate skin and axillary measurements. It is important to recognize the value of using core monitoring instead of peripheral assessment. Continuous temperature monitoring is helpful when using a servomechanism warming device for patients with pre-existing hypothermia or hyperthermia or patients with the potential for temperature instability. If temperature differences do occur, peripheral and core temperatures can be monitored at the same time.

REFERENCE
Thomas, K., & Morriss, F.C. (1990). Temperature sensing devices. In D.L. Levin & F.C. Morriss (Eds.). *Essentials of pediatric intensive care* (pp. 783–785). St. Louis: Mosby–Year Book.

11. Answer (**a**). The process of thermoregulation in the infant requires oxygen consumption and calorie or glucose expenditure. To maintain core temperature, infants may deplete glycogen stores. Oxygen consumption rises 10% to 12% in response to a rise in temperature of 1°C, especially in an already compromised patient. Tachycardia resulting from hyperthermia also can compromise cardiac function and increase the need for oxygen. Infants lose heat quickly as a result of sweating because of the surface area to weight ratio, predisposing them to continued temperature instability.

REFERENCES
Allen, E. (1990). Abnormalities in temperature regulation. In J. L. Blumer (Ed.). *A practical guide to pediatric intensive care* (3rd ed., pp. 126–128). St. Louis: Mosby–Year Book.
Engler, A., & Rushton, C. (1996). Thermal regulation. In M.A.Q. Curley, J.B. Smith, & P.A. Moloney-Harmon (Eds.). *Critical care nursing of infants and children* (pp. 449–467). Philadelphia: W.B. Saunders.

ANSWERS ■ CASE 23-3

1. Answer (**c**). Measuring the core temperature and central temperature assists in determining peripheral perfusion. A difference of greater than 2°C between peripheral and core temperatures is associated with severely compromised cardiac output. Blood supply to peripheral areas is regulated by arterioles in the cutaneous vascular plexus. Circulation to these areas depends on sufficient cardiac output. In the event of poor perfusion related to cardiac failure, regulation of vasoconstriction or vasodilation in response to the delivery of core temperature blood to the periphery is impeded, and the peripheral temperature cannot be adequately assessed.

REFERENCES
Brink, L.W. (1990). Abnormalities in temperature regulation. In D.L. Levine & F.C. Morriss (Eds.). *Essentials of pediatric intensive care* (pp. 175–185). St. Louis: Mosby–Year Book.
Schlein, C.L., Setzer, N.A., McLaughlin, G.E, & Rogers, M.C. (1992). Postoperative management of the cardiac surgical patient. In M.C. Rogers (Ed.). *Textbook of pediatric intensive care* (2nd ed., pp. 467–531). Baltimore: Williams & Wilkins.

2. Answer (**b**). Factors that contribute to hypothermia in the postoperative cardiac patient include the use of muscle paralytics during anesthesia, which prevent the patient from using shivering or voluntary muscle movement to generate heat. Another factor is the environmental temperature of the operating room, which is generally lower and prone to cause radiant heat loss, especially in the infant. The open thoracic cavity also responds to radiant heat loss. A fourth factor contributing to heat loss is the cardiopulmonary bypass circuit. A temperature difference can result from cooling blood before its return to the body, which causes a lower core temperature.

REFERENCES
Engler, A., & Rushton, C. (1996). Thermal regulation. In M.A.Q. Curley, J.B. Smith, & P.A. Moloney-Harmon (Eds.). *Critical care nursing of infants and children* (pp. 449–467). Philadelphia: W.B. Saunders.
Schleien, C.L., Setzer, N.A., McLaughlin, G.E., & Rogers, M.C. (1992). Postoperative management of the cardiac surgical patient. In M.C. Rogers (Ed.). *Textbook of pediatric intensive care* (2nd ed., pp. 467–531). Baltimore: Williams & Wilkins.

3. Answer (**b**). A basic nursing intervention for maintaining a stable thermal zone in the postoperative patient is to use dry linens and to keep the patient covered consistently. These methods help to pre-

vent heat loss through conduction, evaporation, and convection.

REFERENCE

Harjo, J., & Jones, M.A. (1993). The surgical neonate. In C. Kenner, A. Brueggemeyer, & L.P. Gunderson (Eds.). *Comprehensive neonatal nursing: A physiologic perspective* (pp. 903–913). Philadelphia: W.B. Saunders.

4. Answer (a). Anesthesia can contribute to hypothermia through several mechanisms. The muscle paralysis prevents shivering, and depression of the hypothalamic thermoregulatory center causes vasodilation and a decreased metabolic rate, which reduce heat production and increase heat loss.

REFERENCE

Engler, A., & Rushton, C. (1995). Thermal regulation. In M.A.Q. Curley, J.B. Smith, & P.A. Moloney-Harmon (Eds.). *Critical care nursing of infants and children* (pp. 449–467). Philadelphia: W.B. Saunders.

5. Answer (b). An infant receiving heat through the use of a warmer bed or overbed heat light should have frequent temperature monitoring and intake and output monitoring to assist in determining fluid status. One of the disadvantages of the warmer bed is insensible water loss. An infant may need a 10% to 20% increase in maintenance fluid administration to account for this loss.

REFERENCES

Brueggemeyer, A. (1993). Neonatal thermoregulation. In C. Kenner, A. Brueggemeyer, & L.P. Gunderson (Eds.). *Comprehensive neonatal nursing: A physiologic perspective* (pp. 247–263). Philadelphia: W.B. Saunders.
Merenstain, G.B., Gardner, S.L., & Blake, W.W. (1989). Temperature regulation. In G.B. Merenstain & S.L. Gardner (Eds.). *Handbook of neonatal intensive care* (pp. 91–125). St. Louis: Mosby–Year Book.

6. Answer (b). Hypothermia can stimulate tachypnea secondary to increased oxygen consumption. This may produce respiratory alkalosis. Hypothermia can also cause metabolic acidosis related to the decreased metabolic rate and the increased production of carbon dioxide.

REFERENCES

Allen, E. (1990). Abnormalities in temperature regulation. In J.L. Blumer (Ed.). *A practical guide to pediatric intensive care* (3rd ed., pp. 126–135). St. Louis: Mosby–Year Book.
Engler, A., & Rushton, C. (1996). Thermal regulation. In M.A.Q. Curley, J.B. Smith, & P.A. Moloney-Harmon (Eds.). *Critical care nursing of infants and children* (pp. 449–467). Philadelphia: W.B. Saunders.

7. Answer (b). An infant or small child has a greater capacity to lose heat than an older child or adult because of the large body surface to mass ratio or body surface to weight relationship and because of decreased fat insulation.

REFERENCE

Corneli, H.M. (1992). Accidental hypothermia. *The Journal of Pediatrics,* 120 (3), 671–678.

8. Answer (b). Malignant hyperthermia is often triggered by the use of inhalation anesthetics and depolarizing neuromuscular blocking drugs, such as succinylcholine. Malignant hypertension does have an autosomal dominant mode of transmission in 50% of cases, and in about 3% of cases, there is associated myopathy in these families. Interviewing patients or parents before surgical procedures about previous sudden deaths of family members in the operating room assists in identifying patients at potential risk for developing malignant hyperthermia.

REFERENCES

Brandom, B.W. (1992). Malignant hyperthermia. In B.P. Fuhrman & J.J. Zimmerman (Eds.). *Pediatric critical care* (pp. 1281–1290). St. Louis: Mosby–Year Book.
Spagnuolo, S.E.T. (1990). Malignant hyperthermia. In J.L. Blumer (Ed.). *A practical guide to pediatric intensive care* (pp. 655–659). St. Louis: Mosby–Year Book.

9. Answer (a). Signs and symptoms of malignant hyperthermia include a rapid rise in body temperature, combined metabolic and respiratory acidosis, tachycardia, tachypnea, arrhythmias, muscular rigidity, hyperkalemia, and disseminating intravascular coagulopathy. The earliest signs of malignant hyperthermia after injection of succinylcholine include unexplained tachycardia, elevation in end-tidal CO_2, and premature ventricular contractions. Fever commonly is a later manifestation of malignant hyperthermia and may not occur at all if other symptoms are treated early.

REFERENCE

Spagnuolo, S.E.T. (1990). Malignant hyperthermia. In J.L. Blumer (Ed.). *A practical guide to pediatric intensive care* (pp. 655–659). St. Louis: Mosby–Year Book.

10. Answer (d). Dantrolene, a hydantoin derivative, is a skeletal muscle relaxant used in treating spastic muscle disorders. It prevents the release of calcium from storage sites in muscle tissue, and it can prevent the muscle contractions caused by massive calcium release into the muscle cell during a malignant hyperthermic crisis. Dantrolene should be given at an initial dose of 2 mg/kg body weight and infused rapidly. Subsequent doses are based on clinical symptoms, and it is often used prophylactically for at least 24 hours after an acute event. Sodium bicarbonate is often used as an immediate response to acidosis, and various methods are used to provide cooling for high fever in cases of malignant hyperthermia.

REFERENCES

Spagnuolo, S.E.T. (1990). Malignant hyperthermia. In J.L. Blumer (Ed.). *A practical guide to pediatric intensive care* (pp. 655–659). St. Louis: Mosby–Year Book.

Wlody, G.S. (1989). Malignant hyperthermia: Potential crisis in patient care. *AORN Journal,* 50 (2), 286–298.

CHAPTER 24

Skin Integrity

JANIECE MALONEY, RN, CETN
BETSY FISHER, RN, BSN, MA, CETN

CASE 24-1

J., an 18-month-old boy with a recent diagnosis of long-segment Hirschsprung's disease, is admitted for a colon resection and probable ascending colostomy. His abdomen is distended, his arms and legs are thin, and he is small in stature. His mother has attempted to manage his chronic constipation at home with diet, suppositories, and enemas. During preoperative teaching, J.'s mother appears anxious and overwhelmed.

Two days after the surgery, J.'s stoma appears pink and moist. The drainable pediatric pouch placed postoperatively frequently fills with dark green liquid stools.

1. In the postoperative period, the nurse should
   a. Call the physician to report the stoma color and frequent stooling.
   b. Send a stool sample for *Clostridium difficile* culture and ova and parasite analysis.
   c. Monitor stoma color and the pouch seal and record output.
   d. Check the medications to determine if there is a sensitivity.

After discussions with the mother, it is determined that the current drainable pediatric pouching system is appropriate for J. Postoperative teaching includes cutting the opening in the pouch 1/16 to 1/8 inch larger than the stoma, providing a normal diet for J.'s stage in growth and development, and

discussing normal stoma function and appearance, local ostomy suppliers, and signs of possible complications. After an uneventful hospital course, J. is discharged home.

J. returns to the pediatric clinic for routine follow-up. J.'s mother is unable to keep a pouch on J. for more than 8 hours. On close inspection, the nurse notices a circumferential area of red, weeping skin approximately 3/4 inch wide around the stoma.

2. The nurse discusses with J.'s mother that the skin appearance is indicative of
   a. Sensitivity to the backing on the pouch.
   b. Normal appearance of the peristomal skin.
   c. Infection of the peristomal skin.
   d. A pouch opening that is too large.

3. The nurse explains to J.'s mother that the best intervention at this time is to
   a. Obtain a culture so that appropriate medication can be ordered.
   b. Apply a pectin-methylcellulose powder and apply a new pouch with a smaller opening.
   c. Leave the area untouched, because the discoloration should disappear within 2 weeks.
   d. Leave the pouch off and expose the skin to air.

J.'s mother states that she thinks the colostomy is closing on its own, because she noticed small amounts of brown discoloration in the posterior portion of his diaper.

4. The nurse tells her that
  a. The brown discoloration is mucus, which is normal because his rectum is still intact.
  b. The pouch must have leaked into the diaper, and it should be changed.
  c. The doctor should be called, because J. may have developed a rectal fistula.
  d. The colostomy is closing on its own and further surgery may be required.

J. returns to the hospital for closure of the colostomy and re-anastomosis of the colon after 8 months. J. is now eating a normal diet for his age group. His abdomen is no longer distended, and he has gained muscle mass. He is having four to five soft unformed stools per day. Preoperative teaching is initiated by the primary nurse.

Postoperatively, J. progresses well; however, frequent loose stools cause his perianal area to become denuded. J. cries every time he stools or urinates. He also has developed a red rash with small pustules and widespread satellite lesions in his groin and perineal area.

5. These symptoms indicate
  a. A possible drug reaction.
  b. Sensitivity to the diaper.
  c. Yeast.
  d. Diaper rash.

6. The nurse should
  a. Apply an antacid to the denuded areas to alter the acid mantle and leave the diaper off to expose the buttocks to air.
  b. Apply an antifungal cream to the buttocks and groin, followed by a thick layer of zinc-based barrier cream.
  c. Use a blow dryer set on cool to assist in drying the perirectal area before applying a zinc-based barrier cream.
  d. Clean the area well, apply a cornstarch-based powder, and cover tightly with a diaper.

After appropriate treatment, J.'s rash and denuded perirectal area heals, and he is discharged.

CASE 24-2

L., a 17-year-old girl, is admitted with a history of flu-like symptoms and progressive weakness for several days. She is unable to move any extremities, and her breathing is shallow. A diagnosis of Guillain-Barré syndrome is made. L. has been bedridden for the past 5 days because of extreme weakness; as a result, her hydration and nutritional status are poor. Admission blood work reveals an albumin of 2.4 g/dL, white blood cell count of 14,300/mm^3, red blood cell count of 5.1 × 10^6/mm^3, hemoglobin 13 g/dL, and hematocrit 38%.

The arterial blood gas determinations for L. include hydrogen ion concentration (pH), partial pressures of oxygen (Po$_2$) and carbon dioxide (Pco$_2$), bicarbonate (HCO$_3^-$) level, and oxygen saturation (SaO$_2$):

pH: 7.29   HCO$_3^-$: 28 mEq/L
Po$_2$: 70 mmHg   SaO$_2$: 90%
Pco$_2$: 65 mmHg

During the initial assessment, the nurse discovers a large stage 3 sacral ulcer with soft grayish tissue and foul-smelling drainage. The ulcer is 3 × 4 cm and is approximately 0.5 cm deep. There is an area of tunneling at the proximal wound edge, with a depth of 2 cm. A wound culture is obtained.

L. is immediately intubated and admitted to the pediatric intensive care unit (PICU). She is hemodynamically unstable and desaturates when turned manually. Chest x-rays reveal bilateral basilar infiltrates. Because L. is incontinent of urine, a Foley catheter is placed to assist in monitoring output. L. is also incontinent of stool. A fecal bag cannot be placed because of the location of the pressure ulcer.

A surgical consultation is obtained for debridement of the pressure sore. A wet to dry normal saline dressing is placed until debridement is accomplished. When the ulcer is debrided, the wound extends into the muscle, and the dimensions increase to 8 × 1 cm.

1. This wound is now stage
  a. 2.
  b. 3.
  c. 4.
  d. 5.

The surgeon orders a half-strength hydrogen peroxide and normal saline irrigation, followed by full-strength povidone-iodine packing every 4 hours because the wound culture is positive for *Staphylococcus aureus*.

2. The nurse discusses concern about the dressing regimen with the physician because
  a. Hydrogen peroxide destroys fibroblasts; full-strength povidone-iodine is cytotoxic and can be absorbed when used in a large, open wound.
  b. A dry sterile dressing should be used because this is a surgical wound.

c. An antibiotic ointment should be used because the wound was positive for *Staphylococcus aureus*.

d. The dressing regimen should be changed more frequently because of potential fecal contamination.

3. The nurse knows that the appropriate dressing regimen for L. is
   a. Normal saline wet to dry gauze dressing.
   b. Hydrocolloid wafer.
   c. Gel with a composite polymeric dressing.
   d. Calcium alginate with a polyurethane film.

The physicians have ordered a specialty bed for L.

4. The most appropriate specialty bed is
   a. Static air mattress.
   b. Air-fluidized bed.
   c. Continuous lateral rotation bed.
   d. Gel/water–filled mattress.

L. has been in the PICU for several days. Tube feedings are started in the morning. During the morning assessment, the nurse discovers that her heels, ankles, and ears are beginning to redden. All of the areas are intact but nonblanchable. Laboratory values reveal that her albumin level has decreased to 2.0 g/dL.

5. The described areas are stage
   a. 2.
   b. 1.
   c. 4.
   d. 3.

6. What nursing intervention would be the most appropriate?
   a. Massage all bony prominences every 4 hours and apply heat to the affected areas.
   b. No intervention is necessary, because L. is already on a specialty bed.
   c. Allow L.'s head to rest on the bed surface, elevate the heels and ankles off the bed, and obtain a nutrition consultation.
   d. Contact the surgeons to place the patient on an air-fluidized bed.

7. Which risk factor or factors did not contribute to L.'s initial and subsequent skin breakdown?
   a. Poor nutrition and hydration.
   b. Immobility and incontinence.
   c. Presence of infectious process.
   d. Age and diabetes mellitus.

L. progresses well and is able to be extubated. Her pressure ulcer is granulating but is still 7×0.8 cm. L. is transferred out of PICU to the pediatric unit, although she still has some paralysis in her lower extremities. Her albumin level is now 2.5 g/dL, and she is tolerating a soft diet.

8. Changes that the nurse can recommend in L.'s therapy at this point are
   a. Change to a hydrocolloid dressing for the ulcer and put her on a static air mattress.
   b. No change is necessary; this therapy is continued until L. is discharged.
   c. Continue lateral rotation bed and use a composite polymeric dressing.
   d. Discontinue the lateral rotational bed, place on a low air-loss bed, and continue current dressings.

L. continues to progress well and is able to be transferred to a rehabilitation hospital for further therapy.

CASE 24-3

R., a 12-year-old boy with a history of Crohn's disease for a number of years, is admitted to the PICU after excision of a perirectal fistula. R.'s mother states that he is sensitive to tape, and a skin sealant is used under all intravenous dressings. R. has been on long-term, high-dose steroid therapy and exhibits several side effects, including fragile skin, bruising, and small stature. He is having 10 to 12 liquid stools per day and cries out when he must be cleaned.

A specialty bed has been ordered for R.

1. The most appropriate specialty bed for R. is
   a. Air fluidized.
   b. Low air loss.
   c. Continuous lateral rotation.
   d. None; a specialty bed is inappropriate.

2. The most appropriate dressing for R. is
   a. Normal saline wet to dry dressings.
   b. Gel and gauze.
   c. Calcium alginate and a polyurethane film.
   d. Hydrophilic paste and a hydrocolloid wafer.

R. is unable to tolerate any dressing on the wound because of the pain experienced during dressing changes. He expresses embarrassment when his perineal area must be exposed for cleaning or dressing changes. Sitz baths are ordered to assist in perineal cleansing; however, they are too painful. He is placed on a low air-loss bed with a wound irrigation feature (i.e., Clensicair Bed, Hill-Rom, Batesville, In.), which allows him to irrigate his wound each time he stools.

Although R.'s wound stays fairly clean, healing is slow because of frequent stooling. He refuses to eat because of the pain associated with stool in the open wound. The physician decides to perform an ileostomy to divert the stool away from the wound and allow R. to eat normally. An ostomy pouch is placed over the stoma in the recovery room. When the ostomy pouch is changed 3 days later, blistering is seen under the pouch seal, approximately 2 inches away from the stoma.

3. A potential cause of the peristomal blistering is
   a. Stool that has leaked under the pouch seal.
   b. Sensitivity to the pouch tape.
   c. Development of another fistula.
   d. Development of a yeast rash.

4. The nurse should
   a. Leave the pouch off and expose the skin to air.
   b. Leave the pouch off and apply a thick layer of zinc-based barrier cream.
   c. Apply an antacid to the skin, allow to dry well, and apply the pouch in the usual manner.
   d. Trim all tape from the pouch and apply; do a patch test for product sensitivity.

After a patch test is done, R. is found to be sensitive to the tape on the pouch. He shows no sensitivity to pectin-based powders, skin sealants, karaya paste, or solid barriers. The peristomal skin continues to be moist and weeping.

5. The nurse should
   a. Apply a thin layer of tincture of benzoin to the area and allow to dry well before applying the pouch.
   b. Apply a thin layer of karaya paste all over the weeping areas and apply a pouch.
   c. Apply a pectin-methylcellulose powder to the area, wipe away the excess, and apply a pouching system without a tape border.
   d. Clean the area with tepid water, dry well, and apply an alternative barrier.

R. is able to eat a regular diet after a few days, which he tolerates well. He continues to irrigate the wound several times a day and improves slowly. R. learns to care for his ostomy and is sent home to finish the healing process.

6. Appropriate discharge instructions for R. to irrigate his wound at home are to
   a. Use a hand-held shower head to direct the water into the wound.
   b. Use a portable sitz bath, followed by a hand-held shower.
   c. Avoid irrigating the wound at home and return to clinic once each week.
   d. Irrigate the wound with a syringe while lying in bed.

R. returns to the hospital for a split-thickness skin graft to the perineal wound after 3 months. The perineal wound bed is pink and shiny, with a small amount of serous drainage. On return from surgery, R. has a pressure dressing on the perineal area and an impregnated gauze dressing on the donor site on his right thigh. R. pulls off the thigh dressing and refuses to allow the impregnated gauze to be used because it is too painful.

7. In caring for the donor site, the nurse should
   a. Apply a wet to dry normal saline dressing and change it every 8 hours and as needed.
   b. Apply antimicrobial ointment and a Telfa dressing and change it every 12 hours and as needed.
   c. Apply a hydrogel sheet and change it every 3 days and as needed.
   d. Use a blow dryer set on cool to dry the area and allow scab formation.

R. rejects 25% of his graft. On the day of discharge, the area of rejection appears moist, with a small amount of yellow slough and exudate. He still experiences a moderate amount of pain with wound care.

8. The nurse gives the following discharge instructions to R. and his mother
   a. Continue with the shower irrigations until the area heals.
   b. Apply wet to dry normal saline dressings twice each day.
   c. Apply wet to dry Clorpactin dressings once each day.
   d. Apply a hydrocolloid dressing and leave it on for at least 24 hours.

ANSWERS ■ CASE 24-1

1. Answer (**c**). An ascending colostomy is expected to function several times each day. Early in the postoperative period, it is normal for an ostomy to produce green liquid stool. After normal diet and activity resume, the stool should thicken to a more pasty consistency. Stool color is related to the color and type of foods ingested. The frequency, consistency, and amount of stool should be monitored to ensure that the stoma is functioning properly.

REFERENCES

Adams, D.A., & Selekof, J.L. (1986). Children with ostomies: Comprehensive care planning. *Pediatric Nursing,* 12, 429–433.
Dudas, S. (1982). Postoperative considerations. In D. Broadwell & B. Jackson (Eds.). *Principles of ostomy care* (pp. 341–368). St. Louis: C.V. Mosby.

2. Answer (**d**). Because of perioperative manipulation of the bowel, stoma edema is normal. As the swelling resolves, the stoma diameter becomes smaller, and adjusting the size of the opening becomes necessary. The opening in the pouch should be 1/16 to 1/8 inch larger than the stoma. If the opening is too large, the surrounding skin is exposed to effluent and breaks down. As the child grows, the stoma size will change, and adjustment of the pouch opening will be needed.

REFERENCES

Adams, D.A., & Selekof, J.L. (1986). Children with ostomies: Comprehensive care planning. *Pediatric Nursing,* 12, 429–433.
Hagelgans, N., & Whitney, D. (1996). Skin integrity. In M.A.Q. Curley, J.B. Smith, & P.A. Moloney-Harmon (Eds.). *Critical care nursing of infants and children* (pp. 510–531). Philadelphia: W.B. Saunders.

3. Answer (**b**). Applying the powder helps to obtain a dry surface for the pouch to stick. Excess powder should be brushed away before pouch application. By adjusting the pouch opening to be only 1/16 to 1/8 inch larger than the stoma, the peristomal skin can be protected from the stool, and the irritated skin can heal.

REFERENCES

Adams, D.A., & Selekof, J.L. (1986). Children with ostomies: Comprehensive care planning. *Pediatric Nursing,* 12, 429–433.
Hagelgans, N., & Whitney, D. (1996). Skin integrity. In M.A.Q. Curley, J.B. Smith, & P.A. Moloney-Harmon (Eds.). *Critical care nursing of infants and children* (pp. 510–531). Philadelphia: W.B. Saunders.

4. Answer (**a**). Although the rectum has been isolated from the rest of the bowel, it continues to produce mucus. As the mucus in the rectal stump collects, J. must evacuate it.

REFERENCE

Rothenberger, D., & Orrom, W. (1991). Anatomy and physiology of defecation. In D. Doughty (Ed.). *Urinary and fecal incontinence: Nursing management* (pp. 169–188). St. Louis: Mosby–Year Book.

5. Answer (**c**). Yeast typically appears as a prickly red rash with small pustules and widespread satellite lesions. Yeast proliferates in warm, moist, dark regions.

REFERENCES

Esposito, Y. (1982). Readmission needs of ostomy patients. In D. Broadwell & B. Jackson (Eds.). *Principles of ostomy care* (pp. 399–408). St. Louis: C.V. Mosby.
Levene, G., & Goolamali, S. (1991). *Diagnostic picture tests in dermatology.* London: Wolfe Medical Publications.
Wysocki, A., & Bryant, R. (1992). Skin. In R. Bryant (Ed.). *Acute and chronic wounds: Nursing management* (pp. 1–31). St. Louis: Mosby–Year Book.

6. Answer (**b**). An antifungal cream should be applied to the affected areas to treat the yeast rash. The zinc-based barrier cream protects the perianal region from further exposure to stool and urine, allowing the denuded areas to heal.

REFERENCES

Colburn, L. (1990). Early intervention for the prevention of pressure ulcers. In D. Krasner (Ed.). *Chronic wound care* (pp. 78–88). King of Prussia: Health Management Publications.
Kramer, D., & Honig, P. (1988). Diaper dermatitis in the hospitalized child. *Journal of Enterostomal Therapy,* 15 (4), 167–170.
Levene, G., & Goolamali, S. (1991). *Diagnostic picture tests in dermatology.* London: Wolfe Medical Publications.

ANSWERS ■ CASE 24-2

1. Answer (**c**). According to the recommendations of the National Pressure Ulcer Advisory Panel, a stage 4 ulcer involves full-thickness skin loss with extensive destruction, tissue necrosis, or damage to muscle, bone, or supporting structures.

REFERENCE

National Pressure Ulcer Advisory Panel. (1989). Pressure ulcer: Incidence, economics, risk assessment. Consensus development conference statement. *Decubitus,* 2 (2), 24–28.

2. Answer (**a**). Irrigation with hydrogen per-

oxide at any concentration is cytotoxic and slightly bacteriostatic. Hydrogen peroxide also destroys fibroblasts, which are the cells most closely associated with the granulation phase of healing. No therapeutic effects are derived from the use of povidone-iodine in open wounds. This solution is cytotoxic and can be systemically absorbed through the wound bed, causing iodine toxicity. Numerous dressing changes necessitate frequent manual turning of an already compromised patient. Removing taped dressings several times each day can cause skin stripping. A skin sealant can be used under the tape to reduce skin trauma; however, this increases the cost of the dressing. If a systemic infection is present, topical antibiotic ointments do little to suppress infection; oral or parenteral antibiotics are recommended. Dry dressings are contraindicated, because the wound bed may become dry, causing epithelialization.

REFERENCES

Alvarez, O., Rozint, J., & Meehan, M. (1990). Principles of moist wound healing: Indications For chronic wounds. In D. Krasner (Ed.). Chronic wound care (pp. 266–281). King of Prussia: Health Management Publications.
Glugla, M., & Mulder, G. (1990). The diabetic foot: Medical management of foot ulcers. In D. Krasner (Ed.). Chronic wound care (pp. 223–239). King of Prussia: Health Management Publications.
Hess, C. (1990). Alert: Wound healing halted with the use of povidone-iodine. In D. Krasner (Ed.). Chronic wound care (pp. 290–294). King of Prussia: Health Management Publications.
Zink, M., Rousseau, P., & Holloway, G. (1992). Lower extremity ulcers. In R. Bryant (Ed.). Acute and chronic wounds: Nursing management (pp. 164–212). St. Louis: Mosby–Year Book.

3. Answer (**d**). Calcium alginate covered with a polyurethane film is the most appropriate dressing. Calcium alginates can absorb wound exudate, transforming the alginate into a gel. This gel promotes moist wound healing and autolytic debridement, and it is atraumatic on removal. Most alginates are safe for use in infected wounds; however, the manufacturer's recommendations should be consulted before use. The polyurethane film provides an occlusive environment and protects the wound from any stooling that may occur.

REFERENCES

Alvarez, O. (1988). Moist environment for healing: matching the dressing to the wound. Ostomy/Wound Management, Winter, 65–83.

Hagelgans, N., & Whitney, D. (1996). Skin integrity. In M.A.Q. Curley, J.B. Smith, & P.A. Moloney-Harmon (Eds.). Critical care nursing of infants and children (pp. 510–531). Philadelphia: W.B. Saunders.
Krasner, D. (Ed.). Chronic wound care (pp. 415–430). King of Prussia: Health Management Publications.
Oot-Giromini, B., Morris, E., & Feather, J. (1990). The economics of chronic wound care: An overview. In D. Krasner (Ed.). Chronic wound care (pp. 31–46). King of Prussia: Health Management Publications.

4. Answer (**c**). Continuous lateral rotational therapy provides a low air-loss surface for pressure reduction and therapeutic turning for assistance with pulmonary toileting and tissue perfusion. Tables 24–1 and 24–2 present suggested placement and removal criteria. This type of bed therapy can increase secretion clearance. Although lateral rotational therapy can be expensive, the number of days a patient is intubated may be reduced, thus decreasing the hospital stay.

REFERENCES

MacIntyre, N., Fink, M., Kelley, R., Sahn, S., & Wunderink, R. (1990). Continuous lateral rotational therapy in critical care. In N. MacIntyre (Ed.). Proceedings of a roundtable discussion (#A603). Charleston: Health Education Technologies for Support Systems International.
Summer, W., Curry, P., Hoponik, E., Nelson, S., & Elston, R. (1989). Mechanical turning of ICU patients shortens length of stay in some diagnostic related groups. Journal of Critical Care, 4, 45–53.

5. Answer (**b**). According to the National Pressure Ulcer Advisory Panel, stage 1 pressure ulcers are areas of intact skin with nonblanchable erythema.

REFERENCE

National Pressure Ulcer Advisory Panel (1989). Pressure ulcer: Incidence, economics, risk assessment. Consensus development conference statement. Decubitus, 2 (2), 24–28.

6. Answer (**c**). Allowing her head to rest directly on the low air-loss surface reduces interface pressure below the capillary closing level (32 mmHg). Pressure-reducing surfaces, such as a low air-loss bed, does not negate the use of additional pressure-relieving devices. Heels and ankles should be elevated off of the bed surface to prevent further skin breakdown. Poor nutritional status can be a major factor in the development of pressure ulcers. When the serum albumin level is below 3.3 g/dL, supplemental nutrition is required to promote healing and prevent further breakdown. Massaging bony prominences is contraindicated, because it can cause further tissue trauma.

TABLE 24-1.   Criteria for Placement on Continuous Lateral Rotation

Criterion	Parameter*
Pulmonary	
Disease or condition	Acute respiratory distress syndrome
	Pneumonia
	Crushing chest trauma
	Failure to wean
	Atelectasis
	Pulmonary infiltrates
Laboratory values	Pao_2 79 mmHg or less
	$Paco_2$
	34 mmHg or less
	46 mmHg or more
	O_2 saturation 94% or less
Hemodynamic	
Disease or condition	Anasarca
	Inability to tolerate manual turning as evidenced by rapid drop/elevation in blood pressure or pulse
Cardiac	
Disease or condition	Crushing chest injury
	Need to decrease cardiac work load (e.g., unstable postoperative open heart)
	Congestive heart failure
Renal	
Disease or condition	Renal failure
	Anasarca
	Nonresponsive to diuretics
Laboratory values	BUN 16 mg/dL or more
	Creatinine 1.6 mg/dL or more
Orthopedic	
Disease or condition	Crushing pelvic injury
	Unstable total hip replacement
	Any unstable skeletal fracture
Integument	
Disease or condition	Non-healing pressure ulcer or wound extending into the subcutaneous tissue or bone
Nutrition (healing potential)	
Disease or condition	Morbid obesity
Laboratory values	Albumin 2.5 g/dL or less
	Total protein 4.5 g/dL or less
	Prealbumin 10 mg/dL or less
	Transferrin 200 mg/dL or less
	Hemoglobin
	Male: 10 g/dL or less
	Female: 9 g/dL or less
	Hematocrit
	Male: 35% or less
	Female: 30% or less
	WBC count: $11,000/mm^3$ or less
	Platelets: $150,000/mm^3$ or less

* The patient should meet at least two parameters before he or she qualifies for placement on continuous lateral rotation.

REFERENCE

Colburn, L. (1990). Early intervention for the prevention of pressure ulcers. In D. Krasner (Ed.). *Chronic wound care* (pp. 78–88). King of Prussia: Health Management Publications.

7. Answer (**d**). Poor nutritional status can be one of the leading factors contributing to skin breakdown, especially if the serum albumin level is below 3.3 g/dL. With the patient's paralysis, she is unable to shift position to redistribute the pressure on bony prominences, which may lead to tissue destruction. Tissue maceration can result from constant contact with moisture, which can hasten and facilitate skin breakdown. As skin hydration decreases, the barrier function of the skin becomes impaired, allowing bacteria to enter. Although increased age and diabetes mellitus may be risk factors contributing to skin breakdown, L. is young and is not a diabetic.

TABLE 24–2. Criteria for Removal From Continuous Lateral Rotation

Criterion	Parameter
Pulmonary	Steady improvement of chest x-ray films
	Successful ventilator weaning
Hemodynamic	Able to tolerate manual turning
	Resolving anasarca
Cardiac	Resolving congestive heart failure
Renal	Adequate diuresis
	Resolving anasarca
Orthopedic	Fracture stability
Length of therapy	Two weeks of lateral rotation without improvement
	Deterioration of patient's condition with no hope for survival

REFERENCES

Bryant, R., Shannon, M., Pieper, B., Braden, B., & Morris, D. (1992). Pressure ulcers. In R. Bryant (Ed.). *Acute and chronic wounds: Nursing management* (pp. 105–163). St. Louis: Mosby–Year Book.
Colburn, L. (1990). Early intervention for the prevention of pressure ulcers. In D. Krasner (Ed.). *Chronic wound care* (pp. 78–88). King of Prussia: Health Management Publications.
Hill, M. (1994). Color atlas of the skin. In M. Hill (Ed.). *Skin disorders* (pp. 1–11). St. Louis: Mosby–Year Book.

8. Answer (**d**). Lateral rotational therapy is meant to be a short-term treatment to provide pulmonary toilet. A less expensive intervention would be to discontinue the lateral rotational therapy and place on a low air-loss surface for appropriate pressure reduction. Table 24–3 provides information about criteria for placement on a low air-loss or air-fluidized bed.

REFERENCES

Colburn, L. (1990). Early intervention for the prevention of pressure ulcers. In D. Krasner (Ed.). *Chronic wound care* (pp. 78–88). King of Prussia: Health Management Publications.
Summer, W., Curry, P., Hoponik, E., Nelson, S., & Elston, R. (1989). Continuous mechanical turning of ICU patients shortens length of stay in some diagnostic related groups. *Journal Of Critical Care,* 4, 45–53.

ANSWERS ■ CASE 24–3

1. Answer (**b**). R. is at high risk for further skin breakdown because of his long-term steroid use and poor nutritional status. He also has a large perineal wound that requires pressure relief. A low air-loss bed provides the necessary pressure reduc-

tion and allows him to get out of bed to use the bedside commode.

REFERENCES

Colburn, L. (1990). Early intervention for the prevention of pressure ulcers. In D. Krasner (Ed.). *Chronic wound care* (pp. 78–88). King of Prussia: Health Management Publications.
Hagelgans, N., & Whitney, D. (1996). Skin integrity. In M.A.Q. Curley, J.B. Smith, & P.A. Moloney-Harmon (Eds.). *Critical care nursing of infants and children* (pp. 510–531). Philadelphia: W.B. Saunders.

2. Answer (**c**). A calcium alginate dressing provides moist wound healing and absorption of wound exudate, and it is atraumatic on removal. The polyurethane film helps to maintain a moist environment and protects the wound from stool contamination.

REFERENCES

Alvarez, O. (1988). Moist environment for healing: Matching the dressing to the wound. *Ostomy/Wound Management,* Winter, 65–83.
Turner, T. (1990). The development of wound management products. In D. Krasner (Ed.). *Chronic wound care* (pp. 31–53). King of Prussia: Health Management Publications.

TABLE 24–3. Criteria for Placement on Low Air-Loss or Air-Fluidized Bed

Criterion	Parameters*
Nutrition (healing potential)	
Integument	Non-healing pressure sore of wound extending into subcutaneous tissue, muscle or bone
	Morbid obesity
	Uncontrolled pain
	Overwhelming sepsis
	New graft over sacrum or hips
	Large, deep burn or tissue loss
	Stevens-Johnson syndrome
	Anasarca
	Immobility
Nutrition	Poor skin turgor
Laboratory values	Albumin: 2.5 g/dL or less
	Total protein: 4.5 g/dL or less
	Prealbumin: 10 mg/dL or less
	Transferrin: 200 mg/dL or less

* The patient should meet at least two parameters before he or she qualifies for placement on an air-fluidized or low air-loss bed. Other considerations include the presence of contractures, tube feedings, cancer with metastasis, intractable pain, radiation therapy to posterior body surfaces, and respiratory distress. Patients requiring constant head elevation should be placed on air-fluidized beds with head elevation units or low air-loss beds. It is important to consider frequent patient transfers when determining a specialty bed. Friction, shear, and trauma from the bed frame could cause further injury. Re-evaluation of patients on specialty beds should be done often as changes in status occur.

3. Answer (**b**). Before surgery, the patient's mother stated that he was sensitive to tape. The cause of the peristomal blistering is most likely a reaction to the barrier.

REFERENCE

Hill, M. (1994). Diseases of epidermal origin. In M. Hill (Ed.). *Skin disorders* (pp. 27–38). St. Louis: Mosby–Year Book.

4. Answer (**d**). Because R. is known to be sensitive to tape, it can be cut off from around the barrier until a patch test is done to determine if he has any further sensitivities. Skin patch testing is a useful tool to differentiate sensitivity from other causes. Small pieces of questionable products are placed on a nonhairy area of the abdomen, thigh, or back, away from the peristomal area. Patch test materials are removed if a reaction occurs within 48 hours, and the skin is inspected for irritation.

REFERENCE

Watt, R. (1982). Pathophysiology of peristomal skin. In D. Broadwell & B. Jackson (Eds.). *Principles of ostomy care* (pp. 241–253). St. Louis: C.V. Mosby.

5. Answer (**c**). The pectin-methylcellulose powder assists in providing a dry surface for pouch adherence. A pouching system that the patient is not sensitive to, such as a Flextend (Hollister) or Stomahesive (Convatec) wafer with a snap-on pouch, should then be applied.

REFERENCES

Adams, D., & Selekof, J. (1986). Children with ostomies: Comprehensive care planning. *Pediatric Nursing*, 12, 429–433.

Watt, R. (1982). Pathophysiology of peristomal skin. In D. Broadwell & B. Jackson (Eds.). *Principles of ostomy care* (pp. 241–253). St. Louis: C.V. Mosby.

6. Answer (**a**). Wound cleaning is essential for removal of contaminants and necrotic material. R. may be more compliant with his wound care if he can do his own care at home. Using the hand-held shower head allows him to direct the flow of water into the wound bed without the discomfort of a sitz bath.

REFERENCE

Klein, L., & Iles, R. (1990). Topical treatment for chronic wounds: An overview. In D. Krasner (Ed.). *Chronic wound care* (pp. 263–265). King of Prussia: Health Management Publications.

7. Answer (**c**). A hydrogel sheet dressing promotes moist wound healing, is atraumatic on removal, and provides an occlusive barrier. Occluding the donor site also reduces pain.

REFERENCE

Alvarez, O., Rozint, J., & Meehan, M. (1990). Principles of moist wound healing: Indications for chronic wounds. In D. Krasner (Ed.) *Chronic wound care* (pp. 266–281). King of Prussia: Health Management Publications.

8. Answer (**a**). Because R. is unable to tolerate any dressing on the area, continuing wound irrigation at home allows the wound to be cleaned of exudate and necrotic materials.

REFERENCE

Klein, L., & Iles, R. (1990). Topical treatment for chronic wounds: An overview. In D. Krasner (Ed.). *Chronic wound care* (pp. 263–265). King of Prussia: Health Management Publications.

CHAPTER 25

Pain Management

SUSAN J. SENECAL, RN, MSN

CASE 25-1

S. is a 14-year-old postoperative patient who was admitted to the pediatric intensive care unit (PICU) for a posterior spinal fusion from T-4 to T-12. S. arrived with an intact epidural catheter at L-4. She received a bolus dose of Duramorph (0.05 mg/kg) and was started on a continuous drip of Duramorph at 0.01 mg/kg per hour before leaving the operating room at 4:00 P.M. On arrival to the PICU at 4:30 P.M., S. is sleepy but arousable. She has a heart rate of 92 beats per minute (bpm), a respiratory rate of 20 breaths per minute, and O_2 saturation of 99%. Her weight is 60 kg.

1. Based on this information, Duramorph was chosen as S.'s epidural analgesia pain management because Duramorph is
   a. Ten times more potent than morphine.
   b. Hydrophilic and rostrally flows to attach to opiate receptors.
   c. The preferred drug of choice for all thoracic and abdominal surgeries.
   d. Less likely than fentanyl to cause side effects such as pruritus and respiratory depression.

2. As the critical care nurse continues the patient assessment, a check is made of the electrical cold pack directly overlaying the surgical site dressing. The purpose of the cold pack is to
   a. Promote temperature stability in the patient.
   b. Promote a reduction of any pruritus.

   c. Promote reduction of surgical-site edema.
   d. Promote healing by decreasing blood flow and circulation to the surgical area.

3. At 9:30 P.M., S. seems to be sleeping soundly. She has a heart rate of 62, respiratory rate of 11, and O_2 saturation of 93%. Which of the following are the most immediate appropriate actions?
   a. Give 6 mg of naloxone intravenously over 30 to 60 seconds, repeating as needed; start O_2; arouse S. and tell her to breathe; and stop the infusion of epidural Duramorph.
   b. Arouse S. and tell her to breathe; stop the infusion of epidural Duramorph; start O_2; give 0.06 mg of naloxone intravenously over 30 to 60 seconds, repeating as needed; and start a continuous naloxone infusion if needed.
   c. Stop the infusion of epidural Duramorph; start O_2; give 0.06 to 0.3 mg of flumazenil (Romazicon) intravenously over 30 to 60 seconds, repeating as needed; and start a continuous infusion of flumazenil to reverse any respiratory depression.
   d. Start to bag S. with 100% O_2; give 6 mg of naloxone intravenously over 30 to 60 seconds, repeating as needed; and give flumazenil at low doses to reverse any further respiratory depression.

4. How do opioids manage pain when given epidurally?
   a. Opioids decrease prostaglandin production at the site of injury.
   b. Opioids diffuse into the cerebrospinal fluid (CSF), cross the dura, and bind to opiate receptors.
   c. Opioids anesthetize the nerve roots as the nerve roots exit the spinal cord.
   d. Opioids are absorbed into the blood stream and decrease the production of neurotransmitters.

S. stays in the PICU on epidural analgesia for 3 days. Before she is transferred to the medical-surgical unit, her epidural catheter is removed. She is started on an equianalgesic dose of immediate-release oral morphine for pain.

5. Calculate the amount and frequency of oral morphine S. would receive based on her weight of 60 kg.
   a. 6 mg every 2 hours, as needed.
   b. 14 mg every 3 hours, as needed.
   c. 18 mg every 4 hours, as needed.
   d. 36 mg every 6 hours, as needed.

6. The difference in the dosing of oral or intravenous morphine results from the phenomenon of
   a. Potential liver toxicity.
   b. First-pass metabolism.
   c. Respiratory depression longevity.
   d. Decreased renal clearance.

7. When S. is awake, alert, and responding appropriately, the most appropriate pain assessment tool to use for her age would be the
   a. Eland Color Tool.
   b. 0 to 10 scale.
   c. Oucher Pain Scale.
   d. Wong-Baker Faces Scale.

CASE 25-2

M., a 2-day-old, 4-kg term infant girl, is admitted postoperatively to the PICU after an extensive Blalock-Taussig shunt. She has a left thoracotomy incision, chest tube, central venous line, and an arterial line. On arrival she is orally intubated on a fraction of inspired oxygen (FIO_2) of 0.4 mmHg to maintain O_2 saturations greater than 80%, rate 40 breaths per minute, positive end-expiratory pressure (PEEP) of 4 cmH_2O, and a positive inspiratory pressure (PIP) of 20 cmH_2O. Vecuronium (Norcuron) is infusing at 0.4 mg/

hour, and fentanyl is infusing at 4 μg/hour. She has a heart rate of 140 to 144 bpm, systolic blood pressure of 78 to 80 mmHg, and O_2 saturation of 84%. She is pale, and her breath sounds are equal and clear.

Within 24 hours, the vecuronium drip has been discontinued, and M. has become restless. Her ventilatory settings include an FIO_2 of 0.25 mmHg to maintain an O_2 saturation of more than 80%, a rate of 34 breaths per minute, PEEP of 4 cmH_2O, and PIP of 20 cmH_2O. She has a heart rate of 170 to 180 bpm, systolic blood pressure of 93 to 99 mmHg, and O_2 saturation of 79%. She is still pale, and her breath sounds are clear and equal.

1. What is the initial intervention?
   a. Start vecuronium drip at 0.1 mg/kg per hour.
   b. Change to morphine boluses at 0.3 mg/kg every 3 to 4 hours.
   c. Check oxygen and ventilatory support system settings.
   d. Start a midazolam (Versed) drip at 0.06 mg/kg per hour.

2. After the previous intervention, her vital signs remain the same, and the O_2 saturation is 80%. M. remains restless. What is the next intervention?
   a. Change to morphine boluses at 0.1 mg/kg every 3 to 4 hours.
   b. Start vecuronium drip 0.1 mg/kg per hour.
   c. Bolus of fentanyl at 2 μg/kg and then increase the fentanyl drip to 2 μg/kg per hour.
   d. Bolus of midazolam at 0.1 mg/kg and then begin a midazolam drip at 0.06 mg/kg per hour.

After 36 hours postoperatively, M.'s chest tube, central venous line, and arterial line are still intact. She is on an opioid, as needed, and is being weaned off the ventilator. Her respiratory rate is 24 breaths per minute, the CO_2 level is within prescribed parameters, and she is breathing synchronously with the ventilator with no spontaneous respirations.

3. The next intervention would be to
   a. Discontinue all opioids.
   b. Increase ventilatory support.
   c. Give naloxone to reverse respiratory depression.
   d. Give a fentanyl bolus.

M. is successfully weaned from the ventilator. However, over the next 3 weeks, M. returns to surgery twice because of postoperative complications. During the next 3 weeks, M.'s opioid pain medication dose is increased.

4. The opioid is increased because
   a. Opioids have no ceiling effect.
   b. M. developed an addiction.
   c. The effectiveness of opioids diminish as pain diminishes.
   d. M. developed a tolerance.

M. has remained on her pain medication for 4 weeks. It has been 6 days since her last emergency surgery, and she has stabilized medically.

5. One of the next courses of treatment is to
   a. Wean her off intravenous opioid medication during the day and transfer her to the floor the following day.
   b. Stop the opioid pain medication, because M. is addicted, and start her on acetaminophen at a dose of 40 mg every 4 hours, as needed.
   c. Stop her intravenous pain medication and start her on chloral hydrate for any irritability or restlessness.
   d. Wean her off intravenous pain medication decreasing it by one half at first and then by 10% per day.

6. Which of the following are withdrawal or abstinence symptoms of opioid dependency?
   a. Sugar cravings, overeating, diarrhea, hyperactivity, irritability, burping, poor feeding, and sneezing.
   b. Diarrhea, hyperactivity, irritability, vomiting, hiccuping, burping, poor feeding, and sleepiness.
   c. Sugar cravings, overeating, hyperactivity, irritability, sneezing, hiccuping, burping, and sleepiness.
   d. Diarrhea, hyperactivity, irritability, sneezing, coughing, vomiting, hiccuping, and poor feeding.

7. Infants younger than 3 months of age receive a lower dose (one-fourth to one-third dose) of opioids because
   a. Neonates and young infants do not feel pain the same way adults do because of the lack of myelinization of all nerve fibers.
   b. Neonates and young infants do not remember the pain, and the increased risk of opioid side effects should be avoided.
   c. Neonates and young infants commonly experience respiratory depression.

   d. Clearance of opioids is prolonged in neonates and infants younger than 3 months of age.

8. An appropriate pain assessment tool to use for assessment of M.'s pain is
   a. Postoperative Comfort Score by Attia and colleagues.
   b. Eland Color Tool.
   c. Oucher Pain Scale.
   d. Wong-Baker Faces Scale.

CASE 25-3

J. is a 9-year-old boy diagnosed with acute lymphocytic leukemia. During the last year, he has received many chemotherapy drugs, including vincristine and methotrexate. He weighs 50 kg.

1. During his last hospital admission, J. complained of a burning, tingling, shooting pain in both feet. This type of pain is called
   a. Neuralgic pain.
   b. Neuropathic pain.
   c. Lancinating pain.
   d. Radicular pain.

2. If opioids are ineffective, the safest, most effective, and least invasive method for treating the type of pain that J. is experiencing is
   a. Large doses of steroids.
   b. Low doses of benzodiazepines.
   c. Tricyclic antidepressants.
   d. Nonsteroidal anti-inflammatory drugs (NSAIDs).

J. has undergone many bone marrow aspirations for treating and evaluating his cancer. All of these procedures have occurred in the physician's office or hospital treatment room with his physician, nurse, and mother present.

3. Which of the following methods of pain management would be the safest and most effective in this setting?
   a. Pre-procedural preparation by Child Life, EMLA cream at the injection site, and 30 mg of ketamine administered intravenously and titrated to effect.
   b. Pre-procedural preparation by Child Life, EMLA cream at the injection site, and 150 mg of pentobarbital (Nembutal) administered as an intravenous push.
   c. Pre-procedural preparation by Child

Life, EMLA cream at the injection site, a lidocaine and sodium bicarbonate mixture (10:1) administered by deep intramuscular injection, and 25 μg of fentanyl and 2.5 mg of midazolam administered intravenously and titrated to effect.
  d. Pre-procedural preparation by Child Life, EMLA cream, 50 μg of fentanyl, and 5 mg of midazolam administered as an intravenous push.

4. An appropriate pain assessment tool to use to assess J.'s pain when he is awake, alert, and responding appropriately is the
  a. Oucher Pain Scale.
  b. Childrens Hospital Eastern Ontario Pain Scale (CHEOPS).
  c. Eland Color Tool.
  d. Postoperative Comfort Score by Attia and colleagues.

CASE 25-4

L. is a 4-year-old boy who was severely burned with hot water on his chest, abdomen, and legs. He is suffering from second- and third-degree burns over 40% of his body. He weighs 20 kg.

On admission to the PICU, L. is very agitated and crying. He has a heart rate of 150, respiratory rate of 36, blood pressure of 120/82 mmHg, temperature of 38.4°C, and O₂ saturation of 97% to 99%.

1. After the admission procedure is complete and intravenous fluids are started, which of the following interventions may decrease his agitation?
  a. Start a continuous intravenous opioid drip; obtain his favorite toy, which mom brought from home; allow the parents at the bedside; and start ibuprofen around the clock.
  b. Obtain his favorite toy, which mom brought from home; give a bolus dose of an opioid, then start the continuous drip; allow the parents at the bedside; and start ibuprofen around the clock.
  c. Start a continuous intravenous opioid drip; obtain his favorite toy, which mom brought from home; allow the parents at the bedside; and give chloral hydrate.
  d. Give a bolus dose of an opioid, then start the continuous drip; obtain his favorite toy, which mom brought from

home; allow the parents at the bedside; and give chloral hydrate.

2. An appropriate pain assessment tool to use to assess L.'s pain when he is awake, alert, and responding appropriately would be
  a. CHEOPS.
  b. Oucher Pain Scale.
  c. Postoperative Comfort Score by Attia and colleagues.
  d. Visual Analogue Scale.

L.'s medical condition has stabilized. Physical therapy has several sessions of muscle strengthening during the day, for which L. needs to be awake and alert. However, there are two whirlpools each day in which dead scar tissue is removed from L.'s wounds. During these whirlpools, a physical therapist, an aide, and a critical care transport nurse are with him. The pain management goals during this treatment are analgesia, amnesia, and anxiolysis.

3. Choose the medication combination that would best achieve these goals given the circumstances of personnel and patient activity.
  a. Morphine and diazepam (Valium).
  b. Morphine and ketamine.
  c. Fentanyl and midazolam.
  d. Fentanyl and ketorolac (Toradol).

4. During a case conference for L., his pain management is discussed. The resident suggests increasing L.'s ibuprofen to 500 mg every 6 hours. Is this an appropriate or inappropriate action?
  a. An appropriate action, because NSAIDs like opioids have no ceiling effect.
  b. An appropriate action, because increasing the dose of an NSAID will continue to decrease the production of neurotransmitters without increasing the side effects of the NSAID.
  c. An inappropriate action, because an increase in the dose of an NSAID can inhibit opioids from attaching to opioid receptors.
  d. An inappropriate action, because increasing the dose of an NSAID, which has a ceiling effect, only increases its side effects.

5. L. has been using opioids for pain relief for about 1.5 months. His painful procedures and surgical interventions are complete, and his opioids will be weaned. To avoid

withdrawal symptoms, which medication would be used to wean him from opioids?
  a. Pentazocine (Talwin).
  b. Nalbuphine (Nubain).
  c. Methadone.
  d. Butorphanol (Stadol).

6. In what instance might an agonist-antagonist opioid be preferable to a pure agonist opioid?
  a. A 16-year-old patient who needs to be weaned from a ventilator.
  b. A 6-year-old patient with terminal cancer.
  c. A 17-year-old patient who needs to be weaned from opioids.
  d. An infant with hypoplastic left lung after abdominal surgery.

7. Combining NSAIDs and opioids for pain management is more effective because
  a. Opioids potentiate the effect of NSAIDs.
  b. NSAIDs and opioids modulate pain in two different ways.
  c. Both NSAIDs and opioids modulate pain by attaching to opiate receptors in the substantia gelatinosa of the spinal cord.
  d. Both NSAIDs and opioids modulate pain by decreasing prostaglandin production.

ANSWERS ■ CASE 25-1

1. Answer (**b**). Duramorph is preservative-free morphine. Morphine is less lipophilic than fentanyl. When given epidurally, morphine flows rostrally in the CSF, attaching to opiate receptors in the spinal cord and blocking pain impulses.

REFERENCE

Bragg, C.L. (1989). Practical aspects of epidural and intrathecal narcotic analgesia in the intensive care setting. *Heart & Lung*, 18 (6), 599–608.

2. Answer (**c**). Providing a mild degree of analgesia and reducing swelling can be accomplished with the use of ice and other surface-cooling devices.

REFERENCE

Cohen, D. (1993). Management of postoperative pain in children. In N.L. Schechter, C.B. Berde, & M. Yaster (Eds.). *Pain in infants, children and adolescents* (p. 376). Baltimore: Williams & Wilkins.

3. Answer (**b**). Because of morphine's slow

absorption epidurally, the sedative and potential respiratory depression effects may appear as late as 4 to 6 hours after injection and last as long as 24 hours. It is possible to arouse the patient, encourage breathing and administer blow-by O_2. Because the potential respiratory depression effects may last for such a long time, naloxone should be administered in low doses first. The low dose (0.001 mg per kg) of naloxone reverses side effects before reversing analgesic effect. Because the half-life of naloxone is less than 60 minutes, a continuous infusion should be started after the initial boluses.

REFERENCE

Yaster, M., & Maxwell, L.G. (1993). Opioid agonists and antagonists. In N.L. Schechter, C.B. Berde, & M. Yaster (Eds.). *Pain in infants, children, and adolescents* (p. 166). Baltimore: Williams & Wilkins.

4. Answer (**b**). When opioids are injected into the epidural space, they diffuse into the CSF, cross the dura, and bind to opiate receptors in the spinal cord. Because morphine is less lipophilic, it flows with the CSF, binding to opiate receptors along the spinal cord. An opioid like fentanyl is very lipophilic and does not usually flow rostrally but binds immediately to opiate receptors in the spinal cord.

REFERENCE

Schryer, N. (1989). Epidural catheters: Pain management in the child. *Critical Care Nursing Techniques*, 8 (6), 347–355.

5. Answer (**c**). Equianalgesia means the relative analgesic potency. This is the ratio of two analgesics to produce an equal analgesic effect. It is also the ratio of one analgesic given two different ways, (i.e., orally or intravenously). Based on research, a dose of morphine given orally should be three to six times the intravenous dose.

REFERENCE

McCaffery, M., & Beebe, A. (1989). *Pain: Clinical manual for nursing practice* (p. 78). St. Louis: C.V. Mosby.

6. Answer (**b**). First-pass metabolism is an effect which occurs with drugs that are intended to be absorbed in the stomach but are metabolized in the liver. This metabolism reduces the amount of drug that is available for absorption.

REFERENCE

Whaley, L.F., & Wong, D.L. (1991). *Nursing care of infants and children* (p. 1153). St. Louis: Mosby–Year Book.

7. Answer (**b**). The 0 to 10 scale is a pain assessment scale used with school-age children, teenagers, and adults who understand the relativity of numbers. The nurse explains to the patient that 0 equals no pain and that 10 equals the worst pain ever felt. The nurse then asks the patient what number the pain feels like.

REFERENCE

Foster, R., & Stevens, B. (1994). Nursing management of pain in children. In C.L. Betz, M. Hunsberger, & S. Wright (Eds.). *Family-centered nursing care of children* (2nd ed., pp. 882–914). Philadelphia: W.B. Saunders.

ANSWERS ■ CASE 25-2

1. Answer (**c**). Restlessness and agitation may be caused by factors such as pain, environmental stimuli, or respiratory insufficiency. Although oxygen saturation is usually low, 80% to 85%, in a patient with a Blalock-Taussig shunt, respiratory status should always be assessed first. After the respiratory status is assessed and evaluation of interventions is complete, assessing for pain and environmental stimuli follows.

REFERENCES

Castaneda, A.R., Jones, R.A., & Mayer, J.E. (1992). Surgery for infants with congenital heart disease. In D. Fyler (Ed.). *Nadas' pediatric cardiology.* St. Louis: Mosby–Year Book.

Gordon, P.C. (1990). Assessing and managing agitation in a critically ill infant. *MCN; American Journal of Maternal Child Nursing,* 15 (1), 26–32.

2. Answer (**c**). Fentanyl remains the opioid of choice because of its minimal hemodynamic and cardiovascular effects. A bolus is given before the continuous infusion to achieve an immediate therapeutic range of drug efficacy. Otherwise, a therapeutic range usually occurs after five drug half-lives. A continuous method is used to achieve constant analgesia because fentanyl's duration of action is 0.5 to 1 hour.

REFERENCE

Yaster, M., & Maxwell, L.G. (1993). Opioid agonists and antagonists. In N.L. Schechter, C.B. Berde, & M. Yaster (Eds.). *Pain in infants, children and adolescents.* Baltimore: Williams & Wilkins.

3. Answer (**d**). A chest tube and thoracotomy incision can be very painful because of increased innervation in the pleura and surrounding tissues. Increased discomfort may occur with each respiration. Because of the increased pain, infants may "splint" and not breathe effectively. An appropriate dose of an opioid may relieve the pain with a subsequent increase of inspiratory effort.

REFERENCES

Bell, S. (1994). The National Pain Management Guideline: Implications for neonatal intensive care. *Neonatal Network, 13* (3), 9–17.

Cohen, D.E. (1993). Management of postoperative pain in children. In N.L. Schechter, C.B. Berde, & M. Yaster, (Eds.). *Pain in infants, children and adolescents.* Baltimore: Williams & Wilkins.

4. Answer (**d**). Tolerance to an opioid occurs when, after repeated doses, the dose begins to lose its efficacy to manage the pain. To achieve the same effective pain relief, the dose must be increased. Because opioids have no ceiling effect, this increase is safe and may be effective. As patients become more tolerant to an opioid's analgesic effect, they also become more tolerant to the side effects.

REFERENCE

Franck, L.S., & Gregory, G.A. (1993). Clinical evaluation and treatment of infant pain in the NICU. In N.L. Schechter, C.B. Berde, & M. Yaster (Eds.). *Pain in infants, children and adolescents* (p. 527) Baltimore: Williams & Wilkins.

5. Answer (**d**). To avoid withdrawal symptoms, the nurse should slowly decrease the amount of opioids given to the patient. The scheduled decrease can begin with decreasing the dose by one half and then decreasing by 10% per day or by one fourth to one fifth every 3 days. If withdrawal symptoms occur, the opioid dose can be slightly increased to relieve withdrawal symptoms, after which weaning begins again.

REFERENCE

Howe, C.J., Mason, K., & Gordon, P.C. (1996). Pain and aversive stimulation. In M.A.Q. Curley, J.B. Smith, & P.A. Moloney-Harmon (Eds.). *Critical care nursing of infants and children* (pp. 532–554). Philadelphia: W.B. Saunders.

6. Answer (**d**). Signs of opioid withdrawal include coarse tremors, diarrhea, excessive diaphoresis, hyperactivity, irritability, poor feeding, sleeplessness, sneezing, fever, hiccups, nasal stuffiness, salivation, seizures, tachypnea (with respiratory alkalosis), vomiting, and yawning. These signs have all been associated with abstinence syndrome.

REFERENCE

Franck, L.S., & Gregory, G. A. (1993). Clinical evaluation and treatment of infant pain in the NICU. In N.L. Schechter, C.B. Berde, & M. Yaster (Eds.). *Pain in infants, children and adolescents* (p. 527). Baltimore: Williams & Wilkins.

7. Answer (**d**). Neonates and infants less then 2 to 3 months of age should receive a lower dose (one-fourth to one-third dose) of opioids because of prolonged drug clearance in the immature kidneys.

REFERENCE

Lynn, A.M., & Slatter, J.T. (1987). Morphine pharmacokinetics in early infancy. *Anesthesiology, 66,* 136–139.

8. Answer (**a**). Although no one behavior correlates directly with pain, pain assessment tools have attempted to cluster the infant's behavior variables to create a useful clinical format. Through clinical trials, Attia and colleagues have developed a pain assessment tool specifically for infants. This tool includes 10 behavior variables which correlate with infant pain and discomfort, which is scored from 0 to 20.

REFERENCE

Attia, J., Amirl-Tison, M.D., Mayer, M.N., Schnider, S.M., & Barrier, G. (1987). Measurement of postoperative pain and narcotic administration in infants using a new clinical scoring system. *Anesthesiology, 67,* p. 632.

ANSWERS ■ CASE 25-3

1. Answer (**b**). Neuropathic pain is described as a burning, tingling, shooting pain. It is elicited by damage to nerves in the periphery or central nervous system. It can be caused by diabetes, alcohol or heavy metal ingestion, human immunodeficiency virus infection, and neurotoxic drugs such as vincristine.

REFERENCE

Miser, A.W. (1993). Management of pain associated with childhood cancer. In N.L. Schechter, C.B Berde, & M. Yaster (Eds.). *Pain in infants, children and adolescents* (p. 417). Baltimore: Williams & Wilkins.

2. Answer (**c**). Tricyclic antidepressants can effectively manage neuropathic pain. Neuropathic pain conditions are associated with injury, dysfunction, or altered excitability of portions of the periphery or central nervous system. Tricyclic antidepressants manage pain by altering the reuptake of serotonin, a neurotransmitter.

REFERENCE

Olsson, G., & Berde, C.B. (1993). Neuropathic pain in children and adolescents. In N.L. Schechter, C.B. Berde, & M. Yaster (Eds.). *Pain in infants, children and adolescents* (p. 473). Baltimore: Williams & Wilkins.

3. Answer (**c**). Pre-procedural preparation is essential to help children cope with pain, especially for repeated painful procedures. EMLA cream is a topical anesthetic that anesthetizes the skin for invasive procedures. However, EMLA does not anesthetize to the depth of a deep intramuscular injection. A mixture of lidocaine and sodium bicarbonate (i.e., the sodium bicarbonate neutralizes the sting of lidocaine) injected deeply, including the periosteum of the bone, helps anesthetize the area for 3 to 4 hours after the bone marrow biopsy. Fentanyl (0.5 μg/kg) and midazolam (0.05 mg/kg) are titrated to effect and used to decrease pain and anxiety for the patient. The combination of opioid analgesics and benzodiazepines dramatically potentiate each other, especially side effects such as respiratory depression. For this reason, each is given in small doses, usually 25% to 50% of the total dose, and titrated to achieve the desired effect. Continual and ongoing assessment during each procedure is necessary so that changes in pain and anxiety management can occur. However, the practice may be different in different institutions. Combining all of these modalities to assist the patient through repeated painful procedures is an essential aspect of care for the oncology patient.

REFERENCE

Zeltzer, L.K., Altman, A., Cohen, D, Lebaron, S., Manuksela, L., & Schechter, N.L. (1990). Report of the subcommittee of the management of pain associated with procedures in children with cancer. *Pediatrics,* 86 (5), 826–834.

4. Answer (**c**). The Eland Color Tool is a child's body outline, which is used to document the intensity and location of the child's pain. The child chooses three colors to represent: mild pain (a little hurt), moderate pain (more hurt), and severe pain (worst hurt). The child then colors different parts of the body the specific color which represents the amount of pain he or she feels. The school-age child in particular seems to prefer this tool.

REFERENCE

Allen, J., Jedlinsky, B.P., Wilson, T.L., & McCarthy, C.F. (1993). Physical therapy management of pain in children. In N.L. Schechter, C.B. Berde, & M. Yaster (Eds.). *Pain in infants, children and adolescents* (p. 320). Baltimore: Williams & Wilkins.

ANSWERS ■ CASE 25-4

1. Answer (**b**). Familiar and favorite toys, objects, and persons such as parents can effectively diminish fear and anxiety in preschool-age children. Burns of all degrees are very painful. To help relieve that pain, the combination of continuous opioid analgesia and ibuprofen, an NSAID, is indicated. NSAIDs affect nociceptive transmitters, such as prostaglandin, and opioids block pain transmission.

REFERENCE
Carr, D.B., Osgood, P.F., & Szyfelbein, S.K. (1993). Treatment of pain in acutely burned patients. In N.L. Schechter, C.B. Berde, & M. Yaster (Eds.). *Pain in infants, children and adolescents*. Baltimore: Williams & Wilkins.

2. Answer (**b**). The Oucher Pain Scale can be used with children 3 to 6 years of age. It has culturally specific (i.e., Anglo-Saxon, Hispanic, and African-American) pictures of children in various degrees of distress. The child chooses which picture represents his or her pain and hurts.

REFERENCE
Knott, C., Beyer, J., Vellarrvel, A., Denyes, M. Erickson, V., & Willard, G. (1994). Using the Oucher: Developmental approach to pain assessment in children. *MCN; American Journal of Maternal Child Nursing*, 19, 314–320.

3. Answer (**c**). The short durations of action of fentanyl and midazolam make them an ideal choice for painful procedures of short duration. Titrating to effect is important for adequate analgesia and to avoid potential respiratory depression.

REFERENCE
Carr, D.B., Osgood, P.F., & Szyfelbein, S.K. (1993). Treatment of pain in acutely burned patients. In N.L. Schechter, C.B. Berde, & M. Yaster (Eds.). *Pain in infants, children and adolescents*. Baltimore: Williams & Wilkins.

4. Answer (**d**). NSAIDs have a ceiling effect. This means that any increase in effectiveness of the drug that might occur with an increased dose is far outweighed by an accompanied increase of side effects.

REFERENCE
Coyle, N. (1987). Analgesia and pain: Current concepts. *Nursing Clinics of North America*, 22 (3), 727–741.

5. Answer (**c**). Methadone is a long-acting opioid that has been successfully used to wean patients from opioids. Oral methadone is easily absorbed and taken every 12 hours. The remaining medications—pentazocine, nalbuphine, and butorphanol—are agonist-antagonists that might precipitate withdrawal symptoms in a patient who has been on opioids longer than 2 weeks.

REFERENCE
Yaster, M., & Maxwell, L.G. (1993). Opioid agonists and antagonists. In N.L. Schechter, C.B. Berde, & M. Yaster (Eds.). *Pain in infants, children and adolescents*. Baltimore: Williams & Wilkins.

6. Answer (**a**). Agonist-antagonist opioids were manufactured to provide pain relief and decrease the side effects of agonist opioids. There are fewer problems with respiratory depression, constipation, and urinary retention. Nalbuphine (Nubain) can increase a patient's respiratory drive. Agonist-antagonist opioids attach to the kappa and sigma receptors in the brain and spinal cord, and the pure agonist opioids attach to the mu and kappa receptors in the brain and spinal cord. Although both provide analgesic action, agonist-antagonist opioids have a ceiling effect and should be used for moderate to severe pain. Some of the side effects of agonist-antagonist opioids include hallucinations, euphoria, and psychomotor stimulation. Because of these side effects, caution is used in dosing children.

REFERENCE
Yaster, M., & Maxwell, L.G. (1993). Opioid agonists and antagonists. In N.L. Schechter, C.B. Berde, & M. Yaster (Eds.). *Pain in infants, children and adolescents*. Baltimore: Williams & Wilkins.

7. Answer (**b**). NSAIDs modulate pain by decreasing the production of prostaglandins and other neurotransmitters of pain impulses. Opioids modulate pain by attaching to opiate receptors in the spinal cord, central nervous system, and periphery and blocking pain impulses.

REFERENCE
Coyle, N. (1987). Analgesics and pain: Current concepts. *Nursing Clinics of North America*, 22 (3), 727–741.

ACKNOWLEDGMENTS
I would like to thank my colleague Susan Givens Bell, RN, BSN, for her thought-provoking evaluation of these questions and her participation on our Pain Management Team.